Equine Surgery
Advanced Techniques

Equine Surgery
Advanced Techniques

C. WAYNE MCILWRAITH, B.V.SC., M.S., Ph.D., M.R.C.V.S.

Diplomate American College of Veterinary Surgeons; Professor of Surgery. Department of Clinical Sciences, College of Veterinary Medicine and Biomedical Sciences, Colorado State University, Fort Collins, Colorado

A. SIMON TURNER, B.V.SC., M.S.

Diplomate American College of Veterinary Surgeons; Professor of Surgery. Department of Clinical Sciences, College of Veterinary Medicine and Biomedical Sciences, Colorado State University, Fort Collins, Colorado

Illustrations by

TOM MCCRACKEN, M.S. *and* JOHN DAUGHERTY, M.S.

Office of Biomedical Media, Colorado State University, Fort Collins, Colorado

LEA & FEBIGER · 1987 · PHILADELPHIA

LEA & FEBIGER
600 Washington Square
Philadelphia, PA 19106-4198
U.S.A.
(215) 922-1330

Library of Congress Cataloging-in-Publication Data

McIlwraith, C. Wayne.
    Advanced techniques in equine surgery.

    Includes bibliographies and index.
    1. Horses—Surgery. I. Turner, A. Simon (Anthony
Simon) II. Title. [DNLM: 1. Horses—surgery.
SF 951 M478a]
SF951.M46 1986   636.1′089′7   86-20083
ISBN 0-8121-1055-2

PRINTED IN THE UNITED STATES OF AMERICA

Print No.   4   3   2   1

To Nancy and Ann and their horses

Preface

This book follows the excellent response to our previous textbook *Techniques in Large Animal Surgery*. Because of the popularity of that format and the requests that more advanced techniques be similarly presented, this book has been produced. Again, the techniques are designed to be brief, and each discussion is accompanied by appropriate illustrations. The book is not meant to replace more detailed treatises on pathogenesis, clinical signs, and treatment alternatives published elsewhere.

In general, the surgical procedures are more complex than in the previous book and demand more surgical expertise and specialized training. Some techniques that have evolved since the last book or have not reached the stage of being "time honored" are simple, however. With a fair degree of consistency, we have presented techniques that are currently being performed. Some readers will be disappointed that certain procedures are not presented (two examples are cleft palate repair and esophageal anastomosis). Such procedures were omitted usually because follow-up results raised questions of how often they were of real value. On the other hand, some of the techniques presented may be abandoned in the future as results are evaluated more critically and better alternatives are found. In some procedures, a certain amount of expertise is assumed regarding basic approaches and principles presented in our previous text.

All of the drawings in the book are original and based on rough sketches and photographs taken at various points during actual surgery. Dissections on cadavers were also performed in some instances.

To try best to represent techniques currently performed and favored, we have asked and received critical review of these procedures from a number of colleagues. These people include Dr. Ted Stashak and Dr. Gayle Trotter, our surgical colleagues at Colorado State University, as well as Dr. Larry Bramlage, Dr. Charlie Boles, Dr. Joe Foemen, Dr. Peter Haynes, Dr. Doug Herthel, Dr. Tom Montgomery, Dr. Jim Robertson, Dr. Mike Shires, and Dr. John Stick. We are also grateful to our colleagues Dr. Robert Kainer for checking the manuscript and illustrations with regard to nomenclature, Dr. Richard Park for help with radiographs, and Dr. Robert Jones for his help and expertise in the sections on prophylactic antibiotics and nosocomial infections.

Of primary importance, we wish to acknowledge the work of Tom McCracken and John Daugherty, who have provided us with the excellent illustrations. We also would like to thank Al Kilminister for taking photographs during the various procedures and dissections to aid the art work. We also wish to thank Ms. Helen Acevedo for typing the manuscript.

The idea for this book was conceived in 1983 based on requests and encouragement from Mr. George Mundorff, executive editor, Lea & Febiger, and Mr. Christian F. Spahr Jr., veterinary editor of Lea & Febiger. We appreciate their continuing assistance.

C. WAYNE McILWRAITH

A. SIMON TURNER

Fort Collins, Colorado

Contents

1

Case Selection, Client Communication, and Insurance Policies for Equine Surgical Patients

Good surgical principles and skillful technique are important to successful equine surgery. State-of-the-art techniques are paramount to maintenance of standards. Two other principles, however, are equally important to a successful surgical practice: surgical judgment and client communication. We need to be much more than good technicians. There is a wide divergence of opinion about whether certain conditions should be surgically treated. Some of this divergence is based on differing experiences and some on a lack of prospective and retrospective data to give us definitive results. Unfortunately, closed-mindedness on the part of some clinicians is a factor in some situations. Divergence of opinion among competent and experienced surgeons regarding important surgical decisions is real and needs to be accepted. Surgical decision making is not an exact scientific process, and it is unreasonable to expect exact answers to clinical problems.

Case Selection

Analyses of second opinion programs in human surgery have indicated that the number of consultants needed to provide a reliable clinical decision probably exceeds those who are logistically available and whom the patient is willing to visit.[2] Many aspects of surgical decision making are subjective because of the absence of controlled data. Differences among surgeons regarding their inclination to operate are associated with a number of factors, and some of these differences are not easily resolved. On the other hand, a surgeon *who has had experience* with a particular condition might consider a certain treatment clearly appropriate or inappropriate. "Reinvention of the wheel" is still a problem with some surgical residents and clinicians who are overaggressive, inadequately supervised, or whose skills are not sufficiently updated or trained. There are too many good training programs, continuing education courses, textbooks, and published papers available today to justify many of the needless or futile surgical interventions that take place. The old cliches "If in doubt, cut it out" and "A chance to cut is a chance to cure" are still with us, and both of us would admit guilt to having used these at times to justify surgical intervention. It should be recognized, however, that any surgical intervention should be based on good judgment rather than on a mere enthusiasm to perform surgery.

On the other hand, conservatism based on ignorance or closed-mindedness is equally unacceptable. The statement "Surgery won't do any good," which is often heard when the speaker has had no experience with the technique, has never handled such a case, or is unaware of data supporting the given technique, is also unfortunate and sometimes prevents horses from receiving the best chance they deserve. A surgical decision should be based on data of cases handled up to the present time. When such data are not available, the decision to operate should be based on an open-minded evaluation of the options. This entails not only an awareness of what has been done in the past, but also, in many cases, consultation with other surgeons. In addition, no individual should be defensive about obtaining a second opinion, whether he seeks it himself or the client requests it. Adherence to the above principles not only is conducive to optimal standards, but is increasingly important for protection from litigation.

Client Communication

Along with the foregoing principles, communication with clients (owners or trainers) is critical to ensuring that one's practice is both successful and free of litigation. Many, including ourselves, believe that legal problems are commonly related to poor communication between clinicians and clients. This includes communication with owners and trainers regarding options, costs, prognosis, likely complications, and recommendations. In addition, communication regarding postsurgical care is critical and should be accelerated when complications develop. Good communication must be linked to good judgment if problems are to be minimized. Any communication should be as realistic and as honest as possible. All clients need to be warned of potential problems, but exaggerating the difficulty of surgery or the gravity of the potential consequences to protect oneself, or to make oneself look good when a successful result is obtained, is inappropriate.

Direct communication with the person paying the bill is ideal, as is keeping written records of the quoted fees. Providing written aftercare instructions is also a good practice and later minimizes the time spent in telephone contact. Such principles are part of an increased need for written documentation of everything we do, as reflected by the adage

"If it isn't written down, it hasn't been done." We must be "business-like" to some extent. These communications become easier as the clinician acquires depth of experience in both his clinical expertise, surgical judgment and interaction with clients.

Insurance Policies and the Equine Surgeon

The increasing problem with malpractice claims is well recognized and becomes particularly evident as our premiums rise each year. The legal profession continues to make us "malpractice defensive." Adherence to the principles outlined previously in this chapter as well as throughout the book can help prevent some malpractice claims, but cannot protect us completely. Subsequent chapters provide relevant material for our optimal performance and do not give further consideration to the subject of malpractice.

Several insurance policies are available to the horse owner, but the ones that principally concern surgeons are equine mortality insurance, loss of use insurance, and surgical insurance. Loss of use policies are uncommon. Surgical insurance policies have been offered in the past few years, but exclusions are starting to appear as insurance companies recognize categories with a high rate of claim. If available, they can be an appropriate investment, depending on the particular function of the horse.

Equine mortality insurance policies affect equine surgeons most directly and should be addressed. Recent guidelines published by the American Association of Equine Practitioners (AAEP) help clarify a number of points and are a useful source of information and reference.[1] Equine mortality insurance policies provide coverage for loss from accident or disease. The policy does not cover minor injuries, depreciation of value, or failure of an animal to perform certain functions. Destruction due to unsuitability for a particular use is not covered. Three areas are relevant to our role as equine surgeons.

1. THE VETERINARY EXAMINATION FOR MORTALITY INSURANCE. The veterinarian's responsibilities in conducting an examination prior to a horse's being insured are well laid out in the recent AAEP guidelines. These responsibilities to the insurance company include identifying the animal beyond a reasonable doubt, noting sex, color, breeding, age, markings, tattoos, and brands. The veterinarian is required to report the medical facts to the best of his knowledge and belief by answering all questions on the application, but he is not required to attest to the insurability of the horse or to its current value. Despite an owner's reluctance, the examination should be thorough. Looking at a horse in the horse trailer, for example, does not constitute a legitimate examination.

2. THE PERFORMANCE OF SURGERY ON AN INSURED HORSE. Insurance companies have several options regarding elective surgery to be performed on an insured animal. The client must first notify the insurance

company, which in turn may (1) permit the surgery and issue a premium charge for the additional exposure, (2) permit the surgery, issuing no premium charge and accepting no liability for the surgical procedure, or (3) permit the surgery, issuing no premium charge but accepting liability for the surgical procedure. Deciding which of these options to follow is the concern of the insurance company and the client. The surgeon's concern is that permission for surgery has been obtained, and that the insurance company is aware that the surgery to be performed is elective. We feel that it is always up to the client to perform this notification.

The situation for emergency surgery is somewhat different. Virtually all insurance companies will support a veterinarian's decision to proceed with surgery, or even euthanasia subsequent to the surgery, if necessary. It is important to make a positive identification of the animal, however, and communicate with the insurance company if possible.

3. The Performance of Euthanasia on Humane Grounds. This area can create difficult decisions for the equine surgeon. We have all found ourselves in the situation of treating a valuable horse that is rendered useless for its proposed career and being pressured by the owner when the need for euthanasia on humane grounds is debatable. In this regard, the guidelines for recommending euthanasia set up by the AAEP Equine Insurance Committee, with the concurrence of all insurance industry representatives, are highly useful. The committee suggests that the following criteria be considered in evaluating the immediate necessity for intentional destruction of a horse: (1) Is the condition chronic and incurable? (2) Does the immediate condition have a hopeless prognosis for life? (3) Is the horse a hazard to himself or his handlers? (4) Will the horse require continuous medication for the relief of pain for the remainder of his life? If these guidelines are followed, difficult decisions can be made more easily.

Another problem regularly arises. On some occasions, a condition may be present that potentially could be treated by surgery; however, this surgery has a debatable prognosis, and its success or failure may not be evident for some time in the future. To complicate matters, the insurance policy is shortly due to expire and the animal may be found insufficiently acceptable for insurance renewal beyond a 30-day extension clause. For example, one of us has been confronted with a horse having comminuted fracture of the various carpal bones following a race. Although such a horse could be potentially salvaged for breeding by attempting primary repair with lag screw fixation augmented by cast immobilization, it was known that this operation could be unsuccessful, and a continued collapse of the carpus might occur several months later, requiring euthanasia of the horse. In such a case, expiration of the insurance policy in one month allows insufficient time for a fair decision to be made. Such situations still pose problems, and it is important that the veterinarian knows what can be done and that the prognosis represents the interests of the parties concerned. It would be unfortunate, in such situations, if euthanasia were performed on a horse because of a lack of assurance from the insurance company that the insurance policy would not be lapsed before the situation was resolved.

References

1. American Association of Equine Practitioners: The Veterinary Role in Equine Insurance. Golden, CO, 1985.
2. Rutkaw, I.M., Gittelsohn, A.N., and Zuidema, G.D.: Surgical decision making. The reliability of clinical judgement. Ann. Surg., 190:409, 1979.

2

General Considerations in Preparing the Equine Surgical Patient

Numerous steps are involved in preparing a horse for surgery. Guidelines rather than hard and fast rules are presented, because each case must be treated individually and because protocols vary, depending on whether surgery is emergency or elective. In emergency cases, certain procedures in the preoperative preparation must be omitted.

Food Restriction and Grooming

In elective cases, all food (but not water) should be withheld. The duration of withholding varies, depending on the case. We withhold feed for 12 hours in cases of simple, relatively short procedures, such as arthroscopic surgery and cryptorchidectomy. The night before surgery, the animal is muzzled. Some procedures require a longer period of food restriction (e.g., 24 hr) to produce more complete emptying of the intestinal tract, but such a requirement is rare in our experience.

Although food restriction is even more important in the ruminant, it is essential for surgical preparation of the horse. The most frequent problem we have encountered in patients that were not sufficiently withheld from food is tympany of the large colon and cecum. We have seen a few cases where the horse required celiotomy and intestinal decompression because respiratory embarrassment was so severe. Certainly, pressure on the diaphragm and inadequate ventilation represent the biggest threat to the horse's life. To provide a short-term remedy of the situation, the horse is first placed on mechanical ventilation. If bloating is persistent and severe, decompression of the distended large intestine can be achieved by trocharization via the flank. If the small bowel is distended, trocharization is of limited value. It is most useful when the needle (e.g., 18 g, 3 inches) can be placed on a large gas cap of the cecum or large colon. Nasogastric intubation prior to anesthetic induction may be of value in emergency cases where the patient must be anesthetized on a full intestinal tract.

Oral antibiotics have been used in man and small animals to decrease bloating, but they are not used routinely in horses. The risk of altering the flora of the intestinal tract and producing a case of salmonellosis is far too great. The use of preoperative medications, including antibiotics and nonsteroidal anti-inflammatory drugs, is discussed elsewhere throughout the text.

We prefer to muzzle the horse rather than strip the bedding out of the stall. Without bedding, the horse often lies in feces overnight, which makes grooming the next morning a difficult chore. If the horse is muzzled, the muzzle must be applied securely so that the horse does not remove it and feed on the bedding material.

Horses that are dirty or that are shedding a winter coat must be thoroughly groomed before surgery. Some individuals may require a bath to remove dirt and feces from their coats. Vacuuming of the hair coat with one of the commercially available vacuums used for show animals is also useful.

Clipping of the Surgical Site

Unless the horse is unruly or must be anesthetized on an emergency basis, we clip the surgical site the night before surgery. With a busy surgical practice, it may be impractical to clip immediately before surgery, as is recommended for human patients. Clipping has been demonstrated to produce microlacerations of the dermis, which, if inflicted the night before surgery, have a greater opportunity to become colonized by normal skin flora. Clipping a horse prior to surgery requires good technical support and communication between the surgeon and whoever will be clipping. A no. 40 blade is used in most instances, but the procedure can be expedited in horses with a heavy winter coat by using the coarser no. 10 clipper blade initially. The surgical area should always be clipped in a neat square or rectangle with sharp, well-defined edges. (Owners often judge the success of the surgery by the neat clipping job and a neat suture line in the skin incision.) Horses undergoing surgery of the limbs should have hair removed around the limb's entire circumference. Some surgical sites are virtually impossible to clip until the animal has been anesthetized and is in dorsal recumbency. With most horses about to undergo celiotomy, it is possible to do most of the steps involved in clipping the ventral abdomen without anesthesia. Occasionally, depilatory creams are indicated to remove hair. The dense, coarse hair of the mane can be removed in patients undergoing laminectomy for dorsal decompression of the spinal cord.

Immediately prior to induction of anesthesia, the horse's mouth should be washed out. Catheterization of the jugular vein and cleaning of the feet should also be performed at this time.

Position of the Horse

Once the horse has been anesthetized, the correct positioning of the horse on the operating table is ultimately the responsibility of the surgeon. A good support team, however, that knows not only how to position the horse, but also other little idiosyncratic demands of the surgeon, is invaluable. Such a team allows the surgeon to proceed with scrubbing, gowning, and opening instruments, reducing much of the time the horse needs to be under the anesthetic. The surgeon should check the final position of the horse and suggest any "fine tuning" of the animal's position. The important part of positioning is ensuring that the surgical site does not require the surgical team to adopt an awkward fatiguing position throughout the procedure. Fatigue of the surgeon always compromises technique.

Padding of the horse must be adequate and correctly positioned to avoid pressure-related injuries to dependent muscle groups. We use commercially available water mattresses (made to a size dictated by our table dimensions) for padding while the horse is under anesthesia. Studies using wick catheters to measure intracompartmental muscle pressures have shown that supporting a horse on a water mattress caused the least dramatic pressure elevation of the lower limb muscles (e.g., the triceps muscle), while foam padding produced the most.[5] Careful selection of protective padding therefore reduces the severity of muscle damage.[5] Water mattresses are surprisingly robust, and if cared for will last one or two years. Small holes can be quickly repaired, but they do not withstand the ravages of towel clamps or scalpel blades. The water temperature within the waterbed can be controlled. Foals, especially those in various degrees of circulatory collapse, can be assisted in maintaining body temperature by using warm water. Adults can have cold water placed in the waterbed.

All areas of concentrated pressure on the horse should be avoided if possible. Limbs overhanging the table edge must be in contact with suitable padding. Horses in dorsal recumbency should not hang off the edge of the table. A standard size of operating table made for a 450- to 500-kg horse may not be suitable for one of the large draft or European breeds. Horses in lateral recumbency should have the upper hindlimb raised by a suitable leg stand so that the medial thigh muscles are not compressed. Raising the upper hindlimb also ensures that venous return is not compromised. The "down" forelimb should be pulled forward in extension, as this reduces intracompartmental muscle pressures to acceptable levels.[5] Triceps and gluteal muscle groups, in particular, should be adequately padded. We have found that diligent padding, positioning, and adequate maintenance of blood pressure during surgery, combined with a short anesthetic time, are the best precautions against postanesthetic rhabdomyolysis ("tying-up").

Skin Preparation

The aim of skin preparation is to remove debris and to reduce the bacterial population to levels that can be handled by the patient's natural defenses.[4] Complete sterilization of the skin is impossible because many bacteria are harbored in the hair follicles. A wide area of skin should always be prepared in case the skin incision has to be lengthened or modified. Limbs subjected to surgery should be scrubbed around their entire circumference. Many methods of applying the numerous germicidal agents have been documented. Little difference has been shown between spraying or painting methods of application. Because of the density of the hair follicles in domestic animals, however, scrubbing with a germicide that has detergent properties has become accepted practice. The actual mechanical scrubbing of the skin is more important than the killing ability of the germicidal agent used.

The choice of germicide is commonly one of personal preference and tradition. At Colorado State University, we use three povidone-iodine scrubs (Betadine scrub) alternated with three (70%) alcohol rinses, performed by a gloved, trained veterinary technician. After each alcohol application, the surgical site is dried with sterile hand towels. Alcohol rapidly kills microorganisms, and it defats the skin at the same time. Defatting the skin helps plastic surgical adhesive drapes adhere better. During their application, both the povidone-iodine and alcohol are applied with gauzes held either in the hand or with sponge forceps. The povidone-iodine is applied by vigorous scrubbing while the alcohol is wiped on with firm pressure. In areas near open wounds or mucous membranes of the eye, sterile saline solution can be substituted for alcohol.

If one of the commercially available plastic surgical adhesive drapes is used, the final drying of the alcohol must be thorough; otherwise, the drape will not adhere. Adherence is enhanced by the use of a plastic adhesive spray. If plastic drapes are not being used, the surgical site can be sprayed with a suitable germicidal spray such as povidone-iodine (Betadine).

Surgical Draping

Plastic surgical adhesive drapes are used routinely in large and small animal surgery. Their purpose is to prevent skin bacteria from gaining access to the surgical wound by immobilizing them. Controversy exists as to their actual role in reducing wound infection. The adhesive drapes are useful in surgery of the limbs because surrounding anatomic landmarks can be identified, which is a difficult task if they are buried by an excessive amount of draping material. Some parts of the horse are completely unsuitable for draping with these products because of their uneven configuration or because the hair is too dense and coarse. A major drawback occurs when poor application of the drape allows blood and irrigation fluids to seep under it. We have used the films containing iodophor,* which are used in human surgery, and they seem to adhere better. There have been no controlled studies proving their microbiologic efficacy in the horse.

---

*Ioban, 3M Company, Medical Products Div., Minnesota Mining Co., St. Paul, MN.

When limb surgery is performed in horses, the hoof must be diligently isolated from the surgical field. Several disposable gloves can be stretched over the foot. Plastic adhesive drapes can be used over the gloves to prevent the gloves from becoming dislodged. Alternatively, the plastic adhesive drapes can be used to isolate the hoof.

There are reams of literature regarding the advantages and disadvantages of disposable (single-use) or reusable drapes. The majority of the literature leans in favor of disposable drapes *and* gowns (i.e., a complete system).[1–4,6,7] Regardless of the type of drape used, it must resist penetration by microorganisms. With the large variety of woven and nonwoven materials, the choice is often difficult. The traditional draping material is muslin (140 threads per inch). It is capable of bacterial penetration when it becomes wet with any aqueous fluid, allowing microorganisms to travel freely in both directions.[1–4,6,7] The surgeon must keep this risk in mind, especially in lengthy wet operations such as abdominal surgery or repair of long bone fracture. These findings have prompted a finer type of drape (280 threads per inch) to be produced, but moisture is still a problem.[7] Autoclaved orthopedic stockinette, commonly used by human orthopedic surgeons, does not have the recommended thread density and offers less resistance to bacterial strike than the traditional muslin. In orthopedic cases such as repair of long bone fracture, for which surgical time is long and the extent of surgical manipulation extreme, the use of stockinette as a barrier should be discouraged. Bacterial penetration can occur even with dry drapes, owing to mechanical pressure.

Disposable drapes made of a nonwoven material resembling paper or synthetic polymers should now be accepted as the surgical drape of choice. Many veterinary hospitals now use them exclusively. They are waterproof, they can be sterilized, and many are available prepackaged. Some manufacturers* now cater entirely to the veterinary profession and will design a system that includes all the appropriately sized drapes for a particular operation. We currently have such a system for arthroscopic surgery and abdominal surgery.

One disadvantage of disposable drapes is that they are quite easily torn by towel clamps, as might occur when clamping an x-ray cassette to a limb for intraoperative radiographs.

The actual sequence of draping varies tremendously, depending on how the surgeon was trained. We have both been staggered at the different standards of draping seen at various surgical facilities throughout the world. Because virtually all the surgical procedures discussed in this book must be performed under strict aseptic conditions, *isolation of a sterile field and its maintenance must be given the highest priority*. Although fast skillful surgery makes up for deficits in aseptic technique, such deficits should not be condoned. Before draping, the gowned surgeon should don two pairs of gloves, as a break in aseptic technique is likely to occur at this time in the procedure. The drapes must be firmly anchored so that a small amount of inadvertent move-

*Gepco, General Econopak, Inc., Philadelphia, PA 19122.

ment by the horse does not dislodge them and expose them to contaminated areas. The first drape should cover most of the horse (except for the vicinity of the surgical site). Projecting areas that the surgical team might brush against, such as table edges or the animal's limbs, must be covered.

Careful draping of the limb to be operated on requires good coordination and cooperation between the surgeon and assistants and the operating room personnel. The limb can be suspended by white adhesive tape or a wire attached to an I.V. fluid stand, or it may be supported with a special leg stand that is part of the operating table.

To apply a plastic adhesive drape correctly, a sterile assistant should see that it is seated, without wrinkles, directly on the surgical site. The logical time to place the plastic adhesive drape is after the surrounding drapes are in position. This ensures that fluids are carried across the top of the drapes and are not allowed to flow under them. A method for additional draping, which is useful in long bone fracture repair, is the "toweling-in technique," performed after the skin incision is made. No matter how well plastic adhesive drapes are applied, this method is also required to isolate the skin from the wound. To secure drapes to the skin edge, a simple continuous suture of no. 1 or no. 2 nylon can be used. Michel clips or skin staples are useful as well. Skin staples can also be used to secure skin towels in areas that are difficult to drape.[6]

For abdominal surgery, drapes to protect the wound edges are available. These consist of a flexible plastic ring attached to an opening of similar size in a plastic vinyl drape. After the abdomen is entered and hemostasis is achieved, the drape is spread over the wound, and the ring is inserted into the abdomen and allowed to expand into its circular shape under the body wall. The plastic sheet is then tautly drawn and secured with towel clamps.

References

1. Beck, W.C.: Aseptic barriers in surgery. Arch. Surg., 116:240, 1981.
2. Cole, W.R., and Bernard, H.R.: Wound isolation in the prevention of postoperative wound infection. Surg. Gynecol. Obstet., 133:1, 1967.
3. Ha'eri, G.B., and Wiley, A.M.: Wound contamination through drapes and gowns: A study using tracer particles. Clin. Orthop., 154:181, 1981.
4. Kaul, A.F., and Jewett, J.F.: Agents and techniques for disinfection of the skin. Surg. Gynecol. Obstet., 152:677, 1981.
5. Lindsay, W.A., Pascoe, P.J., McDonell, W.N., et al.: Effect of protective padding on forelimb intracompartmental muscle pressures in anesthetized horses. Am. J. Vet. Res., 46:688, 1985.
6. Morris, D.M.: The use of skin staples to secure skin towels in areas difficult to drape. Surg. Gynecol. Obstet., 159:387, 1984.
7. Moylan, J.A., and Kennedy, B.V.: The importance of gown and drape barriers in the prevention of wound infection. Surg. Gynecol. Obstet., 151:465, 1980.

3

Use of Prophylactic Antibiotics in Equine Surgery

Surgical antibiotic prophylaxis refers to the administration of antibiotic(s) to patients without clinical evidence of infection in the operative field.[9] The objectives of prophylaxis are to prevent naturally occurring organisms in one site from proliferating in a normally sterile site, to prevent organisms that are contaminating a normally sterile site from producing disease, and to prevent infection by exogenous organisms. Antibiotic prophylaxis is indicated in the surgical patient when there is an unacceptable incidence of infection, or when there is a low incidence of infection that could become devastating or lethal.

It is now well recognized that in the majority of situations, the use of antibiotic prophylaxis is unnecessary and may lead to multiple problems. There are no controlled studies in horses to define the differences made by using antibiotics in preventing infection. Clearly, however, the wide use of antibiotics in association with surgery has not eliminated surgical infection as a threat to the patient, and it is suspected that it has not reduced the incidence of such infections in most cases. The deleterious effects are better accepted now, and there is evidence that widespread, and often indiscriminate, use of these antibiotics may be responsible for the changing patterns of bacteria implicated in nosocomial infections, and for the emergence of bacterial species (amphibionts) that were previously considered nonpathogenic. (Nosocomial infections are discussed elsewhere in this book.) The emergence of pathogenic species combined with the selection of resistant organisms is of the gravest concern.

Wound Infections

The first step in the development of an infected wound is bacterial contamination of surgically manipulated tissue. Bacterial contamination, which is a component of every surgical wound, arises from two sources: exogenous contamination from the surgery room, or endogenous contamination from the skin or from the gastrointestinal, respiratory, or urogenital tracts of the patient. Whether the bacterial contamination produces infection depends on the number and virulence of the organisms, the patient's defense mechanisms, and the condition of the disrupted tissue. Exogenous habitats of potential pathogens include water, soil, fodder, fomites, and non-equine animal reservoirs. Obviously, these sources should be restricted in the surgery room. The majority of the microorganisms of veterinary importance are not true free-living organisms. Contaminated water, however, is a common source of enterobacteria, and *Salmonella* persists in tap water for 87 days and in pond water for 115 days.[6] The most noteworthy equine pathogen found to be free-living in many bodies of water is *Pseudomonas aeruginosa*, which is also found in the intestinal tract and on mucous membranes.

For endogenous infection, indigenous microflora are found throughout the GI tract, upper respiratory tract, genitourinary tract, skin, and visible mucous membranes.[6] There is no evidence of permanent resident microflora in muscle, the lower respiratory tract, or organs outside the GI tract.

The risk of staphylococcal infection from the patient's skin, an endogenous source of infection, must be considered. It is of major concern in antibiotic prophylaxis in humans during insertion of implants. Bacteremia also represents a source of infection (it is considered capable of seeding prosthetic materials). Another group of patients of concern are those that have a foci of infection remote to the intended operative site. Three areas that may be infected prior to surgery are the skin, lungs, and genitourinary tract.[10] Patients with infection in these sites have been reported as having three times the normal surgical infection rate.

People are the major source of contamination in the hospital environment, and therefore the shedding potential must be controlled. It has been found that 30% of the population are carriers for *Staphylococcus aureus*.[13] Persons shedding more than 1,000 bacteria per minute are classified as shedders. In a conventional operating room, the more complete the surgical attire worn by everyone in the room, the better the control of shedding potential. This applies to the use of body exhaust equipment for the anesthesiologist and scrub nurse as well as for the surgeon. Other effective environmental controls for preventing wound contamination are laminar airflow systems and the use of ultraviolet light.

Whether a bacterial contamination becomes an infection depends on critical events in the early inflammatory phase following surgery, which is a "decisive period" in wound infection. If the occurrence of inflammation is inappropriate and phagocytosis is overwhelmed, the patient develops an infection. Necrosis, ischemia, hemorrhage, and the presence of debris impair local host defense mechanisms and decrease the number of bacterial organisms required to cause infection. If a host is compromised, there is an increased risk for infection.[9] If an appropriate antimicrobial agent is present in adequate concentrations, a wound infection in the contaminated tissue is less likely. Antibiotics must be present in the tissues in the early decisive period to prevent bacterial invasion and proliferation effectively. If they are given later, when the bacteria are well established, the antibiotics will have no prophylactic effect. For example, in a clinical study involving human patients undergoing gastric, biliary, or colonic surgery, it was found that cefazolin, administered one hour before surgery, significantly decreased the incidence of postoperative infection in comparison with a placebo. If the cefazolin was begun one to four hours after the operation, however, no reduction occurred in the postoperative infection rate.[9]

The probability of surgical wound infection can be ascertained by estimating the microbial density in the wound. Because this method may not be practical for a given surgical procedure, however, a method of clinical classification that predicts the incidence of wound infection has been established.[1]

Classification of Surgical Procedures

Clean surgical procedures are those procedures that are performed on a noncompromised host under ideal operating room conditions. Such procedures are elective, and no entry is made into the oropharyngeal cavity or lumen of the respiratory, alimentary, or genitourinary tracts. Inflammation is not encountered, and there is no break in the sterile technique. Examples of clean surgical procedures in the horse include elective joint surgery for removal of chip fractures and osteochondritis dissecans debridement. Antibiotic prophylaxis should not be used routinely in horses undergoing this type of procedure unless the consequences of infection are likely to be grave. In man, for example, such consequences could result from the insertion of a permanent prosthesis. Although no comparable example can be found in horses, a somewhat analogous case might be the insertion of a screw into a carpal slab fracture in a joint that has recently been treated with corticosteroids.

Clean-contaminated surgical procedures involve entry into the oropharyngeal cavity or the lumen of the respiratory, alimentary, or genitourinary tracts without significant contamination from these sites. This category also includes procedures performed on a compromised host or those in which a major break in the sterile technique occurs. Because the mucosa of the oropharyngeal, respiratory, alimentary, and genitourinary tracts harbor diffuse and dense microbiologic flora, some contamination of the wound is inevitable. Procedures involving the upper respiratory tract are good examples of this situation.

Contaminated-dirty surgical procedures involve traumatic wounds, operative procedures with a major break in sterile technique, and operations into a site of active infection. The infection rate can be high in patients undergoing such procedures. Because infection is already established, some might argue that the term "prophylactic" is inappropriate, and that antibiotic administration is instead "therapeutic." The purpose of antibiotic prophylaxis, however, is to prevent infection in soft tissue planes and wounds previously uncontaminated by the bacteria. Surgery involving open fractures is an example of a contaminated-dirty surgical procedure. The risk of subsequent infection increases with the amount of tissue devitalization, the extent of contamination, and the systemic compromise of the host.

Prophylactic Value of Antibiotics

Recently, a study comparing ampicillin prophylaxis versus a placebo in clean surgical procedures in dogs and cats showed that the infection rates did not differ significantly.[14] Any specific recommendations regarding antibiotic prophylaxis in equine surgery is difficult because of a lack of controlled retrospective studies. The following general principles should be recognized, however.

Effective clinical prophylaxis begins with careful patient evaluation and an assessment of susceptibility to bacterial contamination. The situation of performing joint surgery in the racehorse is of particular concern to us. This procedure is clean, at least theoretically, and therefore, antibiotics are not considered to be indicated.[4] Many of these patients, however, have been recently injected with intraarticular corticosteroids as well as other agents. Whether the use of antibiotic prophylaxis is justified and valuable in such cases is unknown.

The assessment of the effects of antibiotics in surgical procedures is difficult because antibiotic prophylaxis is only one of many factors that can influence recovery. Indeed, antibiotics probably play a minor role in preventing postoperative infection as compared with the surgeon's skill in removing dead tissue and blood clots or in providing adequate drainage, or with the activities of a well-trained epidemiologist in maintaining proper infection control.[12] The surgical procedure should be performed properly and swiftly, and care should be taken to handle the tissues gently and maintain normal physiologic conditions. The use of closed suction drains is recommended for deep wounds in which a dead space is left. In other situations, drains are deleterious because of their potential to cause retrograde infection.

Although one cannot recommend with certainty the amount of time that an antibiotic should be continued when it is used prophylactically, there is evidence that no more than one or two additional antibiotic doses are necessary for effective antibiotic prophylaxis in the normal host.[9] In a retrospective study, no difference in infection rates was observed between patients receiving antibiotics for 1 day after surgery and those receiving antibiotics for 7 days after surgery.[11] This finding is important because antibiotics are expensive, may involve drug-related side effects, and may unfavorably influence the local and hospital microflora. (This last problem is further discussed in the section "Nosocomial Infections" in Chapter 4.) In addition, disturbing the endogenous microflora is considered to be particularly important in the induction of postoperative complications such as salmonellosis in the horse.

Studies in Human Patients

In human orthopedics, most surgical procedures are associated with an extremely low infection rate, and therefore antibiotic prophylaxis is not considered to be appropriate. If antibiotics were used indiscriminately, many patients would be subjected to possible antibiotic complications, and only a small minority would benefit.[3] Many elective musculoskeletal procedures, especially those that are of short duration and involve soft tissue surgery, do not require antibiotics. The one exception, however, is the large group of procedures involving implantation of foreign bodies, for which the results of infection can be catastrophic. Antibiotic prophylaxis is therefore considered justifiable and necessary in such cases. *Staphylococcus aureus* and S. *epidermidis* are the organisms implicated in more than 90% of the infections occurring after implant surgery in humans. Because first-generation cephalosporins are active against most staphylococci, their use is desirable in this situation. Cephalosporins are considered to offer protection equal to that offered by other single agents or antibiotic combinations, and the risk of side effects is minimal. Twenty-four hours or less of a first- or second-generation cephalosporin is often recommended for antibiotic prophylaxis in the normal host for clean and clean-contaminated procedures.[3,9]

Penicillin G is considered to have limited use in human orthopedic surgery because of its relative lack of activity against penicillinase-producing *Staphylococcus aureus* and most gram-negative pathogens. The semisynthetic penicillins (e.g., sodium ampicillin) have enhanced anti-gram-negative activity and are useful for prophylaxis against such organisms as *Escherichia coli*. These factors need to be considered when evaluating the use of prophylaxis in equine orthopedics. Recommendations would require knowledge of the relative incidence of streptococcal versus staphylococcal contamination of surgical sites. (This information is unknown at present.) The lack of adequate randomized double-blind prospective studies of clean orthopedic surgery in humans has led to much controversy in this area.[16]

Some surgeons treating human patients recommend a combination of first-generation cephalosporins and an aminoglycoside for 24 hr or less in the compromised host. Use of the same combination for approximately 4 days is recommended for clean-contaminated procedures. For contaminated-dirty procedures, the antibiotic selection for both the normal and the compromised host may be based on preoperative Gram stain, culture results, or anticipated organisms.[9] In most trauma centers, coverage with two antibiotics is recommended for open fractures because of the difficulty in treating gram-negative microorganisms, which have been found with increasing frequency in post-traumatic wound infections. One author recommends administration of cefazolin and gentamicin for 4 to 5 days, with either benzyl penicillin G or clindamycin added for highly contaminated wounds in which anaerobes are expected.[9]

One classic situation where combination therapy is considered to have an advantage over single therapy occurs when severe sepsis develops from *Pseudomonas aeruginosa*. Therapy with any one antipseudomonas agent (e.g., aminoglycosides, third-generation cephalosporins, or alpha-carboxyl penicillin derivative) is less effective than the combined therapy of an antipseudomonas aminoglycoside and an antipseudomonas beta-lactam antibiotic.[12] When possible, however, the clinician should avoid the use of combination therapy because of the greater liklihood of encountering the following problems: (1) drug interactions at receptor sites, (2) changes in elimination of drugs due to competition for elimination routes, (3) potential for greater disruption of normal flora, (4) adverse drug reactions, and (5) increased costs.[12]

Studies in Equine Patients

The use of perioperative antibiotics for equine gastrointestinal surgery is well established, although their general use in human abdominal surgery has been challenged.[5] Studies in humans have emphasized that they should be used in a sufficient dose to provide coverage of the endogenous or exogenous pathogens anticipated, and that they should be given for short periods only. In general, short-term perioperative antibiotic prophylaxis is felt to be useful.[7] The drugs should provide effective protection against both aerobes and anaerobes. In the horse, sodium ampicillin, aminoglycosides, or trimethoprim-sulfa drugs provide coverage of the aerobes likely to be encountered with gastrointestinal surgery. The penicillins provide good coverage of anaerobes with the exception of *Bacteroides fragilis*. Aminoglycosides or trimethoprim-sulfa drugs are not effective against anaerobes. Short-term sodium ampicillin prophylaxis terminated within 24 hours is an option available for routine gastrointestinal surgery. When minimal or no appreciable surgical contamination has occurred, the use of sodium ampicillin (10 mg/kg I.V.), in one dose or in two doses 6 to 8 hours apart, has been recommended.[2] When contamination is moderate to severe, the use of procaine penicillin G (2,000 IU/kg I.M. b.i.d.) and gentamicin (2 mg/kg I.M. or I.V. t.i.d.) has been recommended.

Aminoglycosides have toxic effects, including neuromuscular blockage, cardiovascular depression, nephrotoxicity, and inhibition of gut motility. The first two of these effects preclude the use of the drug preoperatively and the second two effects are important postoperatively. We do not recommend the use of aminoglycosides for more than 3 days, even with contaminated surgery. In addition to the foregoing side effects, we are also concerned about the effect these drugs have on the normal bacterial population of the gastrointestinal tract of the patient with an acute abdomen and their potential to contribute to postoperative complications such as diarrhea (which may or may not be due to salmonellosis).

Recommendations

The following points are important to consider when choosing prophylactic antibiotics.

1. Prophylaxis should be directed against the most likely pathogens at a specific site. Antimicrobials cannot sterilize all possible pathogens at all sites in the animal. The surgeon must therefore consider (a) susceptibility of the most likely pathogens, (b) activity of the drug, and (c) the pharmacokinetics of the drug.
2. The shorter the duration of antibiotic administration, the broader the range of organisms inhibited. A longer duration of administration is more likely to result in resistant organisms.
3. The dose of the antibiotic must be equal to the therapeutic dose.

We need to define the *appropriate antibiotic, the effective concentration* at the site of bacterial lodgment, and the *critical time* of administration.

The use of local antibiotic treatment and intraoperative wound lavage is controversial in humans and has not been well studied in the horse. The finding that aminoglycosides are chemically and microbiologically suitable for inclusion in polymethomethacrylate bone cements for prevention or treatment of orthopedic surgical infections has led to their use in human orthopedics, particularly in association with implant surgery. The drug has also been incorporated into polymethomethacrylate beads and plaster of Paris pellets.[15] We have not yet used these agents in the horse. The use of antibiotics in the wound lavage solution has shown to be beneficial, even in clean surgical procedures,[8] but their use is not common practice.

References

1. Ad hoc committee of the Committee on Trauma, Division of Medical Sciences, National Research Council, National Academy of Sciences. Postoperative wound infections: The influence of ultraviolet irradiation of the operating room and various other factors. Ann. Surg., 160(Suppl):1, 1964.
2. Brown, M.P.: Antibiotics and the surgical colic. Proc. Equine Colic Research Symposium, University of Georgia, Athens, GA, 1982, p 281.
3. Fitzgerald, R.H.: Cephalosporin antibiotics in the prevention and treatment of musculoskeletal sepsis. J. Bone Joint Surg., 65-A:1201, 1983.
4. Guglilelmo, B.J., Hohn, D.C., Koo, P.J., et al.: Antibiotic prophylaxis in surgical procedures: A critical analysis of the literature. Arch. Surg., 118:943, 1983.
5. Hurley, D.L., Paxton, H., and Hahn, H.H.: Perioperative prophylactic antibiotics in abdominal surgery: A review of recent progress. Surg. Clin. North Am., 59:919, 1979.
6. Knight, H.D., and Hietala, S.: Antimicrobial susceptibility patterns in horses. Proc., 2nd Equine Pharmocol Symp., American Association of Equine Practioners, Denver, 1978, p 63.
7. Lewis, R.T., Allan, C.M., Goodall, G.R., et al.: Discriminate use of antibiotic prophylaxis in gastroduodenal surgery. Am. J. Surg., 138:640, 1979.

8. Lord, J.W., Rossi, G., and Daliana, M.: Intraoperative antibiotic wound lavage: An attempt to eliminate postoperative infection in arterial and clean surgical procedures. Ann. Surg., 185:634, 1977.
9. Mader, J.T., and Cierny, G.: The principles of the use of preventative antibiotics. Clin. Orthop., 190:75, 1984.
10. Monson, T.P., and Nelson, C.L.: Microbiology for orthopedic surgeons: Selected aspects. Clin. Orthop., 190:14, 1984.
11. Nelson, C.L., Green, T.G., Porter, R.A., and Warren, R.D.: One day *versus* 7 days of antibiotic therapy in orthopedic surgery. Clin. Orthop., 176:258, 1983.
12. Quintilani, R., and Nightengale, C.: Principles of antibiotic usage. Clin. Orthop., 190:31, 1984.
13. Ritter, M.A.: Surgical wound environment. Clin. Orthop., 190:11, 1984.
14. Vasseur, P.B., Paul, H.A., Enos, L.R., and Hirsch, D.C.: Infection rates in clean surgical procedures. A comparison of ampicillin prophylaxis vs. a placebo. J. Am. Vet. Med. Assoc., 187:825, 1985.
15. Whelton, A.: The aminoglycosides. Clin. Orthop., 190:66, 1984.
16. Williams, D.N., and Gustilo, R.B.: The use of preventative antibiotics in orthopaedic surgery. Clin. Orthop., 190:83, 1984.

4

Complications of Equine Surgery

Postoperative Rhabdomyolysis

Rhabdomyolysis associated with extended periods of general anesthesia or prolonged recumbency can severely complicate the postoperative convalescence. The condition was originally thought to be a neurologic problem due to nerve compression and dysfunction. Most evidence now supports the hypothesis that the condition is primarily a myopathy caused by local hypoxia of various muscle groups.[4] Although it is referred to as "myositis," this is probably a misnomer, and the word "myopathy" should be used. The condition commonly occurs as a *localized* form, though a *generalized* myopathy involving all muscle groups is occasionally seen.

LOCALIZED MYOPATHY. Localized myopathies related to general anesthesia or recumbency are believed to be due to compression of the muscle groups, which compromises circulation. They have been called "radial paralysis," postanesthetic forelimb lameness, postoperative myopathy, and triceps rhabdomyolysis.[4,5] The muscles involved in postanesthetic myopathy in horses in lateral recumbency include the triceps brachii, quadriceps femoris, hindlimb extensors, masseter, and flank muscles. For horses positioned in dorsal recumbency, the muscles of the back—longissimus, iliocostalis, and gluteal medius—as well as the vastus lateralis muscles are affected.[9] In most cases, the "down" limb is affected. Occasionally, the upper limb is involved, in which case the cause is felt to be compromised circulation. This occurs when the limb overhangs the edge of the table or is allowed to assume a crisscrossed position, resting on the lower limb without being supported by a leg stand. With the weight of the animal pressing against the contact limb and the table, a local tissue hypoxia is the source of the myopathy, as evidenced by lactate levels increasing during anesthesia.[4] Localized swelling of muscles increases pressure within the various fascial envelopes, inhibiting capillary blood flow and allowing continued degeneration of muscle.[4]

A "compartment-like" syndrome develops similar to what has been seen in man, with a resulting rise in intracompartmental muscle pressure. When wick catheters are placed in the triceps brachii muscle, pressures between 30 and 50 mm-Hg and up to 80 mm-Hg have been observed.[4] These pressures also alter nerve transmission and explain some neurologic-like signs. They may also explain why there is often confusion between the terms "triceps brachii rhabdomyolysis" and "radial paralysis." The rise in intracompartmental muscle pressure conveniently explains myopathy in groups of muscles that are under pressure but does not explain the generalized myopathy occasionally seen with general anesthesia. Such a generalized form may be due to the anesthetic agent itself. Some believe there is a relationship between this type of condition and malignant hyperthermia.[7,8] Occasionally a syndrome that resembles malignant hyperthermia can occur when the temperature rises throughout surgery and an intense stiffening of the muscles and fasciculation occurs. It is also accompanied by violent thrashing.[8] Myoglobinuria, renal nephrosis, shock, and death are frequent sequelae. This syndrome may be caused by the actual anesthetic agent itself, resembling malignant hyperthermia rather than purely pressure on affected muscles. More work to establish a definite cause-and-effect relationship of this condition and the anesthetic agent must be done.

The condition is seen in horses following general anesthesia of greater than two hours' duration and in horses positioned in recumbency on hard surfaces.[4] It is also seen following very deep anesthesia for procedures requiring muscle relaxation, such as ovariectomy or ophthalmic surgery. Deep anesthesia reduces blood pressure, cardiac output, and oxygen supply to tissues.[9] Postanesthetic myopathy is seen in heavily muscled breeds, draft breeds, Quarter Horses, and especially in horses taken out of training and placed under general anesthesia for one reason or another (e.g., fracture repair). The position of the horse and the type of padding under it are also involved. Postanesthetic myopathy may severely complicate the recovery from certain conditions, such as long bone fractures. The inability to use one or two limbs results in immediate implant failure if the limb repaired is required to support the animal.

In the "localized" form of postanesthetic myopathy the horse will usually stand after recovering consciousness and is initially unaffected. Either in the recovery stall or back in its stall, however, a syndrome of muscular weakness develops, and the horse adopts a "dropped elbow" appearance if the forelimb is involved. This appears superficially like radial nerve paralysis, but horses usually are able to use the extensors. If the hindlimb is involved, then the fetlock will show knuckling. If the quadriceps femoris is involved, the stifle will drop, and the horse will be unable to stand. Most horses that develop these problems have a protracted recovery time.[4] The discomfort usually persists for 2 to 3 days postoperatively in uncomplicated cases. The affected muscle masses may become hard and swollen. If the condition is very painful, it may invoke fear and pain and produce struggling, which compounds the problem. Struggling can disrupt implants and casts used for fracture repair, loosen bandages, dehisce wounds, and cause a variety of other undesirable things that can lead to the demise of the animal.

GENERALIZED MYOPATHY. In horses with a generalized myopathy there is usually involvement of the limbs that are *not* dependent. We have seen this condition irrespective of the duration of general anesthesia. Muscles become rigid even before the horse has stood up after recovery from the anesthetic. There may be anxiety, sweating, and even signs of colic. The animal may not be able to stand, making management of the condition very difficult. Levels of serum enzymes, creatine phosphokinase (CPK), and aspartate amino transferase (ASAT) are usually elevated due to enzyme leakage from muscle cells. A rise in levels of muscle enzymes is frequently seen without clinical signs of muscle damage and, therefore, rises in serum enzymes must be correlated with clinical signs. Enzymes are useful to evaluate the severity of the muscle damage as well as to establish a prognosis for horses that develop the condition.[4] Decreased serum calcium levels have also been reported.[9]

Treatment

Treatment for postanesthetic myositis must be prompt and vigorous. It is essentially symptomatic. The initial treatment should be directed at preventing further muscle damage. Mild cases require nothing more than observation, whereas more serious cases require nonsteroidal anti-inflammatory drugs such as phenylbutazone or flunixin meglumine. For muscle pain, more potent analgesics such as meperidine may be indicated if the horse appears anxious and near panic that may exacerbate the situation. Acepromazine maleate to produce vasodilation of the affected muscles has also been advocated. It also has a calming effect and can help prevent further struggling, thereby preventing further muscle damage. In addition, the horse should have "support" bandages on the opposite limb and be placed in a stall with good footing. Slinging is indicated in severe cases, but few horses tolerate this method of restraint, and it may, in fact, exacerbate the problem if the horse fights the sling. Since there is no proof that glucocorticoids are of value, they should be avoided because of their ability to potentiate laminitis.[1] Fluid therapy should be instituted in severe cases to promote diuresis and minimize the possibility of a life-threatening myoglobinuric nephrosis. Traditionally, fluid therapy to counteract acidosis has been used, but acidosis is not a consistent finding in clinical or experimental cases.[3,10] Bicarbonate is of little value, therefore, except when there is some evidence to indicate that it may increase the solubility of myoglobin, thus decreasing the chances of myoglobinemic nephrosis. Other questionable modalities include vitamin E/Se preparations and systemic DMSO (dimethylsulfoxide). The key to a quick recovery is good nursing care. For horses that cannot rise we feel the use of waterbeds to distribute pressure on dependent surfaces is most beneficial. The horse should be turned frequently and kept clean and dry to minimize the development of decubital sores. Adequate food and water should be available. Most equine surgeons agree that a lot will depend on the personality of the horse. Despite aggressive and heroic measures some horses tend to "give up" and succumb.

We have already emphasized that probably the most devastating sequelae to postanesthetic rhabdomyolysis are struggling in the recovery stall, inability to use one or more limbs, and general fear and panic. These in turn can lead to broken implants following internal fixation, broken casts, acute disruption of sutured wounds, spontaneous limb fractures, and dislodging of bandages. During the treatment of the myositis itself, the surgeon frequently has to attend to these problems. How to deal with these must be decided upon on an individual basis. Certainly, casts must be immediately repaired, either by "patching" them up while the horse is standing or reanesthetizing the horse and applying a completely new cast. Dislodged bandages on wounds must be replaced as soon as possible. If the complication is hopelessly beyond the "patch-up" stage (e.g., implant failure and refracture of the bone), euthanasia is the only solution.

Prevention of postanesthetic rhabdomyolysis is the only way of effectively dealing with the problem. In our experience the problem should be a rare one if attention is given to certain factors. Adequate padding, ensuring that the surgery time is as short as possible, and maintenance of blood pressure throughout surgery are the most important preventative measures. At Colorado State University a commercially available waterbed is the padding of choice. For horses in lateral recumbency the lower forelimb is pulled forward to reduce muscle pressure on the triceps brachii muscle.[2,4] Good padding will also reduce or distribute the pressure on contact muscles. The uppermost hindlimb should be elevated with a limb stand, which helps prevent pressure on the medial muscle groups of the thigh. Other methods of minimizing postanesthetic myopathy include selection of a balanced anesthetic regimen with minimal hypotensive effects. Barbiturates produce a profound drop in blood pressure, and a more balanced anesthetic regimen is indicated. Maintenance of blood pressure is also one method of ensuring adequate profusion to affected muscles and will require reasonably sophisticated monitoring devices. The direct method of measuring arterial blood pressure utilizes the facial or transverse facial artery. It is relatively simple and produces an accurate continuous record. The noninvasive indirect methods using an inflatable cuff around the tail are more convenient and have been shown to correlate well with intra-arterial measurements.[6] The normal mean (lsd) standing blood pressure in the Thoroughbred has been recorded as 111.8 ± 13.3 mmHg systolic and 67.7 ± 13.8

mmHg diastolic. Under anesthesia some hypotension should be expected, but pressures of 50 mmHg or less require some positive steps to increase them.[6] The modern equine surgical practice doing procedures lasting longer than 1 hour should invest in some form of blood pressure monitoring device to provide optimum patient care and minimize the risk of rhabdomyolysis.

Although it is only a clinical impression, some surgeons feel that exclusion of grain from the diet 24 to 48 hours prior to surgery is indicated. Dantrolene sodium, which inhibits the release of calcium from sarcoplasmic reticulum, has been used with reasonable success for prophylaxis against malignant hyperthermia in pigs. Such therapy is based on the presumption that the myopathy is caused by an anesthetic-induced alteration in metabolism of the muscle cells. Although malignant hyperthermia has been reported in the horse, it may be an oversimplification to relate postanesthetic myopathy with this condition. It is often impossible to predict which horse will succumb to the generalized myopathy, and therefore a controlled study using dantrolene prophylaxis is difficult. Its use in horses for the treatment and prophylaxis of myopathies has not been well documented and should still be considered experimental.

References

1. Eyre, P., Elmes, P.J., and Strickland, S.: Corticosteroid-potentiated vascular responses of the equine digit: a possible pharmacological basis for laminitis. Am. J. Vet. Res. 40:135, 1979.
2. Heath, R.B., et al.: Protecting and positioning the equine surgical patient. Vet. Med. 67:1241, 1972.
3. Koterba, A., and Carlson, G.P.: Acid base and electrolyte alterations in horses with exertional rhabdomyolysis. J. Am. Vet. Med. Assoc. 180:303, 1982.
4. Lindsay, W.A., McDonell, W., and Bignell, W.: Equine postanesthetic forelimb lameness: intracompartmental muscle pressure changes and biochemical patterns. Am. J. Vet. Res. 41:1919, 1980.
5. Trim, C.M., and Mason, J.: Postanesthetic forelimb lameness in horse. Eq. Vet. J. 5:72, 1973.
6. Taylor, P.M.: Techniques and clinical application of arterial blood pressure measurement in the horse. Eq. Vet. J. 13:271, 1981.
7. Waldron-Mease, E.: Postoperative muscle damage in horses. J. Eq. Med. Surg. 1:106, 1977.
8. Waldron-Mease, E., Raker, C.W., and Hammel, E.P.: The muscular system. In Equine Medicine and Surgery. 3rd Ed. Edited by R.A. Mansmann, E.S. McAllister, and P.W. Pratt. Santa Barbara, CA, American Veterinary Publications, 1982, p. 586.
9. White, K.K., and Short, C.: Anesthetic/surgical stress-induced myopathy (myositis). Part II. A postanesthetic myopathy trial. Proceedings of 24th Annual Association of Equine Practitioners, 1978. 107 (1979).

Wound Infection

Wound infection following surgery is an ever present threat regardless of the type of surgery, the duration of surgery, or the experience of the surgeon. The overall effect on the patient will vary from simply an extended time in the hospital to loss of function of a limb (e.g., septic arthritis) or even death (e.g., peritonitis following intestinal anastomosis). We have no figures from our hospital records regarding the cost of wound infection to the client because of increased hospitalization, further bandages, and more antibiotics, but the cost should not be underestimated. An extended hospitalization increases the horse's chance of acquiring a nosocomial infection or acting as a source of infection for other animals. The end result of a wound infection is often a source of client dissatisfaction.

Classification

The surgeon should be aware, through good medical records, of the incidence of infection following operations. Although the number of operations on horses is much less than those on humans, we should constantly monitor infections. If the incidence of infection is unacceptably high, then a thorough analysis of where a "breakdown" occurred is required. For example, was there a break in aseptic technique or a lack of proper sterilization by a malfunctioning autoclave? What constitutes an unacceptably high incidence of infection will vary depending on the type of operation. Operations are classified according to four categories based on an estimate of the wound contamination[4] also discussed earlier in Chapter 3.

I. CLEAN WOUND. No infection is encountered, no break in aseptic technique is discovered and no hollow muscular organs are opened. Examples are arthroscopy, laryngoplasty, internal fixation of a closed fracture.

II. CLEAN CONTAMINATED WOUND. A hollow muscular organ is opened, but minimal spillage of contents occurred. Examples are cystorrhaphy for ruptured bladder and laryngeal sacculectomy.

III. CONTAMINATED WOUND. A hollow muscular organ is opened with gross spillage of contents or, alternatively, acute inflammation without pus formation is encountered. A traumatic wound of less than four hours' duration falls in this group, as do operations associated with a major break in aseptic technique, e.g., large colon resection.

IV. DIRTY WOUND. Pus is encountered at operation or a perforated viscus is found. A traumatic wound of more than four hours' duration is put in this category. An example of a dirty wound is guttural pouch empyema.

Definition

In addition, the surgeon must *define* what is infection. Is an inflamed wound with serous discharge infected or possibly infected? Should the definition of infection include a purulent exudate?

In human surgery, the rate of infection for "clean wounds" using the definition above is 1.5%. In our hospital, the rate of infection of certain clean operations such as arthroscopy, is close to zero.

Prevention

Every aseptic or preventive practice should be viewed as desirable if there is a possibility, albeit slight, that it will lead to the prevention of wound infection. Failure to adopt practices that might conceivably prevent infection should be considered unwise ethically and legally.[9]

Prevention of infection begins on many fronts. To avoid prolongation of operating time, the surgeon should not even attempt the surgery without a working knowledge of the local anatomy and, where applicable, practice on cadaver specimens. It has been demonstrated clinically and experimentally that the infection rate of clean wounds roughly doubles with every hour of surgery.[4] There are four possible explanations: (1) dosage of bacterial contamination increases with time, (2) wound cells are damaged by drying and by exposure to air and retractors, (3) increased amounts of suture and electrocoagulation may reduce the local resistance of the wound, and (4) longer procedures are more likely to be associated with blood loss and shock, thereby reducing the general resistance of the animal.[4]

Failure to observe the fundamental techniques for handling tissue greatly contributes to the risk of infection. These techniques include prevention of serum formation, hemostasis, and adequate debridement. Careful consideration of antimicrobial therapy is important, especially when using prosthetic implants such as mesh for herniorrhaphy or nonabsorbable sutures for laryngoplasty. In a classic study Burke emphasized the need to give prophylactic antibiotics *before* contamination occurs and showed that if administration is delayed beyond a certain point the benefit is lost.[2]

Even simple procedures such as the use of double gloves can reduce the incidence of infection. Double gloving should be employed in *all* orthopedic operations involving fracture manipulation where the risk of perforation is high. We do not advocate double gloving for all equine operations mentioned in this book, but we routinely double glove during the draping procedure, as this is commonly where a break in asepsis occurs. The outer gloves are shed just prior to making the skin incision, or if double gloving will be used throughout the operation, the outer gloves are then changed. Studies show that because more holes occur in the outer gloves than in the inner ones, and contamination of outer gloves is more frequent than of inner ones, frequent changing of the outer gloves during the procedure is an important way of minimizing contamination.[13]

Appropriate operating room conduct *and* attire should be considered as the norm in any of the surgeries described in this textbook. Gown over scrub clothes (not street clothes), caps, and masks are the current standard in modern equine practice.

Draping the wound or surgical site should not be underplayed in equine surgery. We have devoted a section to this to emphasize its importance.

The use of various substances to irrigate the wound during surgery has received extensive clinical and experimental study in human surgery, but controlled studies in equine surgery have not been performed. Certainly the literature is confusing, especially regarding the inclusion of various antiseptics such as povidone-iodine in the flush solution. One study, for example, demonstrated that flushing with povidone-iodine produced favorable results,[15] but another showed no beneficial effects.[5] Another study showed that for high risk cases, the inclusion of a topical antiseptic such as povidone-iodine *with* prophylactic systemic antibiotics may be beneficial.[7] Clinical trials to support or refute these methods to reduce infection in horses are lacking. At the present time we are still of two minds about the use of povidone-iodine as a flush. We certainly have abandoned its use as an abdominal cavity flush and only reserve it for contaminated and dirty wounds. Such flushing is always accomplished by copious volumes of irrigating fluid. The benefit of mechanical rinsing should not be underestimated. When the literature has been carefully analyzed, it appears that the inclusion of antibiotics in flush solutions *is* beneficial. Using penicillin rather than saline solution lowered the incidence of infection in sutured lacerations in people,[12] as did the inclusion of neomycin/bacitracin.[1]

The potentiation of infection by foreign material (e.g., sutures) and devitalized tissue is well recognized. The *type* of suture material selected also can influence the incidence of postoperative infection.[11] Studies have shown that the number of bacteria in a wound needed to establish infection can be reduced 10,000-fold by the use of a silk suture and can be reduced even further if tissue is enclosed in the suture.[6] The *type* of suture material selected also can influence the incidence of postoperative infection.[11]

All wounds contain bacteria regardless of the wound's being accidental or intentional. The source of bacteria in the "clean" surgical wound is the endogenous microbial population of normal skin. Deep within the hair follicles, microorganisms can be as numerous as 10^3 per gram of tissue. It is the normal flora of the skin that constitutes a significant source of infection to all surgical patients. The microtrauma (knicks and abrasions) produced by clippers and safety razors have been shown to increase the infection rate in human surgical patients. Because of the thickness and density of hair in animals, clipping and shaving are unavoidable, but wound infection produced by endogenous skin flora can be minimized by careful skin preparation prior to surgery.

Open traumatic wounds may contain bacteria in sufficient quantities that wound closure will result in infection. The analysis of tissue samples to quantitate the number of bacteria (quantitative wound biopsy) has received considerable application in man and is beginning to be used in veterinary surgery, notably in the horse.[10,14] It is also applicable to skin grafting to ascertain if the graft bed is suitable. We do not use quantitative wound biopsy routinely but would encourage the reader to use it if available. It has been stated that the technique should not replace a thorough physical examination and sound surgical judgment.[10] Wounds can be closed if the number of bacteria per gram of tissue is 10^5 or less. Some sources quote 10^6 as the number.[10,14] Some bacteria may be clinically more significant at much lower levels than have been described.

Treatment

The key to successful treatment of wound infection is early recognition. This, in turn, is related to the standard of patient care that the horse receives. As soon as wound infection is diagnosed or pending wound infection is suspected, a good avenue of communication between the surgeon and the person responsible for the horse must be established. The client should be informed of the seriousness of the infection and the potential consequences.

The surgeon should wear sterile surgical gloves during any treatment of the wound itself. Such treatment should be scheduled *after* the day's surgery to reduce the possibility of spread of infection to other surgical patients.

A bacterial swab should be taken and submitted for both anaerobic and aerobic culture. The appropriate hematology samples should also be submitted when systemic involvement is likely. In the simplest of cases, removal of some ventrally located skin sutures to provide drainage may be all that is required. Other more elaborate measures, such as insertion of closed suction or Penrose drains, may be required. The wound will require daily cleaning, and scalding of the skin should be prevented by applying petrolatum to areas of ventral drainage. Sterile gloves should be worn. For infected wounds on the lower limbs of horses some form of bandaging is usually essential. Not only does a cotton bandage protect the wound from exogenous contaminations with organisms such as *Pseudomonas* spp. and *Proteus* spp., but it will, through capillary action, act like a wick to draw away fluids and exudates. Bandages also reduce formation of edema in the limbs.

The use of topical antimicrobial sprays (usually colored a bright red or yellow) are of doubtful value in the management of an established wound infection. The active ingredient in these sprays is frequently inactivated by tissue fluids and is prevented for the most part from reaching the source of infection.[8] Infected wounds of the limbs of horses are frequently pruritic, and restraint in the form of a neck cradle will be necessary to prevent mutilation and dislodging of bandages and dressings.

Probably because of the large number of prosthetic hips implanted in man, comparatively little has appeared in the veterinary literature regarding the management of infection following the use of implants. Buried polymerized caprolactam (Vetafil) historically has been one of the most common offenders. It is packaged in plastic dispenser bottles, chemically sterilized, and suitable for skin closure. It must be autoclaved before being buried and never used in the presence of infection. If these principles are not followed, chronic drainage and fistulation will occur, typical of infection that has become established around a foreign body. Infection following the use of a nonmetalic prosthesis (e.g., polypropylene for herniorrhaphy) and insertion of metallic orthopedic implants will be discussed in more detail.

Despite the widespread use of various types of suture material for laryngoplasty, little has been written about management of the serious postoperative complication of infection around the prosthesis. The technique of laryngoplasty is discussed in Chapter 6. The principles of prevention of infection previously discussed are all appropriate to laryngoplasty. Management of an infected laryngeal prosthesis must be focused on its eventual removal. It should be removed under general anesthesia when localized swelling and edema have subsided. To salvage the horse and return it to some form of respiratory function will require arytenoidectomy.

The treatment of an infected synthetic mesh used for herniorrhaphy should follow principles similar to those used to treat an infected midline incision. Removal of one or two offending anchoring sutures will occasionally resolve the infection and is always worth a try. If the entire mesh is infected, the surgeon will find discolored, devitalized, and unhealthy tissue immediately adjacent to the mesh. This will be a strong indication that the entire mesh must be removed along with any fistulous tracts. When the wound has sterilized itself (several weeks later), the mesh is reinserted.

Following removal of the infected mesh, the wound can be closed immediately with 18 or 22 g wire in a simple interrupted vertical mattress suture, placed through all layers of the abdominal wall.[17] Prior to such a closure, devitalized infected tissue must be removed by sharp dissection. To reduce the tendency of the wire to cut, 2.5-cm lengths of hard rubber are used in the sections of suture overlying the skin. The sutures are preplaced, and the defect in the abdominal wall is closed by putting simultaneous tension on all sutures. Closure of the skin is optional[15] and will depend on the amount of drainage required to avoid abscessation. This method of midline closure is also applicable to an infected midline incision that has occurred *without* mesh implantation. Similar principles are followed, including removal of all previous sutures, sharp dissection of devitalized infected tissue, removal of fistulous tracts, and apposition of the body wall using the suture pattern described.[16]

Infection following internal fixation of a fracture (osteomyelitis) is caused by contamination of an open fracture or contamination at the time of open reduction. Contamination may occur during surgery despite antibiotics and strict aseptic technique, especially if the operation is long. Broad-spectrum antibiotics should be given to horses with any fracture in which internal fixation devices will be implanted. The ideal duration of chemoprophylaxis in animals undergoing orthopedic surgery has not been determined. In man, it has been shown that short-term *perioperative* regimens (24 to 48 hr) are as effective as regimens lasting two to three weeks.[6]

The most striking clinical sign of a horse with osteomyelitis following internal fixation is reluctance to bear weight. The onset of lameness may be sudden. The limb, unless it is protected by a cast, will be hot and painful, there will be leukocytosis, and there may be fever. There is usually retarded wound healing over the implants or even fistula formation. Radiographically, there will be lysis at the fracture site as well as around the implants (along the screw threads), under the plate, or along the pin if one is used. Sequestra may be evident.

The treatment of osteomyelitis following internal fixation requires more than the administration of antibiotics. Culturing a sinus tract may be useful (a bone sample is preferable), not so much from the standpoint of what antibiotic is to be used, but to give the surgeon an idea as to the epidemiology of the infection. Antibiotics are useful if systemic signs of infection exist.

An infected fracture must be made stable at all costs if it is to heal. It has been shown repeatedly that a stable infected fracture is better than an unstable infected fracture.[3] Bone union must occur before the sepsis can be overcome. In some cases the internal fixation devices (e.g., bone plates) must be removed and replaced by another more stable device. The existing internal fixation devices may be left in place as long as they are providing stability. Some wound infections require excision of fistulous tracts, sequestrectomy, and bone grafting. If the bone graft is used, it should be inserted in a viable bed with an abundant blood supply; otherwise, the survival of the graft is severely compromised. External coaptation to aid in achieving stability of the fractures is often required.

Suction drains or ingress/egress systems are sometimes of value, although the technical problems associated with the proper maintenance of such systems in an uncooperative horse make their value questionable.

Treatment of infection following internal fixation is often much more expensive than postoperative infections after other surgical procedures mentioned in this section. It must be emphasized that any further treatment is usually fruitless if *stability* at the fracture site cannot be achieved.[3]

The potential for peritonitis always exists following abdominal surgery in horses when the lumen of the bowel is entered (e.g., enterotomy anastomosis). Other contributing factors are poor technique (leaks in anastomosis), excessive handling of tissues, and overzealous use of chemically irritating antiseptics (e.g., 10% povidone-iodine). Both anaerobic and aerobic bacteria are usually present. Anaerobic bacteria have been traditionally underestimated because of inadequate sampling methods at the time cultures are taken. Acute peritonitis is characterized by shock, ileus, abdominal distention, and nasogastric reflex (stomach tube). The animal may be febrile, the refill time will be poor, and there will be hemoconcentration and leukopenia. Plasma protein will decline due to its effective loss from the circulation into the inflamed peritoneal cavity (third spacing of fluid). Abdominal paracentesis following abdominal surgery as a diagnostic aid is of limited value; an invasion as small as an exploratory laparotomy in a normal healthy horse can cause high white counts in abdominal fluid (this normally resolves in a few days). In acute peritonitis, however, the neutrophil is characterized by degenerative changes, and a consistent and continued rise in the count will occur.

An aggressive, energetic attitude is required to treat acute peritonitis. Attention must be given first to fluid replacement, gastric decompression, and analgesia. Antibiotics directed at both anaerobes and aerobes are required. The usual prescription is penicillin in combination with one of the aminoglycosides. In our experience acute wound dehiscence does not seem to be a problem with acute peritonitis unless the horse is in pain and violent and a mechanical disruption of the suture line occurs. Midline incisions seem to heal even in the face of acute peritonitis.

Lavage has been widely advocated in both small animal and human cases of peritonitis, but increasing doubt has arisen over just how long an animal can tolerate continual loss of peritoneal fluid. Application of these methods to horses is logical but fraught with technical problems. Localized flushing through ventrally located catheters is, in our opinion, of questionable value. Instillation of catheters in the flanks and collection through ventrally located catheters also is of limited value because the ingress fluid tends to follow several paths of least resistance without exposing the enormous surface area of the peritoneum to the benefits of the lavage.

The most effective way to lavage the horse's abdomen is to reopen the midline incision under general anesthesia and liberally expose all of the abdomen to large volumes of warmed polyionic solutions. The inclusion of antibiotics is not recommended, especially antibiotics that produce neuromuscular blockade and therefore the potential for respiratory arrest while the horse is anesthetized. The literature abounds with experimental and clinical experiences with the use of antiseptics (especially povidone-iodine) in the abdominal cavity. We have drifted further and further away from using antiseptics in the abdomen, as the literature is tending to discredit them as opposed to the initial enthusiasm toward their use in the early 1970s.

Certainly a horse with acute peritonitis is a poor anesthetic risk, and good clinical judgment is required in deciding *when* lavage under general anesthesia is indicated. Surgery should be timed to occur after stabilization (e.g., treatment of shock, endotoxemia) has been undertaken and it is becoming evident that conservative measures are failing.

References

1. Benjamin, J.B., and Volz, R.G.: Efficacy of a topical antibiotic irrigant in decreasing or eliminating bacterial contamination in surgical wounds. Clin. Orthop. 184:114, 1984.
2. Burke, J.F.: The effective period of preventive antibiotic action in experimental incisions and dermal lesions. Surgery 50:161, 1961.
3. Burri, C.: Post-traumatic Osteomyelitis. Bern, Hans Huber Publishers, 1975.
4. Cruse, P.J.E., and Ford, R.: The epidemiology of wound infection: A 10-year prospective study of 62,939 wounds. Symposium on Surgical Infections. Surg. Clin. North Am. 60:27, 1980.
5. de Jong, T.E., Vierhout, R.J., and Vroonhoven, T.J.: Povidone-iodine irrigation of the subcutaneous tissue to prevent surgical wound infections. Surg. Gynecol. Obstet. 155:221, 1982.
6. Elek, S.D., and Conen, P.E.: The virulence of *Staphylococcus pyogenes* for man. A study of the problems of wound infection. Br. J. Exp. Pathol. 38:573–586, 1957.

7. Fitzgerald, R.H., and Thompson, R.L.: Current Concepts Review: Cephalosporin antibiotics in the prevention and treatment of musculoskeletal sepsis. J. Bone Joint Surg. 65-A:1201, 1983.
8. Gallard, R.B., Heine, K.J., Trachtenberg, L.S., et al.: Reduction of surgical wound infection rates in contaminated wounds treated with antiseptics combined with systemic antibiotics: An experimental study. Surgery 91:329, 1982.
9. Garner, J.S., Emori, T.G., and Haley, R.W.: Operating room practices for the control of infection in U.S. Hospitals. October 1976 to July 1977. Surg. Gynecol. Obstet. 155:873, 1982.
10. Hackett, R.P., Dimock, B.A., and Bentinck-Smith, J.: Quantitative bacteriology of experimentally incised skin wounds in horses. Equine Vet. J. 15:37, 1983.
11. Le Cicero, J., Robbins, J.A., and Webb, W.R.: Complications following abdominal fascial closures using various nonabsorbable sutures. Surg. Gynecol. Obstet. 157:25, 1983.
12. Lindsey, D., Nava, C., and Marti, M.: Effectiveness of penicillin irrigation in control of infection in sutured lacerations. J. Trauma 22:186, 1982.
13. McCue, S.F., Berg, E.W., and Saunders, E.A.: Efficacy of double-gloving as a barrier to microbial contamination during total joint arthroplasty. J. Bone Joint Surg. 63-A:811, 1981.
14. Peyton, L.C., and Connelly, M.B.: Evaluation of quantitative bacterial counts as an aid in the treatment of wounds in the horse. Eq. Vet. J. 15:251, 1983.
15. Sindelar, W.F., and Mason, G.R.: Irrigation of subcutaneous tissue with povidone-iodine solution for prevention of surgical wound infections. Surg. Gynecol. Obstet. 148:227, 1979.
16. Tulleners, E.P., and Fretz, P.B.: Prosthetic repair of large abdominal wall defects in horses and food animals. J. Am. Vet. Med. Assoc. 182:258, 1983.
17. Tulleners, R.P., and Donawick, W.J.: Secondary closure of infected abdominal incisions in cattle and horses. J. Am. Vet. Med. Assoc. 182:1377, 1983.

Nosocomial Infections

The incidence of nosocomial infections in veterinary hospitals is still only in the early stages of investigation; however, they have recently been recognized as a major problem.[6] Although the highest incidence rates are observed in large referral or teaching hospitals, nosocomial infections can occur in any veterinary practice.

Definition

Nosocomial (hospital acquired) infections are those that occur during hospitalization but are not present or incubating at the time of admission. Such infections may become clinically apparent during hospitalization or after discharge from the hospital. As a general rule, new infections occurring after 48 hours of hospitalization can be considered to be nosocomial.[5] Nosocomial infections are frequently caused by endogenous microorganisms inhabiting the patient's flora. Bacteria are the most frequent agents involved in nosocomial infections, but viruses, chlamydia, mycoplasma, fungi, and protozoa can also be involved.

Etiology and Pathogenesis

For a nosocomial infection to develop, a potential pathogen must be transmitted to a susceptible patient. The source of most endemic nosocomial infections is the endogenous flora of the patient.[6,7] The inanimate environment of the patient has minimal influence on the incidence of nosocomial infections that are caused by multiple drug-resistant bacteria. The likelihood that a patient will become infected depends on a complex interaction of four major factors: (1) the virulence of the agent, (2) the patient's susceptibility to infection by the agent, (3) the nature of exposure to the agent, and (4) the effect of antimicrobial therapy. Several factors that are considered to be important in the nosocomial colonization of human beings with multiple drug-resistant bacteria include: (1) patient to patient spread, often facilitated by transient carriage of the organisms on the hands of the attending personnel; (2) direct spread between patients due to environmental contamination; and (3) the effect of antibiotic pressures, including suppression of susceptible flora with sequential colonization by multiple drug-resistant bacteria and selection of resistant subpopulations of bacteria present in the flora.[7] Some factors that are not considered to be important for human beings but that need to be considered for animals include housing conditions, patient hygiene, and behaviorial aspects of feeding and defecation.

The sources of the opportunistic pathogens causing nosocomial infections include people, animals, inanimate objects, air currents, and occasionally insects or rodents. Once bacteria gain entrance to the hospital, they become part of the "normal flora" of animals. Therefore, the patient becomes its own major reservoir for endogenous infections. Common sites of colonization include the upper respiratory and digestive tracts. It is considered that the important source of organisms that infect the patient and sustain an endemic outbreak is the patient's intestinal tract.[6] As an example of this in the horse, a recent study at Colorado State University demonstrated intestinal colonization of horses by multiple drug-resistant (MDR) bacteria during the course of hospitalization. Nineteen horses that had not been hospitalized previously at the Veterinary Teaching Hospital were cultured on admission and on the fourth day of hospitalization.[6] Twelve horses became colonized with MDR organisms. One additional horse included in the study had been released from the hospital 10 weeks prior to readmission. This horse was colonized with MDR organisms at the time of admission. The organisms were identified as *Klebsiella sp.*, *Escherichia coli*, *Enterobacter sp.*, *Salmonella enteritidis* and *Citrobacter freundii*. All these bacterial isolates share a unique pattern of resistance to ampicillin, chloramphenicol, and gentamicin, which, in mating studies, was shown to be readily transferable. This study indicated a conjugate or plasmid was probably responsible for the resistance.

Bacteria may acquire resistance due to the presence of extrachromosomal plasmids, "R Factors," which may be transferred in total between bacteria and may contain genetic elements called transposons capable of moving from one R factor to another. Such transfer of plasmids and transposons allows resistances to spread widely among the bacterial population, crossing species and genera boundaries. Moreover, several resistant determinants may be linked on one plasmid, making it possible for resistance to multiple unrelated antibiotics to emerge together. Bacteria may also acquire resistance by spontaneous chromosomal mutation, which may be selected from a population of sensitive organisms by "antibiotic pressures." The aforementioned study in the horse demonstrated nosocomial colonization of veterinary patients in a manner similar to that observed in human patients. It is also significant that 60 to 87% colonization was detected, using only a single fecal sample of 1 to 2 g from each subject.[6] This common source of multiple drug resistance was considered to be related to an endemic plasmid problem.

Certain types of patients are known to be at a high risk for bacterial colonization or infection. In an investigation of an outbreak of nosocomial *Salmonella Saint-Paul* infection in hospitalized horses at the University of California, Veterinary Medical Teaching Hospital in Davis, it was found that horses receiving parenteral antibiotics were at 10 times greater risk of having S. *Saint-Paul* isolated than were horses not receiving parenteral antibiotics.[4] The organism had an unusual pattern of antibiotic resistance, being sensitive to tetracycline, yet being resistant to most commonly used antimicrobial drugs tested, including penicillin, streptomycin, neomycin, kanamycin, gentamicin, chloramphenicol, sulfa drugs, and ampicillin. Most of the 33 horses from which S. *Saint-Paul* was isolated showed no or minimal signs of salmonellosis. In 23, some degree of clinical signs were found, 2 died with acute S. *Saint-Paul* bacteremia, and 7 others were euthanized following moderate to severe diarrhea.[4] In the horse, association of antibiotics with occurrence of salmonellosis is considered to be caused by selective elimination of the gut flora antagonistic to *Salmonella*. The authors believed that these cases were nosocomial for several reasons. The serotype seldom had been isolated from hospitalized animals at this clinic, and a relatively large number of cases were detected within a short period. In addition, this organism is most often isolated from turkeys and humans and is not commonly isolated from horses. Finally, the organism had an unusual pattern of antibiotic resistance.

Other associated factors were considered to influence the likelihood of infection in this hospital population.[4] Horses intubated with nasogastric tubes, for example, were 3.9 times more likely to have had the organism isolated from fecal specimens than horses not intubated, and horses with a presenting complaint of colic had 2.2 times greater risk of isolation than horses with other presenting complaints. Based on their findings of parenteral antibiotics as an important iatrogenic risk factor in their study, the authors felt that antibiotic use should be carefully evaluated for each patient. It was also noted that further studies may suggest that certain classes of antibiotics were less likely to be associated with an increased risk of nosocomial *Salmonella* infection or disease and that it might be possible to prefer these antibiotics over others for high-risk patients.[4]

With regard to this aspect, a study has been carried out on the bacteriologic fecal flora of horses before and after oral doses of oxytetracycline or of trimethoprim plus sulfadiazine.[9] Administration of oxytetracyclines to horses was followed by large increases in counts of coliforms, *Bacteroides*, and *Streptococcus* species, as well as the appearance of *Clostridium perfringens* organisms in large numbers, and the accumulation of watery fluid in the rectal contents. On the other hand, these changes were not seen following administration of trimethoprim-sulfadiazine, and it was concluded that oral treatment of horses with this combination was unlikely to be accompanied by the same hazardous effect.[9] It is to be noted that in a study of colitis in the horse it was concluded that C. *perfringens* type A, was the principal etiologic agent.[8]

Normally the host and the anaerobic bacterial flora of the digestive tract act synergistically to limit colonization by potentially pathogenic bacteria, a mechanism known as "colonization resistance." Oral therapy with partially absorbed antimicrobials or parenteral therapy with antimicrobials excreted in the intestine in active form may lead to a decrease in colonization resistance if the anaerobic flora is susceptible to the drug. The ability of antimicrobials to affect colonization resistance has been classified for various agents. In addition to suppressing normal flora, the antimicrobial therapy promotes development of antimicrobial resistant bacteria. Resistance to more than one agent frequently occurs and is usually plasmid mediated. Plasmid-mediated resistance is readily transferred between gram-negative bacteria. The antimicrobial therapy therefore may result in the development of an endemic plasmid or resistance factor rather than simply a single endemic strain of bacteria.

Twenty-three isolations of *Serratia* spp. were made from 21 horses at the University of Florida over a 3-½-year period. Possible nosocomial infection, variable antibiotic sensitivity, and a trend toward decreased antibiotic sensitivity after antibiotic administration were noted.

Control of Nosocomial Infections

The initial factor in the control of any nosocomial infection is to identify the reservoirs, which will include colonized and infected patients, as well as sources of environmental contamination. Careful microbiologic surveillance is important to detect many epidemics of two or more similar MDR isolates. Detection of certain resistance patterns, such as gentamicin resistance or multiple drug resistance, indicate nosocomial infection. Gentamicin resistance can be considered a marker for plasmid-mediated multiple resistance.[2] Precautions to control an endemic nosocomial infection include segregation, isolation, the use of gloves, careful hand washing, and asepsis. Susceptible patients need to be separated, and circumstances may sometimes warrant closure of the hospital unit to new admissions. At the same time, the host risk should be modified as much as possible. Hospitalization time should be kept to a minimum. Antibiotic use should be carefully controlled, particularly in surgical prophylaxis (discussed in Chapter 3). Topical antimicrobial therapy rather then systemic therapy could be useful in some instances. Specific antimicrobial therapy against a nosocomial isolate is an area fraught with hazard, and specific recommendations would be premature. While agents such as amikacin and cefuroxime are effective against gentamicin-resistant *Klebsiella*, indiscriminant use of these drugs causes more antibiotic pressure.

In another study of the antibiograms of 408 *Salmonella* species isolated from horses during a 3-year period, the predominant *Salmonella* serotype isolated was Group B and a high percentage of all isolates were resistant to ampicillin and tetracycline. A pattern of increasing resistance to chloramphenicol and gentamicin was also documented for serogroup B isolates. In another group of isolates, there was a decrease in incidence of susceptibility to trimethoprim-sulfamethoxazole, but these changes are not as remarkable as the overall decrease of susceptibility to chloramphenicol and gentamicin. In summary, an increasing level of resistance to ampicillin, chloramphenicol, gentamicin, and tetracycline was observed in isolates from patients during a 3-year period. The report established the presence of serious problems in these patients prior to receiving treatment at the particular hospital, and it was considered that these may have been associated with prior contact with antibiotics via food, prescription, or undirected use of drugs by an owner or manager.[1]

Based on experience with nosocomial salmonellosis, our clinical microbiologist has identified problem areas and set up control measures. Three major areas of concern have been identified: (1) infected animals; (2) physical facilities, and (3) personnel.

Infected animals are the major source of large numbers of salmonellae. Following are some recommendations that should be established as hospital policy.

1. Any animal arriving at the hospital as a possible salmonellosis case should be placed in the isolation barn.
2. Any hospitalized animal with a positive *Salmonella* culture should be moved to an isolation area.
3. Any hospitalized animal with clinical signs consistent with salmonellosis, but without bacteriologic confirmation, may remain in the large animal barn only if all hospital personnel are aware of the case and adequate precautions are established. These precautions should include personnel assignments that limit possible spread of contamination, setting up footbaths, policies for changing clothes, and placement of rope barriers to restrict all traffic from a perimeter area, including adjacent stalls and areas of drainage in hallways.
4. Any animal placed in the isolation areas must remain there until discharged from the premises. If an animal is to be brought back into the barns from an isolation area, it must have three negative fecal cultures (24 or more hours apart) during a period of one week and be free of clinical signs of possible contagious disease during that week.

Physical facilities must be properly cleaned so they do not serve as a reservoir.

1. *All walls and floors must be repaired and sealed* so that they can be cleaned and disinfected.

2. If loose and torn edges of floor coverings are discovered, they must be trimmed away for proper cleaning.

3. All stalls must be cleaned as if contaminated by salmonellae, regardless of the history of the animal leaving the stall.

4. Shovels, forks, and brooms must be cleaned after use in each stall.

5. Drain covers must be removed and drain bowls must be cleaned to prevent reverse flow of contamination.

6. Hard surface stalls that have been cleaned and disinfected can be reassigned the next day. Dirt floors should remain unoccupied for one week.

7. Cleaning personnel should wear rubber boots, which are to be disinfected after cleaning each stall.

Personnel training must continue to be a major part of any control program for nosocomial infections.

1. Boots, footbaths, and scrub brushes should be available and used in all contaminated or potentially contaminated areas. As a precaution, footbaths should be required between major areas of the barn.

2. Traffic in contaminated areas should be restricted.

3. Clothes changes and showers should be required after handling an animal with salmonellosis.

4. Washing of hands and cleanliness should be emphasized.

To facilitate these recommendations at Colorado State University, a full-time Infectious Disease Control Officer has been appointed. This person is a staff member who can direct cleaning crews, assign or restrict stall use, maintain liaison with the bacteriology laboratory, and set up, maintain, and enforce control measures for footbaths, traffic, and relocation of animals.

References

1. Benson, C.E., Palmer, J.E., and Bannister, M.F.: Antibiotic susceptibility of *Salmonella sp.* isolated at a large animal veterinary medical center: A 3-year study. Can. J. Comp. Med. 49:125–128, 1985.

2. Casewell, M.W., and Phillips, I.: Aspects of the plasmid-mediated antibiotic resistance and epidemiology of *Klebsiella sp.* Am. J. Med. 70:459–462, 1981.

3. Colahan, P.T., Peyton, L.C., Connelly, M.R., and Peterson, R.: *Serratia spp* infection in 21 horses. J. Am. Vet. Med. Assoc. 185:209–211, 1984.

4. Hird, D.W., Pappaioanou, M., and Smith, B.P.: Case-control study of risk factors associated with isolation of *Salmonella Saint Paul* in hospitalized horses. Am. J. Epidemiol. 120:852–864, 1984.

5. Jones, R.L.: Control of nosocomial infections. In Current Veterinary Therapy IX. Philadelphia, W.B. Saunders, 1986.

6. Jones, R.L., Fafoutis, D., and McCurnin, D.M.: Nosocomial colonization of horses by multiple antibiotic-resistant enterobacterioceae. J. Am. Vet. Med. Assoc. 187:291–292, 1985.

7. Weinstein, R.A., and Cabins, S.A.: Strategies for prevention and control of multiple drug-resistant nosocomial infection. Am. J. Med. 70:449–454, 1981.

8. Weirup, M.: Equine intestinal clostridiosis. Acta Vet. Scan. (Suppl.) 62:1–182, 1977.

9. White, G., and Prior, S.D.: Comparative effects of oral administration of trimethoprim-sulfadiazine or oxytetracycline on the faecal flora of horses. Vet. Rec. 111:316–318, 1982.

Laminitis in the Postsurgical Patient

Laminitis (founder) as it relates to the equine surgical patient is an ever present threat to the equine surgical patient. All who perform major surgery on horses will have experienced a case of laminitis at one time or another.

Etiology

For the sake of discussion we have divided laminitis into *systemic* and *mechanical* with respect to the etiology of the condition.

SYSTEMIC LAMINITIS. Systemic laminitis involves many body systems, and the chain of events that occurs is complex. Rather than true inflammation, it is now well accepted that there is an ischemia of the sensitive laminae of the digit with arteriovenous *shunting* of blood as a result of peripheral vasoconstriction.

Carbohydrate overload is the most widely recognized cause of laminitis and, despite the advances that have been made in our knowledge of equine nutrition, still occurs. The horse that is most prone to laminitis due to carbohydrate overload is an obese but well-cared for show horse, for example, a Quarterhorse used for halter classes. When this type of patient is admitted to our clinic, we are careful about the amount of concentrate the horse is fed. We prefer to remove all grain or sweet feed from the diet during hospitalization and to feed grass hay only. This regimen is often a source of client discontent, but the loss of 50 kg of body weight is far easier to manage than an acute case of laminitis with rotation of the distal phalanx. This type of patient has been commonly incriminated as being at risk for postanesthetic myopathy. Reduction in the grain in the diet will possibly minimize the chances of this occurring.

The pathogenesis for laminitis due to carbohydrate overload begins with an alteration in gut flora, with proliferation of lactic-acid-producing bacteria. This causes an alteration in pH of the contents (pH 7 to pH 4); killing enterobacteria and liberating the key component of systemic laminitis, gram-negative *endotoxin*. Lactic acid is also produced by certain strains of bacteria. Endotoxin, plasma lactate, and a generalized low flow state ("shock") all contribute to arteriovenous shunting within the vasculature of the digits to produce an ischemic necrosis of the laminae. Necrosis of the laminae disrupts the interlocking of the laminae and horny wall, and the end result is rotation of the distal phalanx.[4] This is an oversimplification of a very complex chain of events within the horse's body, but for the sake of discussion of laminitis as it relates to the equine surgical patient it is probably adequate.

Laminitis following *abdominal surgery* has been described as "one of the most devastating and disheartening complications that can occur after a horse has essentially recovered from colic.[6,11] It is an ever present threat whenever there is strangulation of the bowel with mucosal damage or any degree of stasis of the contents. The underlying cause is production of endotoxin, its absorption through damaged sloughing intestinal wall, and the resulting *endotoxemia*.[7] It is often seen 48 to 72 hours after surgical correction of the underlying cause of the colic.[6] The severity of the laminitis can vary from a mild stiffness and reluctance to move, with no radiographic evidence of rotation, to a severe crippling lameness with marked rotation of the distal phalanx and sloughing of the hoof wall, necessitating euthanasia. The rate of development of the laminitis also correlates with its severity. A rapid onset usually means a severe case will ensue, and early aggressive treatment is essential.

The development of laminitis in cases of gut stasis, bowel strangulation, and mucosal damage is compounded by peripheral vascular collapse "shock" and varying degrees of hypercoagulability (disseminated intravascular coagulation, DIC).

The relationship of laminitis to a *severe soft tissue infection, cellulitis, retained placenta,* and *pneumonia* can all be explained by *circulating endotoxin*. Prevention is the key to successful management, but laminitis often occurs when it is least expected. High doses of broad-spectrum antibiotics, especially those effective against gram-negative organisms, as well as supportive measures such as fluid therapy, are important in the overall prevention of laminitis as a sequela to these conditions. Laminitis should always be kept in the back of one's mind when a case of postoperative salmonellosis occurs. The underlying etiology is, again, circulating endotoxin. In salmonellosis, the ensuing shock and circulatory collapse, DIC, are also part of the pathogenesis. Other less likely conditions with which laminitis can coexist in surgical patients are verminous arteritis, renal disease, and chronic liver disease.[1]

Several drugs have been incriminated in causing laminitis. Quinidine sulfate used to treat atrial fibrillation and the corticosteroids are ones that come to mind. In this latter group, it has been shown hydrocortisone and betamethasone potentiate the vasoconstrictor actions of biogenic amines.[2] Experimentally, betamethasone has been shown to be 10 times as potent as hydrocortisone, although this does not necessarily mean that this factor of potency exists in clinical doses.[2]

Acute laminitis has also been seen as a manifestation of black walnut (*Juglans regia*) toxicosis. Also seen is limb edema. The toxic principle is called juglone. The condition is seen when black walnut shavings are used as bedding, even when they are mixed in low concentration with pine shavings. Obviously in parts of the world where hardwoods are more abundant, the condition will be seen more often.[9]

MECHANICAL LAMINITIS. Mechanical laminitis is seen when a horse bears excessive weight on one limb because of a painful condition in the opposite member. Such conditions are most commonly fractures that, despite internal fixation and external coaptation, cannot provide enough pain-free support to the limb. Mechanical laminitis is essentially a variation on the classic "road founder". There is no real metabolic component to this type of laminitis, rather a mechanical effect of the pull of the deep digital flexor tendon, with the digital cushion as a fulcrum.[4]

Diagnosis

The signs of laminitis when it appears are similar regardless of the underlying etiology. The horse will be reluctant to walk, and there will be a characteristic shifting of the body weight and an abnormal stance. The digital pulse will be increased, and the horse will begin showing increasing periods of recumbency. The two most common signs of laminitis in a limb that is bearing excessive weight are increasing periods of recumbency and an unusual degree of weight bearing on a limb with a normally painful condition such as a healing fracture or luxation. To complicate matters, rubbing and pressure sores or a broken cast may occur. As soon as laminitis is suspected, radiographs (lateral views) of the feet involved (usually front feet, but hindfeet may be involved in severe cases) should be taken. If the horse is unable to ambulate from the stall to another part of the hospital where radiographs are taken, then they should be taken in the stall using a portable x-ray machine. There are two reasons behind taking radiographs immediately: (1) to establish if a pre-existing rotation of the distal phalanx was present, and the current bout is a flare up (chronic exacerbative laminitis and (2) to establish a baseline set of radiographs to monitor the rate and amount of rotation of the distal phalanx. The prognosis for return to athletic soundness has been correlated to the degree of rotation of P3.[11] The degree of rotation can be determined by subtracting the hoof angle from the angle of the dorsal surface of P3 based on lateral radiographs.

Treatment

The various treatment regimens for *acute* systemic laminitis have, through the years, been more varied and controversial than any other aspect of equine medicine. We do not want to discuss every possible mode of therapy that has been described, and we would certainly not question a particular treatment such as padding the feet or applying sole casts if the reader has had consistent and objectively reliable results. Rather we are presenting what has worked well for us and our colleagues at Colorado State University Veterinary Teaching Hospital. Certainly a "shotgun" approach should be discouraged.

First and foremost in the management of laminitis in a surgical patient is client communication. As soon as practical the person responsible for the horse should be contacted and some form of dialogue established, especially to point out the seriousness of the condition and the possible sequelae

We immediately begin making arrangements to get the horse to a stall that has been bedded in sand or similar soft material. Usually sand has to be moved into the stall from a supply we always have on hand. We feel this bedding is important for the overall comfort of the horse, although we are uncertain in our own minds if further rotation of P3 is prevented or at least slowed. Although unlikely in a hospital situation, if there is excessive grain overload, 1 to 2 gallons of mineral oil per os should be administered to delay absorption of endotoxins, as well as to provide a laxative effect. Many antiinflammatory drugs are currently available, but we have found the judicious use of phenylbutazone to be most beneficial. The initial dose should be administered intravenously to achieve blood levels as rapidly as possible. The constant threat of toxicosis (renal papillary necrosis, gastrointestinal ulceration, protein-losing enteropathy) in prolonged administration of high doses of phenylbutazone should not be forgotten. Corticosteroids are contraindicated. Additional therapy for laminitis includes the use of phenothiazine tranquilizers, such as acepromazine, aimed at increasing circulation to the laminae of the hoof by the peripheral vasodilation. Because of the suspected role of disseminated intravascular coagulation (DIC) in the pathogenesis of laminitis, heparin has been used. It is thought to increase blood flow to the capillaries of the digit by preventing formation of microthrombi. Heparin is certainly not a benign drug, and careful monitoring of various clotting parameters is essential. We do not use heparin routinely for laminitis of systemic origin.

The other drug that may be of use in acute laminitis is the peripheral vasodilator, isoxsuprine hydrochloride. The drug has been used successfully in navicular disease.[10] It is a phenylethylamine derivative of epinephrine and is believed to have alpha-adrenergic receptor antagonist and beta-adrenergic receptor agonist properties. It lowers blood viscosity and inhibits platelet agregation when given in high doses. Its direct vasoactive effect on the smooth muscle wall produces vasodilation.[8] We have used this drug in a limited number of cases and, like most treatment regimens for laminitis, it is almost impossible to judge the degree of contribution the drug has to the overall clinical picture and final outcome.

The key to successful management of laminitis due to excessive weight bearing is attention to the primary problem, which is the pain in the opposite limb. Has the fracture become unstable? Have efforts at rigid immobilization of the fracture failed with plates or screws? Has the surgical site become infected? These all must be addressed and will usually require a cast change (if present) and radiographic evaluation of the injury to assess the source of the pain. In this type of laminitis the contribution of the patient to its own successful recovery should never be underestimated. Some horses just refuse to lie down and do not spare the uninjured limb. A "sensible" horse will spend a large time in sternal or lateral recumbency, thereby resting the support limb.

We have had mixed results with the use of the so called "heart bar" shoe, as far as reducing the amount of rotation following an acute bout of laminitis, but this may be related to how the shoe is applied. It unquestionably takes a skilled farrier to apply such a shoe, because excessive pressure of the bar in the wrong area can result in ischemic necrosis of the tissues of the frog and sole. It is critical that the apex of the heart bar contact the frog in front of the insertion of the deep flexor tendon on the distal phalanx. The bar must not touch the sole and must be sufficiently narrow to avoid pressure to the medial and lateral palmar digital arteries as they enter the foramina of the terminal arch, deep to the digital cushion.[1] Chronic laminitis must be explained to the owner as a condition that will require a constant liaison between an experienced, enthusiastic farrier and veterinarian as well as a financial commitment to both.

The prognosis for subsequent athletic ability will vary from case to case, but certainly the degree of rotation of P3 is a fairly good indicator.[11] In a series of 91 cases, horses with less than 5.5 degrees of rotation returned to former athletic function, whereas horses with more than 11.5 degrees of rotation were lost as performance animals.[11]

In summary, the equine surgeon must always be aware of the potential for laminitis in any surgical patient. Those horses at risk (infectious conditions, gut stasis) must be meticulously monitored for the early signs of the condition so that immediate aggressive treatment can begin without delay.

References

1. Coffman, J.R.: Discussant of Chapman, B., and Platte, G.W.: Laminitis. In Proceedings of the 30th Annual Convention of American Association of Equine Practitioners 1984, 1985, p. 110.
2. Eyre, P., Elmes, P.J., and Strickland, S.: Corticosteroid—potential vascular responses of the equine digit: A possible pharmacologic basis for laminitis. Am. J. Vet. Res. 40:135, 1979.
3. Hood, D.M., Amoss, M.S., Hightower, D. et al.: Equine laminitis: Radioisotopic analysis of the hemodynamics of the foot during the acute disease. J. Eq. Med. Surg. 2:439, 1978.
4. Johnson, J.H.: The Foot. In Equine Medicine and Surgery, 3rd ed. Edited by R.A. Mansmann, E.S. McAllister, and P.W. Pratt. Santa Barbara, CA, American Veterinary Publications, 1983, p. 1048.
5. McIlwraith, C.W.: The acute abdominal patient: Postoperative management and complications. In Symposium on Equine Gastrointestinal Surgery. Vet. Clin. North Am. 4:167, 1982.
6. Milne, D.W.: Postoperative complications: Laminitis. In Equine Medicine and Surgery, 3rd ed. Edited by R.A. Mansmann, E.S. McAllister, and P.W. Pratt. Santa Barbara, CA, American Veterinary Publications, 1983, p. 604.
7. Moore, J.N.: Pathophysiology of intestinal ischemia and endotoxemia. Proceedings of 20th Annual Convention American Association of Equine Practitioners 1984, 1985, p. 295.
8. Neligan, P., Pang, C.Y., Nakatsuka, T., et al.: Pharmacologic action of isoxsuprine in cutaneous and myocutaneous flaps. Plast. Reconstr. Surg. 75:363, 1985.
9. Ralston, S.L., and Rich, V.A.: Black walnut toxicosis in horses. J. Am. Vet. Med. Assoc. 183:1095, 1983.
10. Rose, R.J., Allen, J.R., Hodgson, D.R., et al.: Studies on isoxsuprine hydrochloride for the treatment of navicular disease. Eq. Vet. J. 15:238, 1983.
11. Stick, J.A., Jann, H.W., Scott, E.A. et al.: Pedal bone rotation as a prognostic sign in laminitis of horses. J. Am. Vet. Med. Assoc. 180:251, 1982.

Postoperative Salmonellosis

Acute equine salmonellosis has been reported in association with various factors, including hospitalization,[4,5,7,11] general anesthesia,[8,11] transportation,[7,11] surgery[8,11] (particularly abdominal surgery for colic[4,9,11]), anthelmintic medication,[2,3] tetracycline administration,[6,7] and hot, humid weather.[5] The syndrome concerning the equine surgeon is seen during hospitalization of surgical cases and typically following surgery. It can involve a number of these predisposing factors. The source of the pathogen in many cases is not clear. Contaminated environment[4] and subclinical or inapparent infection in the animal[9] may be a source of the pathogen. Environmental contamination may come from horses with enteritis or from subclinical shedders admitted to the hospital for other reasons.[4,11] Alternatively, the animal may have been infected before developing the clinical signs, such as colic, which prompted its admission to the hospital. Stress associated with colic, transport to the hospital, hospitalization, anesthesia, and surgery may all compromise the immunologic status of carrier animals and initiate clinical enteritis.

Recent findings of Palmer et al. confirm the hypothesis that colicky horses may be shedding *Salmonella* organisms at the time of hospitalization even though many of these shedders do not develop other clinical signs of enteritis.[8,9] Studies have shown that apparently normal horses can be Salmonella shedders, and that such animals can develop clinical salmonellosis after entering a hospital. In one study, feces from 1,451 horses entering a veterinary hospital over a 13-month period were cultured for *Salmonella*.[10] A total of 46 horses (3.2%) yielded one or more *Salmonella*-positive fecal cultures. Twenty horses were found to be excreting *Salmonella* in the feces on admission, and 5 of these later had severe diarrhea associated with enteric salmonellosis. Abdominal surgery and other severe stresses were associated with all cases of severe enteric salmonellosis.

It should be noted, however, that stress of transport, hospitalization, or surgery when a horse is excreting *Salmonella* does not necessarily lead to a clinical problem. In one study evaluating the value of early *Salmonella* cultures in predicting the occurrence of acute salmonellosis as a complication following surgery for colic, for instance, it was found that most colic cases that shed *Salmonella* did not develop acute enteritis despite the extremely stressful conditions they were subjected to. Thirteen out of 100 horses cultured positive for *Salmonella*, but only 2 of these had developed clinical signs of salmonellosis.[8] Because 12 out of 13 of the culture-positive horses survived, it was considered that the infection must have been mild (and this should be contrasted with 28 out of 87 culture-negative horses that survived overall).[8] Thus it appears that being stressed while being exposed to *Salmonella* is not sufficient to produce acute enteritis in all cases. Whether this is caused by variability in the host's response to stress, variability in bacterial virulence, or an as yet undefined factor in the host-bacterium interaction is unclear.

Clinical evidence has also been presented to indicate that the potential for a stressed horse, which happens to be a *Salmonella* carrier, to develop diarrhea after stress may be exacerbated by tetracycline therapy.[6,7] The reason for this has been explained in terms of distribution of tetracycline in the body. Tetracyclines are removed from the blood by the liver and excreted in a concentrated form in the bile into the intestines. Biliary levels average at least 5 to 10 times higher than the simultaneous plasma concentration. This biliary concentration is greater than the minimal inhibitory concentration required against strains of *E. coli*, *Proteus*, and *Klebsiella aerobacter*, the most frequently detected bacterial infections of the human biliary system. The amount of tetracycline that reaches the intestine due to concentration by the liver could have a profound effect on the normal aerobic and anaerobic flora. On the other hand, antibiotics such as penicillin, streptomycin, and chloramphenicol are excreted mainly by the kidney and only a small portion is excreted by the liver. These antibiotics are not thought to reach sufficient concentration to cause comparable disturbances to the normal flora in the intestine. Experimental studies also have been performed to demonstrate the combination of *Salmonella* infection, transportation, surgical stress, and tetracycline administration to produce a salmonellosis syndrome.[7]

Various *Salmonella* species have been involved in clinical equine salmonellosis syndromes. The most common isolates have been *Salmonella typhimurium* and *Salmonella anatum*.[1,4,5] *S. enteritidis*, *S. newport*, *S. heidelberg*, *S. agona*, *S. typhimurium* var. *copenhagen*, *S. infantis*, *S. montevideo*, and others have also been involved. Dual infections have also been reported with *Salmonella typhimurium* and *S. anatum* being the most common.

The syndrome of salmonellosis in hospitalized horses was initially described as a rather specific entity with clinical signs of fever and diarrhea and a neutrophil count of less than 3,600 per cubic mm, or a rapid decline in neutrophilic numbers as specific for the disease.[4] The horse apparently has a relatively small leukocyte reserve, and the hemogram was considered to be an important clinical indicator of bacterial infection and endotoxemia. Because of additional clinical and experimental studies, it is now considered that four clinical syndromes should be considered for a horse infected with *Salmonella* in the hospital situation: (1) asymptomatic fecal shedding, intermittently or constantly; (2) fever, depression, and anorexia without colic or diarrhea, and in some cases neutropenia and left shift; (3) severe, acute fulminant diarrhea with fever, depression, anorexia, neutropenia, and dehydration; (4) septicemia, fever, depression, anorexia, neutropenia, and death.[13] From these syndromes it can be seen that some infected horses may show fever, anorexia, and depression without concurrent diarrhea or any other obvious gastrointestinal abnormalities.

It has been suggested, in one report at least, that the degree of temperature rise may provide an indication of the severity of the problem.[5] In this study, horses that had temperatures of 38.9 to 40° C, with diarrhea, had a 50% survival. When the temperature rise was at the 40.6 to 41.1°C level and diarrhea was present, all the patients succumbed.[5] That 9 out of 16 clinically ill patients in this study died is adequate indication of the severity of the problem.

In another study, where salmonellosis was experimentally produced, neutropenia occurred within 24 hours after stress and lasted 5 days, whereas the diarrhea developed between 3 and 9 days after stress. Therefore, neutropenia may not be apparent clinically at the onset of diarrhea. It is also possible for neutrophilia to be detected at the onset of diarrhea which would be misleading.[7] It was considered, by these workers, that if the clinician is aware of stress, regular white blood cell counts will assist in predicting where stress-induced salmonellosis with enteritis and diarrhea are likely to occur. For reasons cited above, however, the association between *Salmonella* infection, stress, and clinical disease is not an absolute one. Confirmation of the disease requires aggressive bacteriologic studies, and up to 5 consecutive negative cultures are considered appropriate before the presence of salmonellosis can be eliminated.

In clinical salmonellosis, fluid and electrolyte therapy is essential. The value of antimicrobial drugs in enteric salmonellosis of horses requires further study. The efficacy of antimicrobial therapy directed towards eliminating the *Salmonella* from the gastrointestinal tract, lymph nodes, and major organs of the host has not been encouraging or consistent. Chloramphenicol was commonly used but is no longer because of the human health hazards. While the isolate may show sensitivity to drugs such as gentamicin sulfate, acquired resistance to such antibiotics by the organisms is a common problem, and the potential to develop nosocomial infections is a real threat. Early identification of the disease and attempts to minimize surgical and medical stresses are important. *When any hospitalized horse develops a temperature with depression, a white cell count and differential is done immediately.* Although the stress of transportation cannot be eliminated in a referral clinic, timely and fast surgery with minimal stress, both preoperatively and postoperatively, is important. The authors feel that surgery should be performed within 48 hours of hospitalization to minimize the acquisition of an infection and that postoperative hospitalization should be kept to a minimum. One group has suggested that surgery should be performed within 24 or 48 hours of hospitalization or delayed for a week.[4] Although some degree of food withholding is important for general anesthesia, it also should be recognized that starvation acts as an additional stress on the gastrointestinal system and could potentially promote the disease. The use of tetracycline in hospitalized surgical patients should be avoided.

Attention must also be paid to minimizing the chance of hospital contamination. Any horse that develops diarrhea is isolated from other patients. A horse is considered nonsuspect after 3 consecutive negative cultures. It is to be remembered that fewer *Salmonella* organisms are needed to produce the disease in a weak animal. *Salmonella* bacteria have a marked ability to survive and remain viable in places where E. *coli* quickly die out. Only a small amount of urine and/or feces in moisture is needed for good growth of *Salmonella*, and the organism will grow better in diluted urine and feces than in the normal excretions.

Vaccines prepared from *Salmonella typhimurium* have been evaluated in horses.[12] At this stage, the lack of specificity of a causative organism means that vaccination is not yet a reality in the horse.

References

1. Bruner, D.W.: Salmonellosis: A continual threat to New York State's cattle and horses. Cornell Vet. 75:93–96, 1985.
2. Baker, J.R.: Salmonellosis in the horse. Br. Vet. J. 126:100–105, 1970.
3. Dimock, W.W., Edwards, P.R., and Bryner, D.W.: The occurrence of paratyphoid infection in horses following treatment for intestinal parasites. Cornell Vet. 30:319, 1940.
4. Dorn, C.R., Coffman, J.R., Schmidt, D.A., et al.: Neutropenia and salmonellosis in hospitalized horses. J. Am. Vet. Med. Assoc. 166:65–67, 1975.
5. Morse, E.V., Duncan, M.A., Page, E.A., and Fessler, J.F.: *Salmonellosis equidae*: A study of 23 cases. Cornell Vet. 66:198–213, 1976.
6. Owen, R. ap R.: Post stress diarrhoea in the horse. Vet. Rec. 96:267–270, 1975.
7. Owen, R. ap R., Fullerton, J., and Barnum, D.A.: Effects of transportation, surgery and antibiotic therapy in horses infected with *Salmonella*. Am. J. Vet. Res. 44:46, 1983.
8. Palmar, J.E., Benson, C.E., and Whitlock, R.H.: Subclinical salmonellosis in horses with colic. Proceedings of Equine Colic Research Symposium. University of Georgia, 1982, p. 1980.
9. Palmar, J.E., Benson, C.E., and Whitlock, R.H.: *Salmonella* shed by horses with colic. J. Am. Vet. Med. Assoc. 187:256–257, 1985.
10. Smith, B.P., Reina-Guerra, M., and Hardy, A.J.: Prevalence in epizootiology of equine salmonellosis. J. Am. Vet. Med. Assoc. 172:353–356, 1978.
11. Smith, B.P.: Atypical salmonellosis in horses: Fever and depression without diarrhea. J. Am. Vet. Med. Assoc. 175:69–71, 1979.
12. Smith, B.P., Hardy, A.J., Reina-Guerra, M.: A preliminary evaluation of some preparations of S. *typhimurium* as vaccines in horses. Proceedings of Equine Colic Research Symposium, University of Georgia, 1982, p. 211.
13. Whitlock, R.H., Morris, D.D., Palmer, J.E., and Becht, J.L.: Differential diagnosis of acute salmonellosis in colic. Proceedings of Equine Colic Research Symposium, University of Georgia, 1982, p. 187.

Infections of the Respiratory Tract

Many of the operations described in this book are performed on racing horses or show horses. Typically, these horses are in contact with a large number of other individuals, all potentially harboring a wide variety of respiratory viruses. Superimposed on viral diseases may be a poorly ventilated stall with dust and ammonia fumes capable of producing a chemical irritation in the respiratory tract. Further compounding this is the inhalation of dirt and blood during strenuous exercise.[4] Endoscopy of horses involved in maximum exercise has confirmed just how "traumatic" racing is to the pulmonary tissues, as evidenced by the high incidence of blood and dirt found in the lower respiratory tract.[1] A further compromise to the respiratory system occurs when a horse's head is tied up for extended periods, removing the assistance of gravity as a method of clearing exudate and debris. This list of insults to the respiratory system is also compounded by the vague syndrome of "stress," such as the stress of racing and training, changes in weather, or transport over long distances to a surgical facility. Pleuritis and pleural effusion are occasionally seen following stress from transport or general anesthesia. In one study of 82 cases of pleuritis due to pneumonia or lung abscess, 20 horses (24.4%) had been *transported* a long distance. Acute pleuritis can also be seen following general anesthesia.

When a horse is unable to lower its head, natural drainage of the respiratory tract is prevented, and secretions and exudates tend to drain back into the lungs. This hypothesis has been supported by numerous anecdotes. When horses with fractures of the long bones are treated in floatation tanks to reduce the effective body weight, they are unable to lower their heads because of the design of the tank. A frequent complication of prolonged inability to lower the head has been termed floatation-induced pulmonary disease.[7] Occasionally a horse must be cross tied to an overhead wire system to prevent it from lying down and disrupting a suture line (e.g., in femorotibial arthrotomy used for approach to subchondral cysts of the distal femur; see Chapter 5 for details). These horses must be watched carefully for signs of bronchopneumonia and pleuritis because of impairment of natural drainage (gravity) of the respiratory tract. If an overt respiratory infection develops, the horse should be untied and allowed hand grazing as frequently as practical, with its head in the natural position, to aid in removal of exudate from the respiratory tract.

Other causes of postoperative respiratory tract infections are any operations to correct abnormalities of the upper respiratory tract such as laryngoplasty or staphylectomy. In these cases the normal function of the larynx is altered, and the chance of inhalation of foreign material is increased, especially during feeding. Surgery in the region of the guttural pouch can cause nerve dysfunction resulting in dysphagia and aspiration pneumonia. The prognosis for recovery from aspiration pneumonia is variable and has to be assessed on an individual case basis. If aspiration pneumonia is suspected, high doses of broad-spectrum antibiotics are indicated.

The presence of a respiratory tract infection in a surgical candidate is exacerbated by the combined effect of the general anesthetic *and* being in sternal or lateral recumbency for extended periods. Most general anesthetic agents, if used in sufficient doses to provide analgesia, will produce varying degrees of depression in respiratory function, including compromise in ciliary function.[3] A horse with an infection of the lower respiratory tract has already lost varying degrees of respiratory reserve. While the horse is in lateral or sternal recumbency there will inevitably be some degree of hypoxia and hypercapnia, both of which will be compounded by atelectasis and edema from an infectious process in the lung.

Hypoxia and hypercapnia can be most severe during induction when there are varying degrees of apnea. To avoid these complications the horse should be intubated immediately and placed on an oxygen-rich gas mixture. This treatment is particularly applicable to the horse with a compromised respiratory system. Intermittent positive pressure ventilation (IPPV) should be considered in the patient at risk. The horse is vulnerable during the postsurgical periods as well, when it has been disconnected from the anesthetic machine and is breathing room air.[3]

Besides the immediate threat to the horse's life if it is anesthetized while it has a respiratory tract infection is the risk of causing an exacerbation or flare-up of the condition. This may produce a life-threatening bronchopneumonia, or pleuritis. In one study of 82 cases of pleuritis, 7 (8.5%) were postsurgical patients.[8] Patients may die or develop permanent respiratory compromise. Invariably, hospitalization time will be increased, which further increases the horse's chance of acquiring other respiratory viruses from hospitalized horses, or even contracting a more serious nosocomial infection such as salmonellosis.

An actual case that was admitted to Colorado State University Teaching Hospital is illustrated in Table 4-1.

All surgical candidates, especially those at risk, should be carefully evaluated preoperatively with respect to the respiratory system. This evaluation should begin with a complete history, including vaccina-

Table 4-1.

	4/4 Day 1 Admission	4/6 Day 3	4/9 Day 5	4/11 Day 7	4/15 Day 11	Day 12
Plasma protein	6.7	6.8	7.0	6.9	7.0	
PCV	39	33	34	33	37	
Hemoglobin	14.3	12.8	12.8	12.6	14.0	
Nucleated cells	14,500	11,300	12,500	11,800	8,400	
Band neutrophils	–	–	–	–	–	
Segmented neutrophils	8,265 (57%)	7,119 (63%)	8,625 (69%)	7,906 (67%)	2,604 (31%)	
Lymphocytes	4,930 (34%)	3,729 (33%)	3,500 (28%)	3,186 (27%)	5,292 (63%)	
Monocytes	1,160 (8%)	339 (3%)	250 (2%)	708 (6%)	252 (3%)	
Eosinophils	145 (1%)	113 (1%)	125 (1%)	–	252 (3%)	
Fibrinogen	300	400	400	600	500	
Body temperature (°F)	101.5	100.4	101.0	102.0	100.0	
Other findings	Nasal discharge Harsh lung sounds		Depressed Thoracic radiographs taken; No significant findings	Depressed Appetite poor	Still depressed More alert but improving Appetite good	Surgery performed
Treatment		Septra*	Septra*	Septra*	Septra*	Septra*

*Trimethoprim-sulfamethoxazole 960.

tion history and history of any prior illnesses. A thorough physical examination is essential. Horses shipped to Colorado State University Clinic for surgery that arrive with a serous or seropurulent nasal discharge and cough are carefully scrutinized. A horse with a slight elevation in temperature (2 to 3° F, 1 to 2° C) with no obvious involvement of *other* body systems is regarded with suspicion. Such horses should have an immediate complete blood count (CBC) performed along with careful auscultation of the lungs and trachea. There may be no involvement of the lower respiratory tract, but only careful clinical examination will determine this. An area of ventral dullness should immediately arouse suspicion of pleuritis with pleural effusion, which will be discussed in greater detail later. A complete blood count from a horse with a respiratory infection will usually show an increased WBC with relative and absolute neutrophilia. There will be a slight shift to the left in some cases.

Chest radiographs are not taken as a routine preoperative workup, but they are done if bronchopneumonia or pleuritis with pleural effusion is suspected. Certainly many practices are limited in their ability to perform chest radiographs because of lack of equipment. Most studies are limited to lateral views, and although anatomic differences exist between horses and small animals, radiographic signs of pulmonary disease are similar.[2] Most lung lesions such as those of bronchitis must become well advanced before becoming recognizable radiographically. Frequently, life-threatening respiratory disease must be accompanied by a completely normal set of radiographs[2] (see case example, Fig. 4-1A). A horse with pleuritis will be stiff and reluctant to

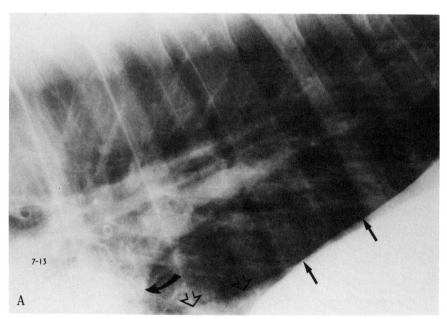

FIG. 4-1A. Lateral radiograph of the horse discussed in the example. No radiographic abnormalities are seen. The diaphragm (solid arrows), dorsal border of the caudal vena cava (open arrow), and caudal dorsal heart border (solid curved arrow) are all distinctly seen.

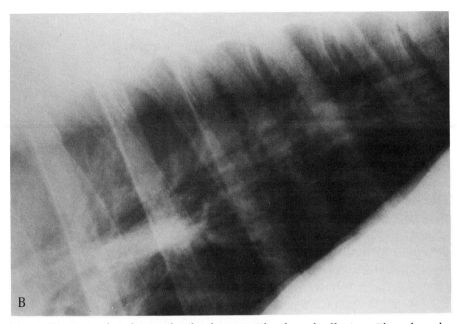

B

FIG. 4-1B. Lateral radiograph of a horse with pleural effusion. The pleural effusion has obliterated a portion of the diaphragm border, the caudal vena cava, and heart border. The fluid has gravitated to the ventral thorax causing the increased opacity.

move, signs resembling those of acute laminitis or even "tying-up." Some appear almost colicky, with an anxious expression.[9] They feel pain when pushed firmly on the ribs and breathe with shallow respirations. Auscultation of the thorax may be unremarkable *early* in the disease, but as the disease progresses, respiratory sounds decrease in the ventral thorax region and normal to harsh airway sounds are heard dorsally. Radiographs may reveal a fluid line, and there may be radiographic signs of a concurrent bronchopneumonia (Fig. 4-1B). If pleuritis is suspected, either in the presurgical evaluation or as a sequela to surgery and general anesthesia, then pleurocentesis is indicated.

Pleurocentesis is performed through surgically prepared skin between the 5th and 7th ribs, immediately dorsal to the costochondral junction.[9] The skin, intercostal muscles, and sensitive parietal pleura are infiltrated with the appropriate local anesthetic solution.[8] Fluid is collected with a sterile 3-inch metal teat cannula or catheter. The fluid should be collected in an EDTA tube for fluid analysis, as well as submitted for culture, cell count, cell type, and protein measurement.[9] Most cases of pleuritis will have a high protein content as well as a high white blood cell count. Pleural fluid can best be considered identical to peritoneal fluid so far as clinicopathologic values are concerned.[10]

Our immediate approach to a case of respiratory disease, either preoperatively or postoperatively, is to inform the owner of the horse of the nature of the condition and discuss the overall plan for management. When the horse arrives for surgery with pre-existing disease, the prudent thing is to delay surgery. Whether to send the horse home (preferably not back to the racetrack) or to hospitalize it until recovery has to be decided on an individual basis, and hard and fast rules cannot be laid down. To subject the horse to a long journey immediately may be more harmful than to monitor the convalescence in your hospital, where it may become exposed to a wider population of viruses. The delay in performing surgery will mean increased hospitalization and certainly more expense for the owner. If there is good client communication, the end result will be a minimum of dissatisfaction and a good understanding of the seriousness of the disease and its sequela if surgery were to be performed. As a general rule, we feel that a horse should be operated on as soon after arrival as possible, provided a physical examination and the appropriate diagnostic tests show that the horse is a good risk. To delay surgery so that the horse "can become accustomed to the hospital" and thereby be "less stressed" is a fallacy. All delay will do is increase the horse's exposure to other viruses and possible nosocomial infections.

We feel that a course of antibiotics is indicated for any animal with respiratory disease that may be subjected to general anesthesia. Certainly, cases of respiratory disease that occur postsurgically need to be evaluated on an individual basis. Which antibiotic to use is a matter of personal choice. Refractory cases are placed on broad-spectrum antibiotics. Too often clinicians change antibiotics after 1 or 2 days because the respiratory disease fails to respond completely. Then another antibiotic is chosen when there is no response. This type of therapy is one of the major factors behind the development of a chronic refractory pneumonia unresponsive to many different potent expensive antibiotics. The first drug used to treat the respiratory condition must be given a chance to be effective before a more potent antibiotic is selected. Serial white blood counts, daily auscultation of the lungs, and twice daily monitoring of body temperature are all necessary to monitor recovery.

If pleuritis is diagnosed, chest drainage may be required daily as well as the appropriate antimicrobial therapy. In the acute painful case, phenylbutazone is useful to relieve the pain, enabling the horse to eat and drink normally.[9]

Case Example: A two-year-old Thoroughbred gelding was admitted to Colorado State University for arthroscopic surgery. The horse arrived late at night by van. A soft cough and purulent nasal discharge were observed during the physical examination. Surgery was delayed because of the respiratory disease. The sequence of events, including hematologic studies, is outlined in Table 4-1.

Arthroscopic surgery was performed (in dorsal recumbency) on Day 12 following admission, and recovery from anesthesia was uneventful. The total time under general anesthesia was 1 hour. Actual surgery time was 30 minutes. The horse's temperature remained normal postoperatively, and the horse was discharged from the hospital 6 days after surgery.

References

1. Arthur, R.M.: Subacute and Acute Pleuritis. Proceedings of the 29th Annual Convention of the American Association of Equine Practitioners 1983, p. 65 (1984).
2. Farrow, C.S.: Equine thoracic radiology. J. Am. Vet. Med. Assoc. 179:776, 1981.
3. Gillespie, J.R., and Amis, T.C.: Respiratory physiology of the surgical patient. In The Practice of Large Animal Surgery. Edited by P. Jennings. Philadelphia, W.B. Saunders, 1984, p. 356.
4. Mansmann, R.A.: The stages of equine pleuropneumonia. In Proceedings of the 29th Annual Convention of the American Association of Equine Practitioners, 1983, p. 61 (1984).
5. Mansmann, R.A.: Pleuritis in Equine Medicine and Surgery. 3rd ed. Edited by R.A. Mansmann, E.S. McAllister, and P.W. Pratt. Santa Barbara, CA, American Veterinary Publications, 1983, p. 774.
6. McAllister, E.S.: Viral Respiratory Infections in Equine Medicine and Surgery, 3rd ed. Edited by R.A. Mansmann, E.S. McAllister, and P.W. Pratt. Santa Barbara, CA, American Veterinary Publications, 1983, p. 732.
7. McClintock, S.A.: Some Clinical and Physiological Effects of Floatation of Horses. MS Thesis, The University of Sydney, 1984.
8. Raphel, C.F., and Beech, J.: Pleuritis and pleural effusion in the horse. In Proceedings of the 27th Annual Convention of the American Association of Equine Practitioners, 1981, p. 17 (1982).
9. Smith, B.P.: Pleuritis and pleural effusion in the horse: A study of 37 cases. J. Am. Vet. Med. Assoc. 170:208, 1977.
10. Wagner, A.E., and Bennett, D.G.: Analysis of equine thoracic fluid. Vet. Clin. Pathol. 11:13, 1981.

5

Orthopedic Surgery

Lag Screw Fixation—Principles

One method to compress a fracture is to use a lag screw, a fundamental technique used routinely by carpenters and engineers. This method is particularly suited to horses with intraarticular fractures where accurate anatomic alignment at the level of the joint surface is essential to avoid secondary degenerative joint disease. Alignment is particularly important for the racing horse who must be 100% sound or the operation is deemed a failure.

General Considerations

A variety of fractures in horses are amenable to lag screw fixation, but the ones described in detail in this book are:

1. Slab fractures of the third carpal bone
2. Sagittal fractures of the proximal phalanx
3. Lateral condylar fractures of third metacarpus or metatarsus

In other fractures in the horse (such as mid-sesamoidean fractures) the indication for lag screw fixation is not as definite because of either inadequate or poor long-term results.

A single lag screw is used alone to repair certain slab fractures of the third carpal bone, but generally speaking two or more are used to prevent *rotation* of the fragment. Lag screws alone are rarely used to repair long, oblique, spiral, or fissure fractures of the tubular long bones such as the femur, tibia, radius, and humerus. Lag screws are often used in combination with bone plates to repair major long bone fractures. In the repair of comminuted fractures, the fracture site is

53

reconstructed with lag screws before applying a neutralization plate or plates. The use of lag screws to reconstruct a comminuted fracture of the third metacarpal bone is discussed in this section.

Two types of lag screws are available: the cortical bone screw and the cancellous screw. Under most circumstances, owing to the density of equine bone, a cortical bone screw is used. To achieve the lag screw principle the thread of the screw must gain purchase only in one fragment. For cortical screws this is achieved by *overdrilling* the fragment next to the screw head to such a size that the screw thread will not gain purchase on this portion of the bone. This hole is termed the *gliding hole*. If it were not overdrilled, then when the screw is tightened, the gap between the fracture fragments would be maintained. Therefore the screw should achieve purchase only in the "far" cortex or transcortex, i.e., away from the head. The hole in this cortex is the *thread hole*. A cortical screw is threaded for its entire length and has a lower ratio between the outer diameter and the core than the cancellous screw.

In certain areas of the musculoskeletal system, particularly in the metaphyseal regions of the bone in foals, bone is too soft for cortical screws and one must use a *cancellous screw* to achieve compression between the fragments. To increase the surface area of contact between the screw and bone, the ratio between the outer diameter and the core is greater than that found in a cortical screw. The cancellous screw has a smooth shank near the head and a threaded portion near the tip. When employed as a lag screw, the smooth shank must pass through one fragment and the threaded portion must gain purchase in the other; thus, as the screws tighten, the fragments are compressed. Cancellous screws have two lengths of thread at the tip, 16 mm and 32 mm. Because maximum holding power is desired during fracture repair in horses, there is little place for screws with small threads, and the cancellous screws with the longer threads (i.e., 32 mm) should be used whenever possible. Recently, cancellous screws that are threaded along their entire length have become available.

Cancellous screws should be used with caution in dense cortical bone. If the surgeon has stripped a cortical screw due to overzealous tightening, however, the only way to achieve compression is to use a cancellous screw in its place or to use a larger diameter (e.g., 5.5 mm) of cortical screw.

During the healing process new bone will form around the smooth shank of the cancellous screw, and consequently if screw removal is necessary, the cancellous thread must be able to cut its way back out of the bone. If the bone around the shank is too dense, then the cancellous screw can break at the screw thread junction. Therefore, cancellous screws are usually used as lag screws only when cortical screws have failed. Repair of fractures in young foals with very soft bone is a possible exception to this rule.

The system of orthopedic implants recommended is the AO-ASIF system (Arbeitsgemeinschaft Fur Osteosynthesefragen—Association for the Study of Internal Fixation). This system of implants has been used most widely in horses and, in our opinion, is the most adaptable.[1]

To exert the maximum amount of interfragmentary compression, a lag screw must be inserted at right angles to the fracture plane.[2] If the bone is under some axial load, however, the screw ideally should be inserted at right angles to the long axis of the bone. Therefore, the ideal direction to achieve maximum interfragmentary compression and resistance to axial load is a direction between these two extremes. This is a somewhat hypothetical solution and is not always feasible in certain equine fractures. For example, in a repair of a sagittal fracture of the proximal phalanx, insertion of the screws either at right angles or parallel to the long axis of the bone usually achieves adequate compression to align the joint surface.

Mechanical testing of the holding power of orthopedic screws has shown that 5.5 mm diameter cortical bone screws provide greater holding power than 4.5 mm cortical bone screws in the diaphysis of foal bone. In addition, the 5.5 mm screw is a suitable alternative to a 6.5 mm cancellous screw.[3] In adult horse bone it has been shown that 5.5 mm diameter screws have greater holding power and greater tensile strength than 4.5 mm cortical screws, and therefore the larger screws should be used when available.[4]

The steps in insertion of a lag screw are illustrated in the technique "Fracture of the Third Carpal Bone." The equipment used for lag screw fixation is listed in Appendix I and is illustrated in Figure 5-1.

References

1. Fackelman, G.E., and Nunamaker, D.M.: Manual of Internal Fixation in the Horse. New York, Springer-Verlag, 1982.
2. Mueller, M.E., Allgower, M., Schneider, R., and Willengger, H.: Manual of Internal Fixation, 2nd ed. New York, Springer-Verlag, 1979.
3. Yovich, J.V., Turner, A.S., and Smith, F.W.: Holding power of orthopedic screws in equine third metacarpal and metatarsal bones. Part I. Foal bone. Vet Surg., 14:221, 1985.
4. Yovich, J.V., Turner, A.S., and Smith, F.W.: Holding power of orthopedic screws in equine third metacarpal and metatarsal bones. Part II. Adult horse bone. Vet. Surg., 14:230, 1985.

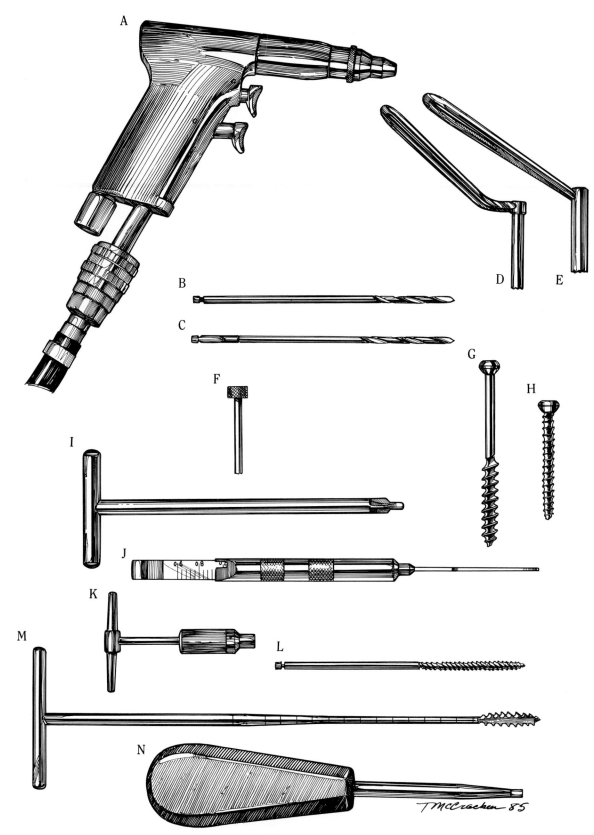

FIG. 5-1. Instruments required for lag screw fixation. A, Air drill; B, 4.5-mm drill bit; C, 3.2-mm drill bit; D, 4.5-mm tap sleeve; E, 6.5-mm tap sleeve; F, 3.2-mm drill sleeve; G, cancellous screw (32-mm thread); H, cortical screw; I, countersink; J, depth gauge; K, tap handle; L, 4.5-mm cortical tap; M, 6.5-mm cancellous tap; N, hexagonal-headed screwdriver.

Repair of Fracture of the Third Carpal Bone

A slab fracture of the third carpal bone is one that extends from one articulation to the next and is most frequently located on the dorsomedial surface of the bone (radial facet) (Fig. 5-2A). The injury is seen most commonly in the fast-gaited horse such as the racing Thoroughbred, Quarterhorse, and Standardbred. Other carpal bones, such as the radial and fourth carpal bones, can sustain slab fractures. The basic principles of repair apply to all, however, but the following description will apply to the more common third carpal bone slab fracture.

A slab fracture of any carpal bone may begin as a hairline fissure fracture that can later displace into a more painful fracture that carries a worse prognosis. Such undisplaced fractures are difficult to diagnose, and various radiographs at oblique angles and skyline views are necessary to delineate the fracture. Prompt diagnosis is essential because continual weight bearing causes micromotion at the fracture site resulting in degenerative joint disease. We and other colleagues feel that many early lesions on the third carpal bone go undiagnosed and with continued exercise develop a displacing slab fracture with a much worse prognosis.[2]

Occasionally, slab fractures of the carpal bones (especially the third) occur in a sagittal rather than in the usual frontal (or nearly frontal) plane. The majority of these are managed conservatively, but some are amenable to lag screw fixation.[5]

Typically, a slab fracture of the third carpal bone is more painful than the more common chip fracture. There is marked pain upon carpal flexion and distention of the midcarpal (intercarpal) joint as well as pain on palpation of the fracture itself.[1] Intraarticular (local) anesthesia is not required for diagnosis unless the fracture is undisplaced.

A complete set of radiographs should be taken: AP, lateral, flexed lateral, APLMO, and APMLO views. The well-known "skyline" or tangential view is mandatory when a slab fracture of any of the carpal bones is suspected.[1–8] This view will show the position of the slab fracture in relationship to the tendon of the extensor carpi radialis and thereby help the surgeon decide on the correct location for the bone screw. It will also demonstrate the thickness of the slab and help the surgeon decide if removal is more appropriate or a smaller screw or even two screws are required. This view can also demonstrate whether the slab is in one or two pieces which would have a profound effect on the prognosis. As with any injury to the carpus in a fast-gaited horse, the contralateral carpus should be radiographed because both joints frequently are involved.[6]

It has been stated regarding the indications for screw fixation of slab fractures of the equine carpus that "any fracture that is radiographically distinct will benefit from surgery".[2] We feel that screw fixation is indicated for all horses that are to be returned to athletic activity and for horses to be used for breeding purposes when displacement occurs. In severe slab fractures when there is imminent

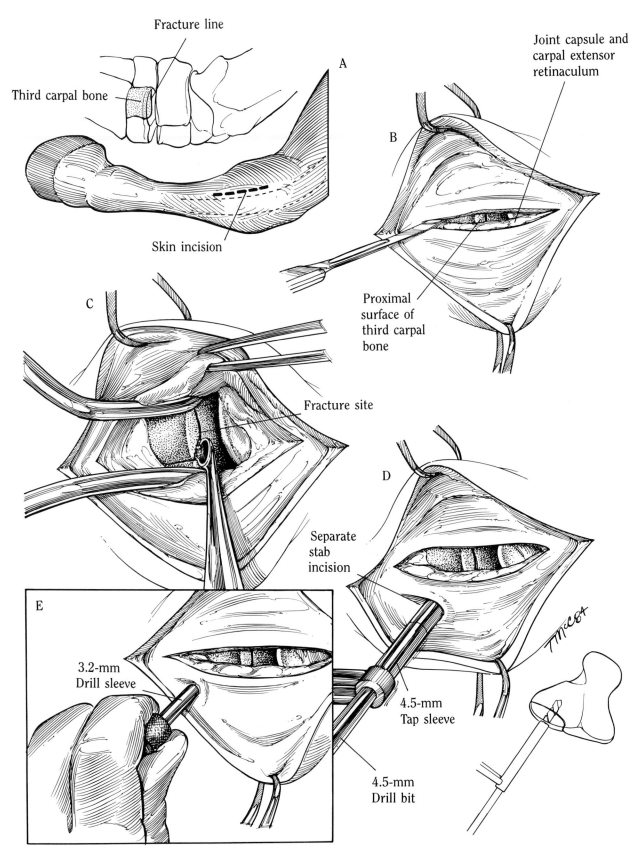

Fig. 5-2A–E. Lag screw fixation of slab fracture of third carpal bone.

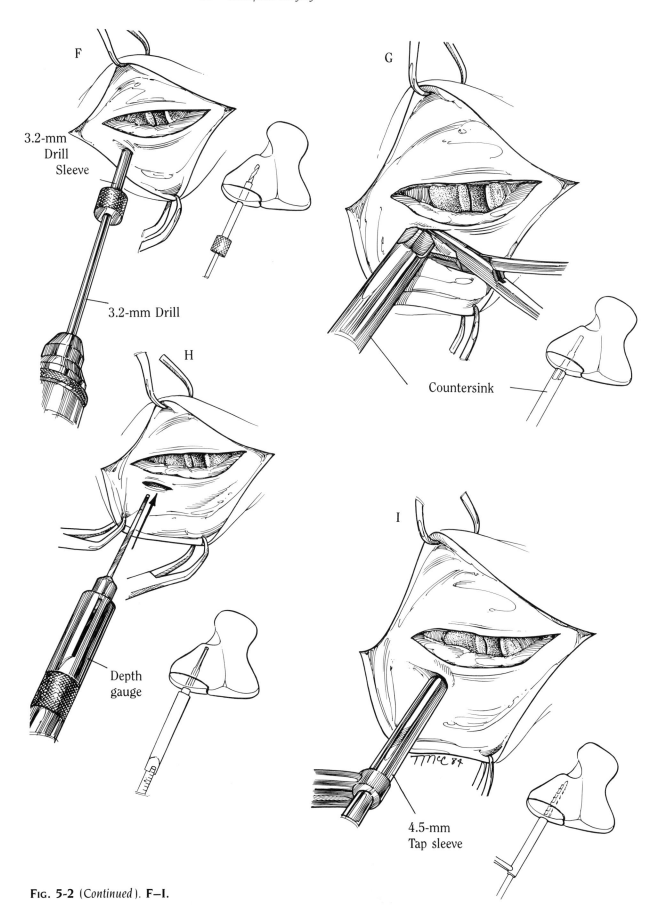

3.2-mm
Drill
Sleeve

3.2-mm Drill

Countersink

Depth
gauge

4.5-mm
Tap sleeve

FIG. 5-2 (*Continued*). **F–I.**

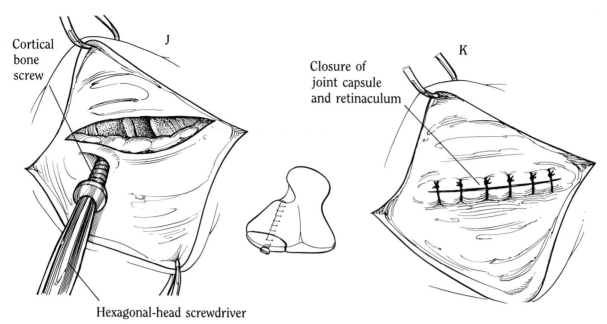

Cortical bone screw

J

Hexagonal-head screwdriver

Closure of joint capsule and retinaculum

K

FIG. 5-2 (Continued). J, K.

collapse of the second row of carpal bones, internal fixation is essential for salvage.

With the advent of arthroscopic surgery it is not unusual to combine this type of surgery with screw fixation of the slab fracture. For example, a slab fracture of the third carpal bone may occur concurrently with chip fractures of the same joint, the radial carpal joint of the same leg, or the opposite carpus. These chip fractures are best treated with arthroscopic surgery rather than subjecting the horse to multiple arthrotomies, which would lower the prognosis. If both screw fixation and arthroscopy are to be performed during the one operation, then it is most advantageous to operate on the horse in dorsal recumbency.

When experience has been gained with the arthroscope in the midcarpal joint of the horse, slab fractures can be repaired by inserting the screw through a stab incision over the fragment and monitoring fracture reduction through the arthroscope.

Anesthesia and Surgical Preparation

The surgical procedure is performed under general anesthesia with the horse placed in lateral recumbency and the affected limb down. Some surgeons prefer to operate with the horse in dorsal recumbency and the limb elevated to take advantage of natural hemostasis. Certainly if both limbs are to be operated (e.g., one for screw fixation with or without arthroscopy and the other for arthroscopy), then we strongly recommend that dorsal recumbency be used. This position allows the surgeon to go immediately to the opposite joint without having to roll the horse over. Prior to induction of anesthesia, the patient's limb is clipped from the coronet to the midradius all the way around the limb. Following induction of anesthesia, the area of surgical excision is shaved, and a routine surgical preparation is performed. By preparing the limb before surgery, the time under anesthesia can be reduced. Perioperative antibiotics are recommended, although some surgeons prefer not to use any at all.

Additional Instrumentation

Lag screw fixation of a slab fracture requires curettes, retractors, periosteal elevators, and a bulb syringe. Arthroscopy equipment should be available if osteochondral fragments are to be removed from either carpal joint or if the slab fracture is going to be fixed arthroscopically. Also required are the ASIF instruments for lag screw fixation (see appendix) and a selection of ASIF cortical bone screws.

Surgical Technique

After draping (the use of sterile plastic adherent drapes is recommended for this procedure), the following structures should be identified: the tendinous insertion of the extensor carpi radialis muscle, the tendon of the extensor carpi obliquus muscle, the antebrachiocarpal joint, and the midcarpal joint. Identification of these structures is facilitated by flexing and extending the carpal joint. An 8-cm straight incision is made parallel and medial to the edge of the tendon of the extensor carpi radialis (Fig. 5-2A). The incision extends from the middle of the face of the radial carpal bone to the middle of the face of the third carpal bone. The skin edges are then reflected from the subcutaneous fascia toward the base. A straight incision approximately 5 cm long is made through the subcutaneous fascia, carpal extensor retinaculum, and joint capsule. The incision is made parallel to the tendon of the extensor carpi radialis muscle, but avoids the tendon sheath (Fig. 5-2B). Synovial fluid will flow from the incision when the joint is entered. Any blood vessels or their visible lumens should be cauterized at this point. Using suitable retractors, the surgeon carefully retracts the edges of the incision in the carpal extensor retinaculum and joint capsule; this retraction will expose the proximal surface of the third carpal bone and the distal surface of the radial carpal bone.

The extent of the fracture is examined, and the approximate center of the fragment (site for screw location) is estimated. Any free fragments of bone and cartilage at the fracture site are removed, as well as any osteochondral fragments on the margin of the "slab" or on the opposite surface of the radial carpal bone. Curettage is performed where necessary (Fig. 5-2C).

Reduction of the fracture usually occurs when the limb is put in flexion. With the limb in this position a 4.5-mm gliding hole is drilled using the 4.5-mm tap sleeve to protect the surrounding soft tissues (Fig. 5-2D). Frequently the screw must be inserted through a separate stab incision through the tendon of the extensor carpi radialis if the site does not coincide with the arthrotomy incision. The stab incision should be made in a direction parallel to the fibers of the tendon.

Direction of the drill bit is critical, and it should be directed perpendicular to the plane of the fracture and parallel to the articular surface. In fractures that are somewhat displaced the surgeon will "feel" when the fracture site has been entered. In the undisplaced hairline or fissure fracture it may be impossible to feel when the 4.5-mm drill bit has arrived at or crossed the fracture site. One technique is to place a ruler on the surface of the bone parallel to the bit and monitor the depth of bone that has been penetrated.[3] Most slab fractures are 6 to 10 mm thick, but the gliding (clearance) hole should be at least 12 mm deep to allow countersinking.[3] Intraoperative radiographs are also useful to see that the drill bit has crossed the fracture line.

A 3.2-mm drill sleeve is inserted into the 4.5-mm gliding hole (Fig. 5-2E). Parting the soft tissues that tend to cover the gliding hole with the tips of a hemostat will facilitate its location. The 3.2-mm thread hole is drilled into the parent portion of the third carpal bone. It is usually not necessary to drill out the palmar surface of the bone, and such drilling should be avoided so that the contents of the carpal canal are not damaged. The drill should be cleaned frequently. A thread hole of 20 to 25 mm is recommended, as this will provide enough length for a 4.5-mm cortical bone screw[3] to provide adequate compression (Fig. 5-2F).

The hole is now countersunk, again using hemostats to part the soft tissues at the entrance to the hole. The hole should be countersunk around its entire circumference. Because the tip of the countersink is 12-mm, a glide hole of adequate length must be provided to allow it to engage the bone. Inadequate countersinking results in excessive protrusion of the screw head into the soft tissues (Fig. 5-2G). Failure to countersink the hole increases the chance of splitting the fragment during tightening. The depth gauge is inserted to determine the appropriate size of screw (Fig. 5-2H). Its length is read off the scale, and 2 mm is subtracted from the measurement.

The 4.5-mm cortical tap is inserted using the 4.5-mm tap sleeve to protect the soft tissues (Fig. 5-2I). Care must be taken not to impact the tap in the blind ending pilot hole because it will strip the threads of bone that have been cut in the parent portion of the bone (Fig. 5-2I).

The appropriate sized screw is inserted and tightened judiciously (Fig. 5-2J). Excessive torque may result in splitting the fragment, which would be catastrophic to the outcome of the surgery. Radiographs should be taken intraoperatively and postoperatively to ensure the correct direction and final placement of the bone screw.

The arthrotomy incision is closed in three layers. The joint capsule and retinaculum are closed with a layer of simple interrupted sutures of absorbable synthetic material or monofilament, nonabsorbable material. The sutures should not penetrate the synovial membrane. Preplacement of the sutures in the joint capsule and extensor retinaculum ensures an accurate apposition and a tight seal (Fig. 5-2K).

Following joint capsule closure, 4 to 5 ml of Ringer's solution are flushed into the joint with a 20-gauge needle. If any leaks are observed through the incision, additional sutures can be placed at this time. The subcutaneous fascia is closed with a simple continuous pattern using synthetic, absorbable sutures. The skin is closed with a simple interrupted or vertical mattress pattern using synthetic, monofilament sutures, and the limb is wrapped with a tight pressure bandage. Control of minute capillary ooze will be possible if the tourniquet is released after the pressure wrap is applied.

Postoperative Management

The limb is wrapped in a firm pressure bandage for three weeks, during which time the bandage is changed several times. If the carpal joint is unstable or if there is some question as to the stability achieved with internal fixation, a full limb cast should be applied to protect the repair while the horse recovers from the anesthetic. For example, horses with multiple slab fractures or a slab fracture causing complete joint collapse should have a cast during recovery from anesthesia as well as during a good portion of the convalescence. The cast may be cut off some weeks later when the soft tissues have healed. Skin sutures are removed at 10 to 12 days. Care must be taken when bandaging the carpal joint so as not to cause a pressure sore on the accessory carpal bone; this can be avoided by cutting a small hole in the back of the bandage over the accessory carpal bone. During convalescence, the horse is kept in a box stall. The convalescence and aftercare will vary depending on the individual case and the severity of the injury to the carpal bone. Generally, it is 6 to 12 months before the horse should return to its athletic activities. Radiographic monitoring of the fracture healing is recommended. Also, the degree of periosteal proliferation can be assessed. Excessive periostitis usually points to a poorer prognosis.

The implants are usually not removed. They are frequently blamed for causing permanent disability when the real cause is concurrent degenerative joint disease.

Comments

For large slab fractures of the third carpal bone, two screws should be used. This is rare in our hospital but should be considered if the indication exists. Two screws can be used in slab fractures of the other carpal bones, such as the fourth carpal bone.[8] When two screws are being used, most surgeons opt for the smaller diameter screws because 2 large 4.5 mm screws may weaken the bone and risk splitting the fragment.[4] If smaller screws are used, then the surgeon must become familiar with a different set of instrument dimensions, as outlined in the following table.

Size of Screw (mm)	Size of Glide Hole (mm)	Size of Thread (Pilot) Hole (mm)	Size of Tap (mm)
4.5	4.5	3.2	4.5
3.5	3.5	2.7	3.5
2.7	2.7	2.5	2.7

One of the smaller diameter bone screws may be used in smaller, thinner slab fractures if the surgeon believes that the larger screw may split the bone.[8] If the slab does split as the screw is tightened, the surgeon has no choice but to remove the slab of bone or to use two screws, one in each portion of the slab. A split slab usually requires considerable dissection of and trauma to the joint. Slab fractures of the third carpal bone also occur in combination with slab fractures of the radial carpal bone.

Multiple fractures of the carpal bones, such as a very large, displaced, slab fracture of C3 with or without involvement of other bones (e.g., C4 and radial carpal bones) result in instability of the joint if unsupported. These injuries do require lag screw fixation of the affected bone(s) to prevent progressive collapse of the joint and a functionless limb. Lag screw fixation of multiple slab fractures greatly enhances the stability of the joint during the convalescence. Such an injury ends the horse's athletic career, but surgery is indicated to salvage the animal for breeding if it is sufficiently valuable.

Frequently a slab fracture requiring internal fixation occurs in a joint that has had a recent injection of corticosteroids. Certainly a risk exists if an arthrotomy is performed, and it has been recommended to delay an elective surgery such as chip fracture removal for two weeks.[2] Radiographs and a clinical examination should be done after the two-week period to evaluate if infectious arthritis or progressive degenerative joint disease has developed.[2] With a slab fracture a delay of two weeks before immobilization of the fragment can mean the end of the horse's career. During the delay there will be continued motion at the fracture site during normal weight bearing and damage to the affected bone (third carpal bone) and opposing carpal bone (radial carpal bone). Therefore the owner should be told the risk of surgery (i.e., infection) and immediate screw fixation should be considered. Broad-spectrum antibiotics should be administered perioperatively.

References

1. Auer, J.A.: Diseases of the carpus. In Vet. Clin. North Am. (Large Anim. Pract.) 2:91, 1980.
2. Bramlage, L.R.: Surgical diseases of the carpus. Vet. Clin. North Am. (Large Anim. Pract.) 5:261, 1983.
3. Fackelman, G.E., and Nunamaker, D.M.: Manual of Internal Fixation in the Horse. New York, Springer-Verlag, 1982, p. 37.
4. Palmer, S.E., and Adams, F.R.: Repair of a slab fracture of the third carpal bone using ASIF small fragment technique: A case report. J. Equine Med. Surg. 3:33, 1979.
5. Palmer, S.E.: Lag screw fixation of a sagittal fracture of the third carpal bone in a horse. Vet. Surg., 12:54, 1983.
6. Park, R.D., Morgan, J.P., and O'Brien, T.: Chip fractures in the carpus of the horse: A Radiographic study of their incidence and location. J. Am. Vet. Med. Assoc. 157:1305, 1970.
7. Turner, A.S.: Large animal orthopedics. In Textbook of Large Animal Surgery. (P. Jennings, ed.) Philadelphia, W.B. Saunders, 1984, p. 810.
8. Vale, G.T., Wagner, P.C., and Grant, B.D.: Surgical repair of comminuted equine fourth carpal bone fractures. Equine Pract. 4:6, 1982.

Repair of a Sagittal Fracture of the Proximal Phalanx (P1)

Longitudinal fractures of the proximal phalanx are seen in horses that perform strenuous activities such as racing, western performance events, trotting and pacing races, and jumping.[1,3–5] These fractures can occur in a variety of configurations ranging from small hairline fissures in the fetlock joint to severely comminuted fractures with many pieces.[1,3–5] Rarely are proximal phalangeal fractures open. All of the different configurations of proximal phalangeal fractures seen in horses will not be discussed in this section. Instead we will illustrate the steps required to repair a simple sagittal fracture of P1 that extends from the metacarpophalangeal joint to the junction of the middle and distal third of P1 (Fig. 5-3A). This is a relatively common configuration and would be a good case to try for a surgeon who has had relatively little experience with the ASIF technique. If there is any doubt, however, the surgeon should always practice screw placement on a cadaver limb.

The clinical signs of proximal phalangeal fractures vary. In severely comminuted fractures there will be severe lameness, and crepitation will be evident. In some fractures, such as the longitudinal fissure commencing in the fetlock joint illustrated in Figure 5-3, the lameness can be quite subtle. Diagnostic nerve blocks or training when such fissures are present can result in complete dehiscence of the fracture and a marked decline in the prognosis for future athletic soundness. A small fissure may develop into a more complicated configuration under normal weight bearing.[8]

For emergency transport to a facility where more elaborate treatment can be performed, the limb should be placed in a large, tight-fitting pressure bandage with support on the opposite limb. The animal will usually protect the limb because of extreme pain. If horses are to be shipped long distances with such a fracture or if the fracture is comminuted and unstable, the attending veterinarian may elect to place the limb in a fiberglass cast prior to transport.[8] At least four radiographic views should be taken (AP, LM, and two obliques). There is often a duplication of the fracture line owing to the different course taken in the dorsal and palmar (plantar) cortices (Fig. 5-3A). This may be mistaken for comminution or even sequestration. For fissures close to the articular surface, the x-ray beam should be directed at such an angle as to eliminate superimposition by the proximal sesamoid bones.

Horses with longitudinal fractures of the proximal phalanx should be considered candidates for rigid internal fixation because failure to re-establish the congruity of the joint surfaces (metacarpophalangeal and proximal interphalangeal) will result in degenerative disease of these joints.[1–5,8] Some surgeons recommend that small fissures that begin at the proximal end of the proximal phalanx and do not progress any farther than 1 to 2 cm be handled conservatively in a cast. It

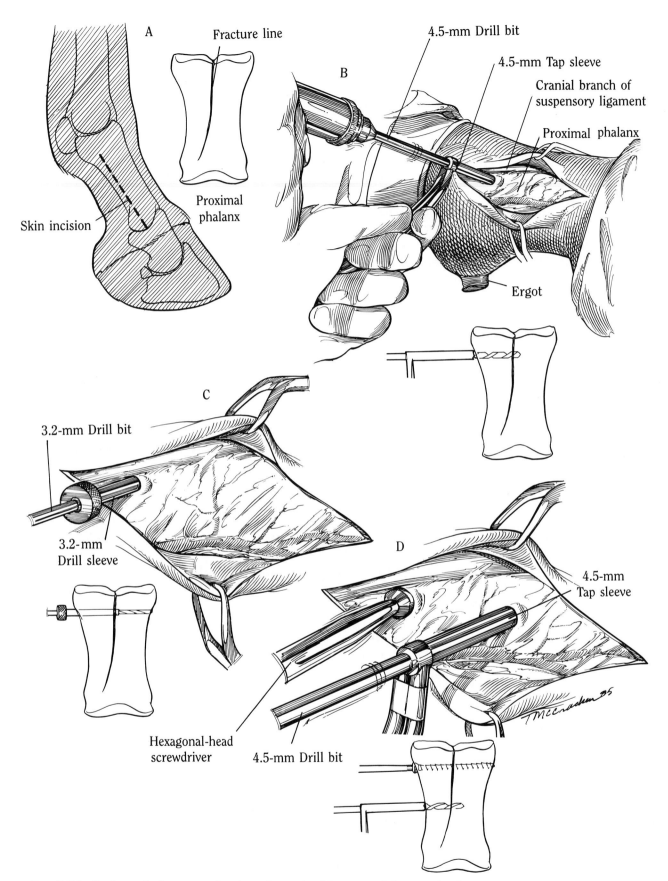

Labels in figure:

A

Fracture line

Proximal phalanx

Skin incision

B

4.5-mm Drill bit

4.5-mm Tap sleeve

Cranial branch of suspensory ligament

Proximal phalanx

Ergot

C

3.2-mm Drill bit

3.2-mm Drill sleeve

D

4.5-mm Tap sleeve

Hexagonal-head screwdriver

4.5-mm Drill bit

FIG. 5-3A–D. Steps in lag screw fixation of a sagittal fracture of the proximal phalanx.

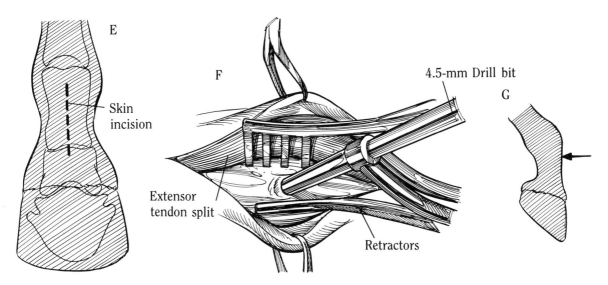

FIG. 5-3 (*Continued*). **E–G.** Steps in lag screw fixation of a frontal fracture of the proximal phalanx.

is our belief that such fissures usually continue further distad at the microscopic level and may dehisce into a fracture with a poorer prognosis. The convalescent period is usually much shorter following internal fixation, and the total expense (including hospitalization) for treatment of the fracture may be less if handled surgically than if cast application is the sole method of therapy.[3]

Periosteal proliferation resembling osselets on the proximal dorsal aspect of the proximal phalanx and demineralization along the fracture line are seen in fissures that have been handled conservatively. Such fractures should be given a guarded prognosis for athletic soundness.[1,4]

Internal fixation of proximal phalangeal fractures consists of insertion of one or more ASIF cortical bone screws using the lag screw principle.[7] It is recommended that the introductory section on the lag screw principle be read now unless the reader has already done so.

Anesthesia and Surgical Preparation

The surgical procedure is performed under general anesthesia with the horse in lateral recumbency. Prior to attempting screw fixation, the surgeon must be thoroughly familiar with the configuration of the fracture as determined by radiographs. Because the plane of the fracture frequently begins at the sagittal groove and spirals down the bone, oblique views are absolutely essential to "map out" the fracture lines.

The horse's limb is positioned with the smaller fracture fragment uppermost; thus, the threaded portion of the screw hole closer to the fetlock joint is as long as possible, enabling the fixation to have the greatest holding power. There are many variations on the location and position of the lag screws, and each fracture should be carefully assessed beforehand to reduce operating time.

To reduce time under anesthesia the area over the fracture can be clipped, shaved, and surgically prepared prior to inducing anesthesia. The limb is then covered with a sterile bandage, which is removed when the horse is positioned. The use of an Esmarch's bandage and tourniquet is optional. We prefer to use both, as they help reduce operating time. A sterile Esmarch's bandage is now applied by the surgeon, and a nurse can apply a tourniquet. Alternatively, the limb can be shaved and prepared as soon as the horse is positioned following application of the Esmarch's bandage and tourniquet.

Proximal phalangeal fractures almost always require intraoperative radiographs to check for screw placement and depth of the gliding hole. It is strongly recommended that the limb be positioned to facilitate this procedure with a minimum of redraping and chance to break aseptic surgical technique. Radiographs must be coordinated with technical staff to avoid time-wasting maneuvers that will prolong anesthesia.

Additional Instrumentation

This procedure requires instruments for lag screw fixation and an assortment of cortical and cancellous bone screws.

Surgical Technique

The surgical approach may be through stab incisions although, if more than two screws are to be inserted, we prefer a more extensive laterally or medially located incision (Fig. 5-3B, C). For fractures in a frontal plane where all the screws will be placed in a cranial to caudal direction an I-shaped incision provides good visualization of the extensor tendon and corresponding branches of the suspensory ligament. Details of this approach are outlined in the section on pastern arthrodesis, although for lag screw fixation the position of the "I" must be moved proximad and the pastern joint should not be opened. If only one or two lag screws are to be placed in a cranial to caudal direction, then a simple longitudinal incision will be adequate.[3]

During initial experiences with lag screw fixation of these fractures, it was deemed necessary to place screws to ensure maximum resistance to shortening and maximal compression of the fracture by "inserting a screw along an imaginary line between a line perpendicular to the long axis of the bone and a line perpendicular to the fracture line."[1] However, with fractures close to a sagittal plane there is little tendency for slippage along the longitudinal plane of the fracture, and placement of screws at right angles to the fracture line or parallel to the metacarpophalangeal joint is technically easier than trying to bisect the angles between these two directions.[8] Lag screws are inserted at the appropriate positions on the bone as dictated by the configuration of the fracture. Reduction of these fractures is generally not a problem, as they usually align themselves as the fragments are compressed. The screw closest to the fetlock joint is usually inserted first, using the cranial branch of the suspensory ligament as a landmark (Fig. 5-3B). Kirschner wires or 2.0 mm drill bits are sometimes used to estimate the anticipated positions of the lag screws.

Repair of a Lateral Distal Condylar Fracture of the Third Metacarpal or Metatarsal Bones

Fractures of the lateral condyles of the third metacarpal and metatarsal bones are seen predominantly in racing Thoroughbreds and Standardbreds. The configuration of the fracture covers a wide spectrum, ranging from a small fissure entering the fetlock joint to complete displacement and separation of the fragment from the parent cannon bone.[1,2,4,10,11] The clinical signs can vary from mild lameness that is exacerbated by exercise in undisplaced fissure fractures to acute lameness with heat, pain, and swelling in displaced fractures. The fractures primarily involve the forelimbs, but occasionally the hindlimbs will be affected, especially in Standardbreds.

Radiographs of the affected fetlock joint should be taken to establish the diagnosis. At least four views should be taken: AP, lateral, and two oblique views. Care should be taken to evaluate the radiographs for concomitant problems. The following conditions are sometimes seen with condylar fractures: (1) axial fractures of the proximal sesamoid bones; (2) apical fractures of the proximal sesamoid bones; (3) osteochondral fractures of the proximal aspect of the proximal phalanx; (4) periarticular osteophytes indicative of degenerative joint disease; and (5) suspensory desmitis (apparent clinically).[1-4,6,10,11] All other injuries associated with condylar fractures should be taken into account prior to surgery. Such injuries may have a significant bearing on the prognosis with respect to return to racing soundness. For example, at the fracture site the presence of undetected erosive (lytic) lesions on the palmar (plantar) region of the condyle and comminution with loose osteochondral fragments should be investigated[1,10] by taking a 125-degree dorsopalmar (dorsoplantar) metacarpal (metatarsal) skyline (125-degree DPMS) projection.[1,10] Occasionally a fracture will involve the medial condyle but propagate in a spiral fashion a considerable distance up the bone to the nutrient foramen.[2,4,9] Multiple radiographic views are necessary to fully define the fracture planes,[4,9] because fractures of this configuration have a tendency to break catastrophically proximal to the region of the fracture site.[9]

Lateral condylar fractures can be handled in a variety of ways, depending on the degree of separation of the fragments and the intended use of the animal. If the animal is to be retired for breeding purposes and there is minimum displacement of the fracture, pressure bandages or a plaster cast in combination with box stall rest for eight weeks may suffice. An additional eight weeks of stall confinement is required if there is considerable displacement of the fracture or the fragment. The convalescent period after a condylar fracture, much like that for fissure fractures of the proximal phalanx, is much shorter following internal fixation, and the total expense (including hospitalization) for treatment may be less if internal fixation is used. If the horse is intended for further athletic performance, the treatment of choice is lag screw fixation with two or more ASIF cortical bone screws.[1-6,9-11]

There are several aims of rigid internal fixation of such fractures: (1) to re-establish the congruity of the articular surface; (2) to minimize the gap that fibrocartilage has to bridge during the healing process; (3) to minimize movement at the junction of the articular cartilage and bone, reducing proliferative changes and subsequent joint stiffness (degenerative joint disease), and (4) to ensure that the original fissure does not enlarge and become displaced to the point of complete dehiscence.[1,4,6,9–11] Such fractures should be repaired as soon as the affected leg has "cooled out," which is generally 24 to 48 hours after the injury.

Anesthesia and Surgical Preparation

The horse is positioned with the affected leg uppermost. The leg is prepared for surgery in a routine manner, and an Esmarch's bandage and tourniquet are applied. To reduce anesthetic time the limb can be clipped, shaved, and surgically prepared prior to inducing anesthesia. The limb is then covered with a sterile bandage, which is removed when the horse is positioned. The use of an Esmarch's bandage and tourniquet is optional. We prefer to use them, as they help reduce operating time. A sterile Esmarch's bandage is now applied by the surgeon and a nurse can apply a tourniquet. Alternatively, the limb can be shaved and prepared as soon as the horse is positioned following applications of the Esmarch's bandage and tourniquet.

Condylar fractures almost always require intraoperative radiographs to check for screw placement and depth of the gliding hole. It is strongly recommended that the limb be positioned to facilitate this procedure, with a minimum of redraping and chance to break aseptic surgical technique. Radiographs must be coordinated with technical staff to avoid time-wasting maneuvers that will prolong anesthetic time.

Additional Instrumentation

This procedure requires instruments for lag screw fixation and an assortment of cortical bone screws.

Surgical Technique

Minimally displaced fractures can be approached through stab incisions in the skin, whereas displaced fractures are best approached through an incision over the lateral collateral ligaments of the fetlock joint. The latter, more extensive incision allows visualization of the proximal end of the fracture, thereby aiding alignment at the joint surface. It also gives better visualization of the configuration of the fracture, as these fractures sometimes spiral cranially or caudally. If the fracture is displaced, then the more extensive incision will enable the surgeon to remove hematoma and bony debris from the fracture site. Some incisions (S-shaped) provide good exposure but may produce skin sloughs at the apices if they are too curved. The displaced fracture must be reduced before screw fixation. To evaluate reduction at the joint surface and remove loose osteochondral fragments at the palmar articular surface, an arthrotomy of the dorsal surface of the fetlock joint must be performed.[1,4] This is done in the same location as one would remove an osteochondral fragment of the dorsal rim of P1 or hypertrophied synovial membrane (villonodular synovitis) and is described in this book (pages 133–136) and other texts.[7] If the condylar fracture has a concurrent loose osteochondral fragment at the palmar articular surface, it is at this point in the procedure that the fragment must be removed. The metacarpophalangeal joint is slightly flexed, and periosteal elevators are used to distract the fractured condyle away from the metacarpus. The fracture site is cleaned of debris, and the typically triangular pieces of bone can be extracted from the palmar aspect of the joint.

To achieve reduction, the large ASIF bone reduction forceps* may be used. The ASIF C-clamp can also be used but is technically more exacting to use. The C-clamp ensures that the screw will be directed across the greater diameter of the bone. When in position, the clamp should be tightened and an AP intraoperative radiograph taken to ensure that the drill will be directed parallel to the joint surface. When the surgeon is satisfied with the reduction of the fracture, the distal screw should be placed 1 to 2 cm proximal to the articular surface. To obtain adequate compression of the fracture site at the level of the articular surface, the more distal screw must be positioned carefully. Preferably this screw should be placed proximad to the collateral ligament to minimize trauma to this structure. On the other hand, in the management of smaller condylar fractures whose fracture lines do not extend very proximad, it may be necessary to place the most distal screw in the depression (fossa) of the most distal aspect of the bone.

Placement of the screw is begun by drilling the 4.5-mm gliding hole in the fracture fragment. Intraoperative radiographs are required to see that the 4.5-mm drill has crossed the fracture site when drilling this and subsequent gliding holes. The bone in this region is quite dense, and it is better to cross the fracture site and shorten the length of the pilot hole[5] (Fig. 5-4A, B).

The 3.2-mm sleeve is placed in the 4.5-mm glide hole, and the pilot hole is drilled without exiting the opposite cortex (Fig. 5-4C). Constant cleaning of the drill bit is essential during the drilling of these and subsequent holes in such dense bone. The depth gauge is used to determine the length of the cortical screw to be used, being careful not to catch the hook of the depth gauge on soft tissues if the pilot hole has been drilled completely through both cortices. If the ASIF C-clamp is being used, the threads will now be cut, keeping the C-clamp in place. Then the depth gauge is used. This is not the normal sequence of lag screw application as recommended by the AO Group,[8] but is necessary if the C-clamp is being used to maintain accurate reduction. Otherwise, tapping is performed after the depth is measured (Fig. 5-4D, E). Using the countersink for the screw hole clos-

---

*Available from Synthes Ltd., Wayne, PA.

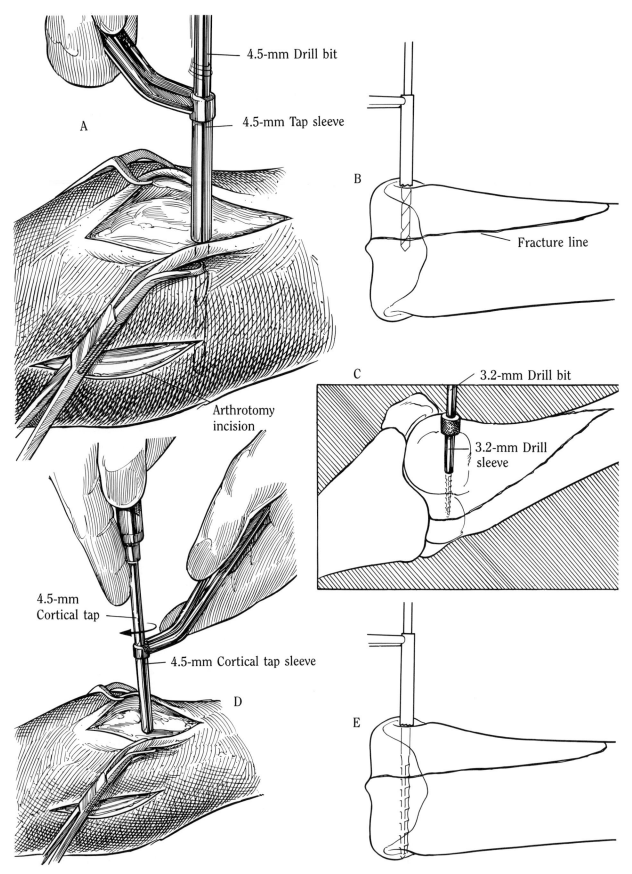

A — 4.5-mm Drill bit

4.5-mm Tap sleeve

Arthrotomy incision

B — Fracture line

C — 3.2-mm Drill bit

3.2-mm Drill sleeve

4.5-mm Cortical tap

4.5-mm Cortical tap sleeve

D

E

FIG. 5-4A–E. Steps in repair of a lateral distal condylar fracture in the meta-carpus or metatarsus.

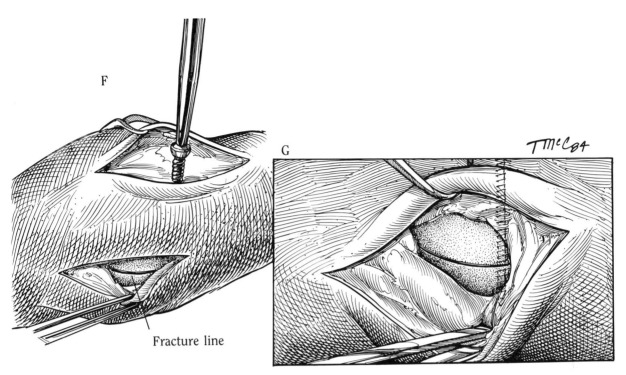

F

G

TMcC84

Fracture line

FIG. 5-4 (*Continued*). F, G.

est to the joint is not necessary and can be potentially injurious to the collateral ligament.

An ASIF cortical bone screw of appropriate length is inserted and tightened, but not excessively (Fig. 5-4F). An intraoperative radiograph is taken at this point to check fracture reduction and ensure that the threaded tip of the screw is not protruding into the opposite collateral ligament.

Once this screw is placed, the ASIF hexagonal-headed screwdriver can be left in place, and the remaining screws inserted "freehand" in a sequence similar to the placement of the first screw. The 4.5-mm gliding hole must extend *beyond* the fracture line and it may be necessary to take intraoperative radiographs to ensure this placement in undisplaced fractures. Screws that are placed more proximally should be countersunk to ensure even pressure on the screw head. Reduction of the fracture site can be monitored through the arthrotomy incision or with the arthroscope (Fig. 5-4G).

The arthrotomy incision is closed by a layer of simple interrupted absorbable sutures of synthetic absorbable or synthetic monofilament nonabsorbable material. The sutures should be preplaced in the joint capsule to facilitate accurate anatomic apposition and a tight seal. The subcutaneous fascia is closed with a simple continuous pattern using synthetic absorbable material, and the skin is closed with simple interrupted or vertical mattress sutures of monofilament nonabsorbable material. The wound through which the screws were placed is closed in two layers: subcutaneous fascia and skin. The tourniquet is then removed, and a sterile dressing is placed over the incision. A fiberglass cast is then applied, encasing the entire foot and extending to the proximal aspect of the metacarpus (metatarsus) to protect the fracture fixation during recovery from anesthesia.

Postoperative Management

Perioperative antibiotics are recommended and tetanus prophylaxis should be provided. The cast can be removed one or two weeks after surgery depending on the individual case and how the horse tolerates the cast. Nonsteroidal anti-inflammatory drugs should be used judiciously during the postoperative period.

Postoperative exercise should be minimal for the first three months. Box stall rest is recommended. After this time hand-walking can be commenced, and the horse eventually turned out. Training should not recommence for six to eight months and not until follow-up radiographs have been taken.

Comments

The prognosis for future athletic soundness is good following internal fixation *if* the fracture is relatively fresh, if concurrent injuries do not exist, and if good alignment of the articular surface was achieved during surgery. It is well recognized that radiographic evaluation of the injury, shortly after the injury, does not give the surgeon an adequate assessment of the trauma sustained to the articular cartilage and joint capsule at the time of injury.

The implants are generally not removed following healing unless lameness can be directly attributed to their presence. If the screws are to be removed, their location is confirmed by radiography with 18-gauge disposable hypodermic needles as markers. At present there is no real argument for or against removing the screws. In one series of cases reported there was no difference in performance between those animals that had the screws removed and those that did not.[6] Some horses do appear to improve following removal of the implants, but an equal number will improve without removing them.[6]

The presence of concurrent injuries appears to be a major factor in determining the future racing performance of the horse. The only way to fully appreciate these concurrent injuries is by performing a meticulous clinical and radiographic examination, including the 125-degree dorsopalmar metacarpal (metatarsal) skyline view.

For an undisplaced condylar fracture, with a concurrent osteochondral fragment in the palmar aspect of the fracture site, removal of this fragment is very difficult without opening up the fracture site. Some cases including those with large fragments would benefit by leaving the fragment in place and not traumatizing the fracture further.[1]

References

1. Adams, S.B., Turner, T.A., Blevins, W.E., et al.: Surgical repair of metacarpal condylar fractures with palmar osteochondral comminution in two Thoroughbred horses. J. Vet. Surg. 14:32, 1985.

2. Alexander, J.T., and Rooney, J.R.: The biomechanics, surgery and prognosis of equine fractures. In Proceedings 18th Annual Convention of the American Association of Equine Practitioners. 1972:1973, p. 219.

3. Barclay, W.P., Foerner, J.J., and Phillips, T.N.: Axial sesamoid injuries associated with lateral condylar fractures in horses. J. Am. Vet. Med. Assoc. 186:278, 1985.

4. Copelan, R.W., and Bramlage, L.R.: Surgery of the Fetlock Joint. Symp. on Equine Orthopedics. Vet. Clin. North Am. 5:221, 1983.

5. Fackelman, G.E., and Nunamaker, D.M.: Manual of Internal Fixation in the Horse. New York, Springer-Verlag, 1982.

6. Meagher, D.M.: Lateral condylar fractures of the metacarpus and metatarsus in horses. In Proceedings 22nd Annual Convention of the American Association of Equine Practitioners, 1976:1978, p. 147.

7. Milne, D.W., and Turner, A.S.: An Atlas of Surgical Approaches to the Bones of the Horse. Philadelphia, W.B. Saunders, 1979.

8. Muller, M.E., Allgower, M., Schneider, R., and Willenegger, H.: Manual of Internal Fixation, 2nd Ed. New York, Springer-Verlag, 1979.

9. Richardson, D.W.: Medial condylar fractures of the third metatarsal bone in horses. J. Am. Vet. Med. Assoc. 185:761, 1984.

10. Rick, M.C., O'Brien, T.R., Pool, R.R., et. al.: Condylar fractures of the third metacarpal bone and third metatarsal bone in 75 horses: Radiographic features, treatments and outcome. J. Am. Vet. Med. Assoc. 183:287, 1983.

11. Turner, A.S.: Large Animal Orthopedics in the Practice of Large Animal Surgery. (P. Jennings, ed.) Philadelphia, W.B. Saunders, 1984, p. 825.

Compression Plating of Simple and Comminuted Fractures of the Third Metacarpal or Metatarsal (Cannon) Bones

Fractures of the cannon bones are common in horses because of their vulnerability. They are also common in foals, especially during halter-breaking accidents or when a mare stands on the foal. Because of the poor soft tissue covering they are frequently open. When the horse is being transported to a facility for further evaluation, radiographic assessment, and possible repair, the injured leg should be in a well-applied splint, Robert Jones bandage, or a fiberglass cast. If not, the fracture will certainly become open if it is not already, and the fracture ends will soon become abraded and smoothed off.

The question whether to repair the fracture with internal fixation or external coaptation alone will depend on the configuration of the fracture, the size of the subject, economics, and the skill of the surgeon. The following section of this chapter is not meant to be a complete treatise on compression plating in horses. We are assuming that the surgeon who is about to attempt repair of such a fracture has been to one of the recognized ASIF/AO courses on internal fixation of fractures held at various centers around the world. This chapter should be regarded as a "refresher" that can remind the surgeon of some of the many details that must be attended to if such a repair is undertaken.

A good radiographic study of the entire bone, including the joint above (i.e., carpometacarpal) and the joint below (i.e., metacarpophalangeal joint) the fracture is mandatory. This should include oblique views, or any other views that may more accurately define the configuration of the fracture. Hairline fissure fractures that extend proximad or distad may be present and will markedly affect the method of repair, location of plate(s) and lag screws, as well as the prognosis. An open fracture should not discourage the surgeon from internal fixation with plates and screws. In fact, it should be a greater indication for internal fixation. One exception to this rule is an open fracture that enters the nutrient foramen of the third metacarpal. This has an extremely poor prognosis and should not be attempted. It has been well demonstrated experimentally in laboratory animals and equally well demonstrated clinically in man and the horse that bone will heal in the face of infection if the right biomechanical situation exists, namely, *stability at the fracture site*.

Although the subject of case selection is important and should not be underestimated, it will not be discussed in great detail here. Obviously a young animal of lighter body weight is going to heal more rapidly than a mature or aged horse greater than 400 kg in body weight.

Anesthesia and Surgical Preparation

The horse (foal) should be started on broad-spectrum antibiotics immediately before surgery. This will ensure the presence of the antibiotic in the hematoma at the time of surgery. Antibiotic coverage should continue for 24 hours after suction drains are removed (see "Repair of a Comminuted Fracture").

Safe general anesthesia is essential. The animal is positioned and suitably padded with the affected limb uppermost. Shortly after induction, two holes are drilled into the hoof wall, and baling wire is looped through the holes and twisted back on itself and held by an assistant. A large-diameter soft rope is threaded around the sternum or groin of the foal and secured to counteract traction that may be exerted on the distal limb. Steady continuous traction is commenced as soon as a suitable plane of general anesthesia has been reached. Surgical preparation must include the entire circumference of the fractured bone and extend from proximal radius to the coronet. Following clipping of the limb, the surgical site is shaved and the entire limb prepared for aseptic surgery.

Draping of cannon bone fractures must be done thoroughly, and a full complement of drapes should be available to do so. The draping should create a sterile field and must maintain such a field despite the handling and manipulation that inevitably occurs during the repair. The drapes should never become dislodged. A sterile adhesive plastic drape should be applied in such a manner that the limb is as free as possible and the surgeon has a constant appreciation of the surrounding anatomy.

The location of the plate to repair a diaphyseal fracture of a cannon bone will depend on the configuration of the fracture. Strain gauge measurements have shown that the third metacarpal bone is axially loaded and the dorsolateral aspect of the third metatarsal bone is under tension during normal weight bearing.[1,7] With the fractures shown in Figure 5-5A to Figure 5-5D the plate could be placed virtually anywhere except the caudal aspect of the bone. Because soft tissue coverage is critical to the outcome of internal fixation of the cannon bones, an approach that splits the lateral digital extensor tendon has been recommended,[3] and it is this approach that is presented here.

Additional Instrumentation

This procedure requires instruments for bone plate application, as well as a complete inventory of ASIF dynamic compression plates of various sizes (see Appendix II). Also required is a suction drain and material for fiberglass cast application.

Surgical Technique

The skin incision is made directly over the lateral digital extensor tendon as shown in Figure 5-5E. As soon as the skin incision has been made, sterile towels are sewn or stapled to the wound edges, incorporating the plastic adhesive drape in the sutures or staples. Stapling the skin towels to the wound edge is an advantage because the application time is shorter than that for suturing the drapes to the limb.[5] The fibers of the tendon are split, dividing the tendon longitudinally

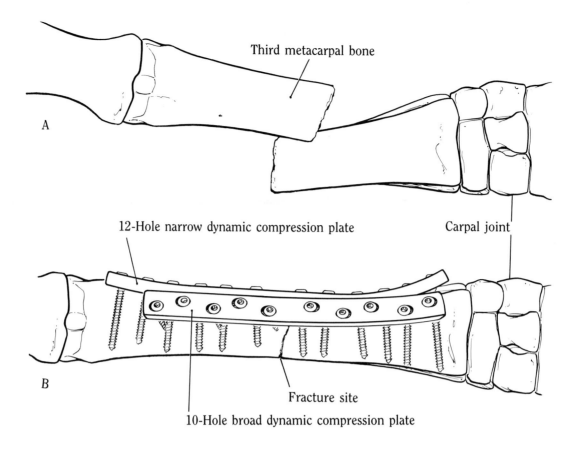

Third metacarpal bone

A

12-Hole narrow dynamic compression plate

Carpal joint

B

Fracture site

10-Hole broad dynamic compression plate

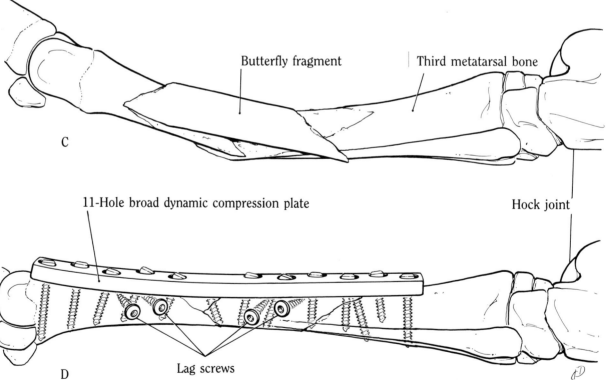

Butterfly fragment

Third metatarsal bone

C

Hock joint

11-Hole broad dynamic compression plate

Lag screws

D

FIG. 5-5. A. Line drawing (from radiographs) of a simple fracture of the third metacarpus (adult). B. Completed repair of the simple third metacarpal fracture in Figure 5-5A. Two bone plates were required to complete the repair. C. Line drawing (from radiographs) of a comminuted fracture of the third metatarsus (foal). D. Completed repair of the fracture in Figure 5-5C. One bone plate and four lag screws were required to complete the repair.

along most of its length into two equal portions. The periosteum is also incised down to the bone, and the periosteum is reflected in preparation for application of the bone plate (Figure 5-5F).

When the surgical site has been exposed, hematoma and tissue debris are removed by suction. Small bony fragments that will not be incorporated in the repair are removed with forceps. Throughout the procedure, tissues should be kept moist but not allowed to become completely waterlogged because of excess flushing.

REPAIR OF A SIMPLE FRACTURE. The fracture is reduced carefully by manipulating the fracture ends as steady judicious traction is applied with the aid of the baling wire held by a nonscrubbed assistant. The fracture must be reduced carefully without damaging the bone ends; otherwise good anatomic interdigitation of the fracture will not occur. Reduction should be such that limb alignment (rotation, angulation) is good. Once the fracture has been reduced, it can be temporarily secured with a lag screw. Inserting the screw is easiest if there is some obliquity to the fracture line as shown in Figure 5-5G but may be impossible if the fracture is a transverse one. This lag screw will provide additional compression at the fracture site. The screw should be a 4.5-mm bone screw of appropriate length. Because the hole is drilled in an oblique direction, it should be adequately countersunk so as to prevent plastic deformation of the head of the screw.

A compression plate of suitable length is selected. Aluminum templates are useful to help select the correct size of the plate as well as to contour it. The plate should span the bone from one metaphysis to the next. The most suitable implant currently available for long-bone fracture repair is the broad Dynamic Compression Plate (DCP). The plate is contoured (bent and twisted) to match the shape of the aluminum template. For the fracture shown in Figure 5-5A a small amount of "prebending" of the plate will help provide more uniform compression opposite the fracture site. This is achieved by providing a 2-mm gap under the plate at the fracture site.[4]

Slight twisting of the plate will be required. We find it easier to do this by holding the plate in the bending press and using *one* of the bending irons to achieve the twist. The surgeon should try to contour the plate as perfectly as possible without excessively prolonging the operating time.

The plate is attached to the bone by inserting the first screw through the plate about 1 cm from the fracture site. The screw is not tightened completely. The plate is then displaced toward the fracture site to bring the shaft of the screw up against the displaced edge of the screw hole. The screw on the other side of the fracture is inserted through the plate using the yellow "load" drill guide. Both screws should engage both cortices of the bone (Fig. 5-5 H, I). When the tap is passed through the plate, it should pass through the 4.5-mm tap sleeve with the plate protector positioned at its end.

The two screws are situated at either side of the fracture site, located eccentrically in the holes in the plate (i.e., in the "load" posi-

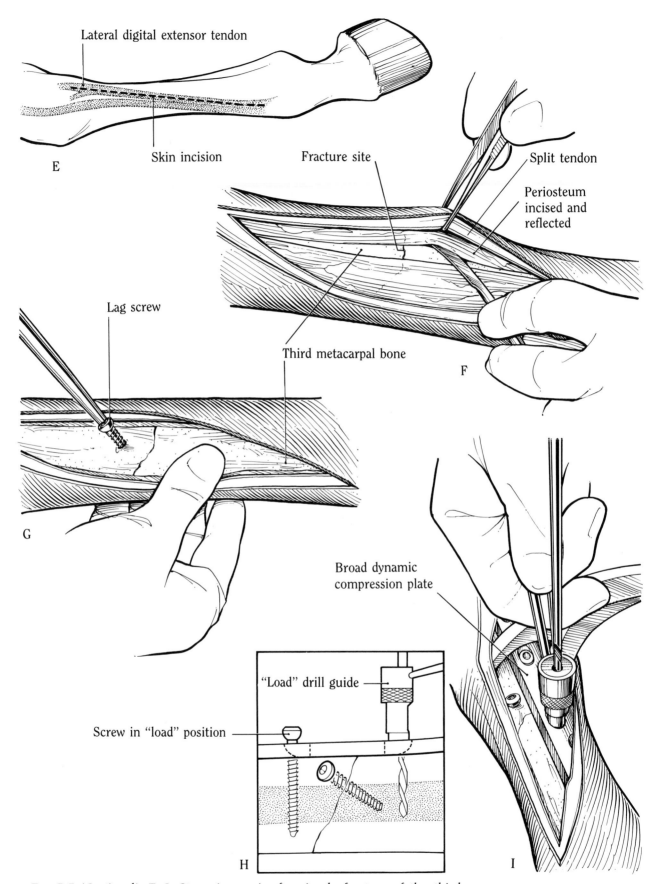

FIG. 5-5 (*Continued*). **E–I.** Steps in repair of a simple fracture of the third metacarpus or metatarsus.

tion). As the two screws are alternately tightened, compression will be observed at the fracture site. The remaining screws are placed in the neutral position using the corresponding neutral or "green" drill guide. As an alternative to placing a lag screw across the fracture prior to fixation, a lag screw can be placed through the plate and across the fracture to provide interfragmentary compression.

The remaining screws should engage in both cortices of the bone and should be angled to cross the bone at its greatest diameter wherever they are located. Cortical bone screws, either 4.5 or 5.5 mm in diameter, can be used for the remaining screws.

If the bone is very soft, such as may be encountered in the metaphysis of newborn foals, either 5.5-mm or 6.5-mm cancellous screws can be used. These larger screws are also useful if the surgeon inadvertently strips the threads of one of the cortical screws.

In certain sized individuals (e.g., >250 kg), an additional plate (broad or narrow compression plate) will be required. This should be situated at 90 degrees to the first plate, with all the screws placed in the "neutral" position. If a second plate is applied, the original lag screw should be removed and, if possible, used as one of the screws in the plate (Fig. 5-5B). Every step of the repair should be aimed at achieving maximum stability at the fracture site.

REPAIR OF A COMMINUTED FRACTURE. The fracture illustrated in Figure 5-5C is comminuted and has a small "butterfly" fragment. It is in three parts and can be converted into a two-part fracture by reattaching the fragment to the parent bone with a lag screw. At this point the fracture is reduced with another lag screw (Fig. 5-5J). The fracture is then repaired as described above for the repair of a simple fracture. The fragment should be positioned *under* the plate as shown in Figure 5-5K. Additional compression could be achieved at the fracture line by placing lag screws through the appropriate holes in the plate and directing them across the fracture plane (Fig. 5-5L).

All holes in the plate should be filled. If a fracture line appears directly under one of the holes in the plate, then rather than leave it void, it should be filled. A glide hole is drilled through the fracture site until the medullary cavity is reached. The 3.2-mm drill sleeve is placed in the hole, and a 3.2-mm hole is drilled and tapped and a 4.5-mm cortical screw of appropriate length is inserted (Fig. 5-5D).

Placement of a suction drain is advisable to evacuate the hematoma at the surgical site (an ideal medium for bacteria). The drain should be placed along the entire length of the incision and then tunneled by means of a trocar through several centimeters of soft tissues. The tube should be under constant vacuum (Fig. 5-5N).

The incision is closed by first apposing the divided lateral digital extensor tendon and using a synthetic absorbable suture material in a simple continuous pattern (Fig. 5-5M). The subcutaneous tissue and skin are closed by the pattern and materials of the surgeon's choice. For adults and yearlings the limb should now be placed in a full-limb fiberglass cast that extends to the proximal end of the radius or tibia,

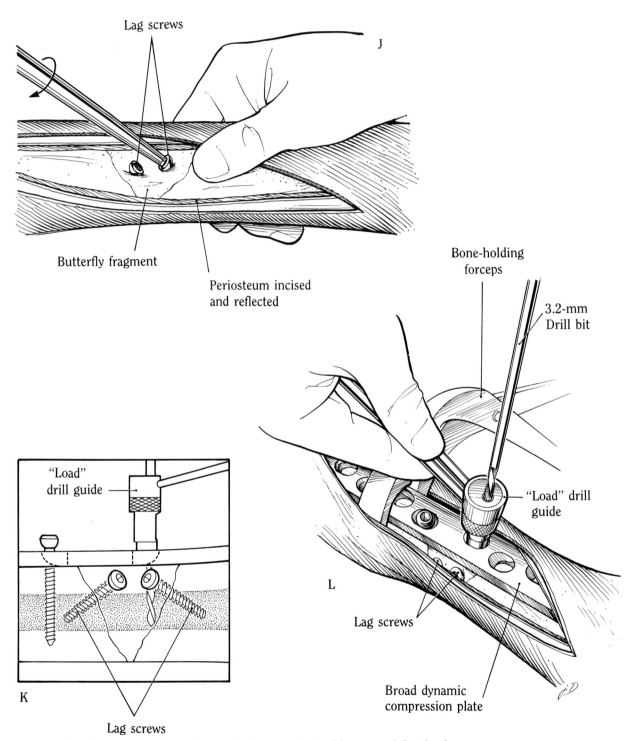

Lag screws

J

Butterfly fragment

Periosteum incised
and reflected

Bone-holding
forceps

3.2-mm
Drill bit

"Load" drill
guide

"Load"
drill guide

L

Lag screws

Lag screws

Broad dynamic
compression plate

K

Lag screws

Fig. 5-5 (*Continued*). **J–L.** Steps in repair of a comminuted fracture of the third
metacarpus or metatarsus.

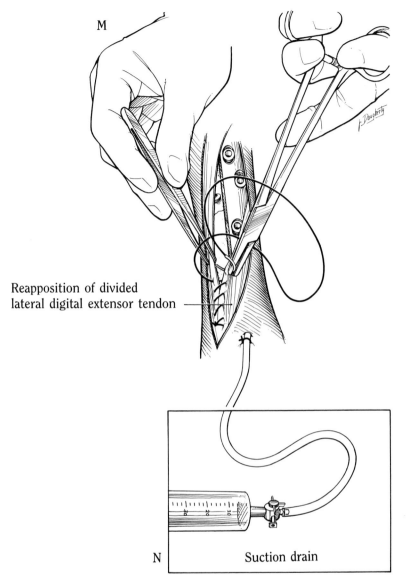

Reapposition of divided
lateral digital extensor tendon

N | Suction drain

FIG. 5-5 (Continued). M, N. Closure of the wound following plate application, showing reapposition of the lateral digital extensor tendon, with use of a suction drain to evacuate blood or serum.

whichever is appropriate. For foals, rather than apply a cast, a well-applied Robert Jones bandage will sometimes suffice in a well stabilized fracture by rigid internal fixation. The suction drain is brought out through the cast. The reservoir (bellows apparatus) should be attended to every hour for the first 12 hours so that as much hematoma as possible is removed. It should never be allowed to back flow, and solutions of any description should not be flushed up the tubing. Antibiotics should be continued until at least 24 hours after removal of the drain. The drain is removed when the collection of fluid is diminished, usually after a clot of blood, fibrin, and tissue debris has formed within the lumen. The cast can be removed any time after 24 hours in young foals and can coincide with drain removal. Older animals require periods of extended immobilization.

The animal is confined to a box stall. As foals are likely to be the most appropriate candidates, a box stall large enough to accommodate the mare and the foal should be available. Shavings or a light bedding of straw is also recommended to enable the foal to ambulate without becoming trapped by deep bedding.

Comments

The surgical approach described for cannon bone fractures provides a maximum amount of soft tissue over the implant, should breakdown of the skin incision occur.[3] If the fracture configuration dictates that a more dorsal (cranial) approach is required, then the common (or long) digital extensor tendon can be split in a similar fashion.

Subperiosteal dissection creates the least amount of trauma to the soft tissues and provides the best postoperative blood supply to the healing bone.[2] In addition, removal of the periosteal layer allows the plate to have more intimate contact with the bone, thereby increasing bone-to-plate friction. For similar reasons, the plate should be contoured with as much precision as time permits. One method to improve friction between the plate and the bone is a technique called plate luting. The fracture is repaired as described; when the repair is complete, all screws passing through the plate are loosened to permit the plate to be lifted off the bone slightly. Polymethylmethacrylate (PMMA) is mixed into the dough stage and then applied to the ventral surface of the plate. The plate is now attached firmly to the bone. The PMMA will form a thin layer between the plate and bone. As the plate is tightened most of the PMMA will be forced to the sides. This excess is removed.

Prebending is another important maneuver to achieve more uniform compression across the fracture site. It would not be possible for a comminuted fracture such as the fracture shown in Figure 5-5C or for a very oblique fracture line, but it would be suitable for the fracture shown in Figure 5-5A.

If comminution does exist, the comminuted region should be placed under the plate and consideration be given to the insertion of a cancellous bone graft. Comminuted fractures repaired with internal fixation must be supplemented with external coaptation, even though both methods are frowned upon in human orthopedics.

Screws with large diameters (5.5-mm cortical) have been recommended to achieve greater holding power.[9,10] One advantage of the larger screws is that they have the same pull-out strength as the partially threaded cancellous screws. A fully threaded screw is preferable to a partially threaded screw, especially if removal of the implants is anticipated when the fracture has healed.

The biggest obstacle to overcome in the surgical repair of cannon bone fractures is preservation of the viability of the soft tissues covering the implants. The energy that caused the fracture has in part been displaced into the soft tissues and overlying skin, making them vulnerable to the additional insult of surgery. On occasion, the insult of surgery is too much, and the skin sloughs over the implants. This sloughing admits infection so that implants eventually loosen and the fracture becomes unstable.

The AO/ASIF Dynamic Compression Plate (DCP) with its uniquely designed screw holes should be used rather than the older round hole plate (Muller plate).

The DCP is more versatile, and the screws can be angled without creating excessive stress on the screw heads. Plate removal is an additional procedure with additional expense involved. It is not routinely recommended unless a specific indication exists. Common indications include drainage and fistula formation, usually due to infection around the implants. If the animal is destined to be used for some form of athletic performance, then implant removal *is* usually necessary because screws placed from the dorsal cortex to the palmar cortex in a sagittal plane in (cranial to caudal) have an "anchoring" effect, not allowing normal flexion of the bone during maximal loading. This results in pain and soreness until the implants are removed.

References

1. Brewener, A.A., Thomason, J., Goodship, A., et al.: Bone stress in the horse forelimb during locomotion at different gaits. A comparison of two experimental methods. J. Biomechanics 16:565, 1983.
2. Bramlage, L.R.: Longbone fractures In Symposium on Equine Orthopedics. Vet. Clin. North Am., 5:285, 1983.
3. Bramlage, L.R.: Fractures of the 3rd Metacarpal and Metatarsal Bones. Paper presented at the 16th Annual Course on Internal Fixation of Fractures and Non-Unions. Columbus, Ohio, 1985.
4. Fackelman, G.E., and Nunamaker, D.M.: Manual of Internal Fixation in the Horse. New York, Springer-Verlag, 1982.
5. Morris, D.M.: The use of skin staples to secure skin towels in areas difficult to drape. Surg. Gynecol. Obstet. 159:387, 1984.
6. Milne, D.W., and Turner, A.S.: An Atlas of Surgical Approaches of the Bones of the Horse. Philadelphia, W.B. Saunders, 1979.
7. Turner, A.S., Mills, E.J., and Gabel, A.A.: In Vivo measurement of bone strain in the horse. Am. J. Vet. Res. 36:1573, 1975.
8. Turner, A.S.: Large animal orthopedics. In Practice of Large Animal Surgery. (P. Jennings, ed.) Philadelphia, W.B. Saunders, 1984, p. 816.
9. Yovich, J.V., Turner, A.S., and Smith, F.W.: Holding power of orthopedic screws in equine third metacarpal and metatarsal bones: Part I, Foal bone. J. Vet. Surg. 14:221, 1985.
10. Yovich, J.V., Turner, A.S., and Smith, F.W.: Holding power of orthopedic screws in equine third metacarpal and metatarsal bones: Part II, Adult horses. J. Vet. Surg. 14:230, 1985.

Plate Fixation of a
Simple Fracture of the Olecranon

Fractures of the olecranon are relatively common, especially in younger horses. A kick from another horse, a sudden fall, and avulsion of a part of the bone by the pull of the triceps brachii muscle are the usual causes of such fractures.[1-3,5-9,11,13,14] A simple olecranon fracture generally responds well to internal fixation if certain principles are followed, and for this reason we felt it would be appropriate to describe the method of repair of such a fracture.

A horse with a fracture of the olecranon will bear a variable amount of weight on the limb, depending on the location of the fracture and the degree of disruption of the triceps-olecranon apparatus. The typical stance of an animal with an olecranon fracture resembles the dropped elbow stance of radial paralysis. Swelling and crepitation may be evident upon palpation, but the amount will depend on the location of the fracture and the degree of comminution and instability.

The diagnosis of a fracture of the olecranon is confirmed with radiographs (craniocaudal and medial-to-lateral views). The lateral view usually shows the fracture configuration most clearly and is best taken with the x-ray beam directed in a medial-to-lateral direction across the cranial aspect of the chest. Olecranon fractures can assume a variety of configurations. Most commonly, the fracture occurs through the semilunar notch of the elbow joint, although other configurations may be seen that range from an avulsion of the epiphysis of foals to severe comminution of the ulna with luxation of the radius craniad (Monteggia type of fracture).[8] Distraction of the proximal fragments is sometimes severe, owing to the pull of the triceps brachii muscle. If the surgeon is new or inexperienced at ASIF compression plating techniques, then it would be unwise to attempt one of the complicated fractures of the olecranon. These would be cases to refer to someone with more experience.

Olecranon fractures have been managed by surgical or nonsurgical methods in different situations. The configuration of the fracture will often determine which method will be chosen. For minimally displaced fissure fractures, treatment with absolute stall rest for six to eight weeks, prevention of "contracted" flexor tendons of the affected limb, and support of the contralateral limb may suffice. Cross tying is sometimes indicated to prevent the animal from lying down and displacing the fracture upon rising. The affected limb should be radiographed periodically to check for distraction or displacement of the fragments, in which case internal fixation is indicated. In extremely comminuted fractures nonoperative management may be the only alternative because of the large numbers of fragments. Economics may also be a deciding factor in the method of repair. Nonoperative treatment, however, should not be regarded as a "conservative" approach because, in our opinion, it has a higher chance of failure than operative treatment. Surgical treatment, when applicable, results in restoration of normal elbow joint mechanics and possible return to athletic soundness. In our experience, this is rarely the case after nonsurgical treatment.[14]

If nonsurgical management is elected, a number of complications can arise, including (1) "contraction" of the flexor tendons of the affected limb with stiffness of joints; (2) severe atrophy of the triceps brachii muscle; (3) failure of fracture union, due to excessive distraction of fragments; (4) permanent pain and stiffness of the elbow joint, due to secondary degenerative joint disease; (5) angular limb deformities (in young animals), such as valgus or varus deformities of the carpus of the contralateral limb, due to excessive compensatory weight bearing; and (6) laminitis in adult horses, due to compensatory overload of the uninjured limb.[14]

The main goal of surgical intervention in olecranon fractures is to offset the distracting forces of the triceps brachii muscle and to reestablish continuity of the articular surface of the elbow joint.[1-3,5-9,11,13,14]

The most satisfactory technique for repair of a fractured equine olecranon is rigid stabilization, using dynamic compression plating along the caudal aspect of the bone, and this method is described. Fortunately, the tension surface of the bone is its caudal aspect because of the pull of the triceps brachii muscle. Pinning and tension band wiring techniques, which are successful on olecranon fractures of small animals and man, have limited application in the horse, owing to the greater body weight of the patient.[14] Because the stability is less with pinning and wiring devices, convalescence is frequently prolonged and weight bearing is delayed.[7] One exception to the preference for plate fixation is the very proximal avulsion fracture of the olecranon process that is impossible to plate because of the lack of bone within the proximal fragment.

Because the plate is subjected to tensile forces, which it resists extremely well, fracture repair is generally not fraught with problems of implant failure that occur in the other tubular long bones of adult horses. Most olecranon fractures respond quite dramatically postoperatively, as early weight bearing and pain-free ambulation occur soon after rigid internal fixation.

Anesthesia and Surgical Preparation

The surgical procedure is performed under general anesthesia with the horse placed in lateral recumbency with the affected limb uppermost.

Prior to induction of anesthesia the entire elbow region is clipped, including a portion of the lateral thorax and forelimb. By clipping the limb before surgery the anesthetic time can be reduced.

Additional Instrumentation

Compression plating of the olecranon requires a full complement of long-bone plating instruments and an assortment of cortical and cancellous screws (see Appendix).

Surgical Technique

The limb is draped, using sterile plastic adherent drapes for the immediate surgical site. A curvilinear skin incision is made as illustrated in Figure 5-6A. Using a muscle separation technique, the bone is approached between the ulnaris lateralis muscle and the humeral head of the deep digital flexor muscle.[10] The ulnaris lateralis muscle is reflected craniad and the humeral and ulnar heads of the deep digital flexor muscle caudad, exposing the caudal aspect of the ulna (Fig. 5-6B).

Olecranon fractures are usually easy to reduce.[14] Bone reduction forceps with points are useful in reduction of fractures that are being treated some time after the original injury. In chronic cases fibrous tissue may be interposed between the fracture fragments, making perfect reconstruction of the fracture impossible. In such cases the bone plate should be applied without extensive debridement because once the fracture is stabilized, ossification usually proceeds rapidly.[12]

The compression plate should be contoured to fit the caudal aspect of the bone (Fig. 5-6C). Some twisting of the plate may be required. A technique has been described in which the distal parent fragment of the olecranon is "shaved" with an osteotome or chisel to aid in seating the plate on the rounded caudal aspect of the bone.[6] This technique is useful for some fresh fractures and may be essential for long-standing injuries when callus and fibrous tissue have produced an irregular surface to the bone.

Application of the Plate

The plate of appropriate length is applied by the techniques and methods outlined by the Association for the Study of Internal Fixation (ASIF).[4,12] A narrow ASIF Dynamic Compression Plate is suitable for most horses. For simple fractures into the semilunar notch without a lot of distraction at the fracture site, the plate is applied in the following sequence. A 3.2-mm hole is drilled about 1 cm proximal to the fracture site (Fig. 5-6D). Because of the proximity of the radiohumeral joint, it is recommended that the screw inserted in this hole be relatively short so as not to invade the articulation. The hole is tapped (Fig. 5-6E). A narrow dynamic compression plate is accurately contoured to the caudal aspect of the ulna and loosely attached to the bone by a cortical bone screw, using the predrilled, pretapped hole. The plate should then be displaced toward the fracture line so that this screw occupies a position on the inclined slope of the hole of the dynamic compression plate.

A second hole is drilled using the DCP yellow "load" guide. The screw in this hole should also be relatively short so as not to invade the articulation (Fig. 5-6F). The hole is tapped (Fig. 5-6G). These two screws are now positioned eccentrically away from the fracture site (Fig. 5-6H). Tightening the screws reduces the fracture and produces compression of the fracture site because of the self-compressing

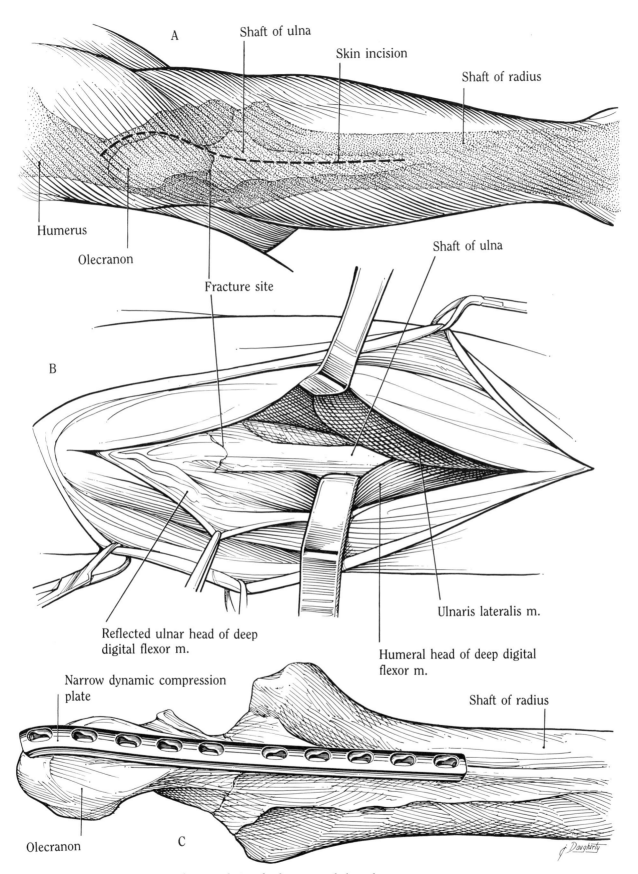

A

Shaft of ulna

Skin incision

Shaft of radius

Humerus

Olecranon

Fracture site

Shaft of ulna

B

Reflected ulnar head of deep
digital flexor m.

Ulnaris lateralis m.

Humeral head of deep digital
flexor m.

Narrow dynamic compression
plate

Shaft of radius

Olecranon

C

FIG. 5-6A–C. Compression plating of simple fracture of the olecranon.

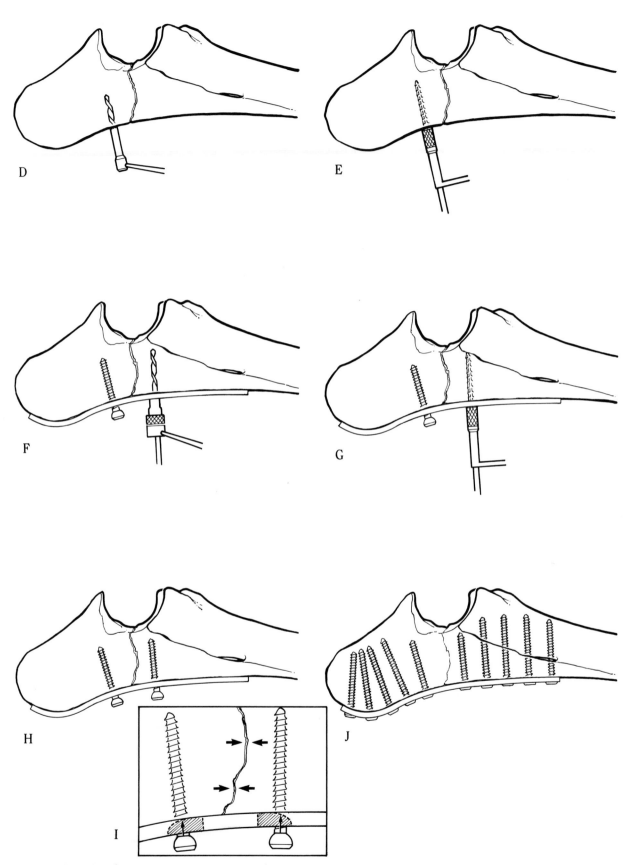

FIG. 5-6 (Continued). D–J.

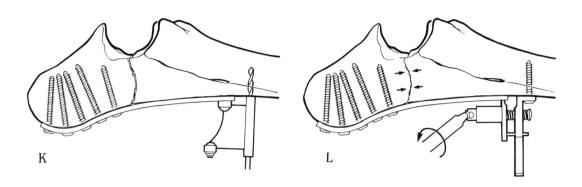

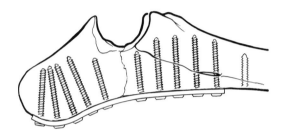

K

L

M

FIG. 5-6 (Continued). K–M.

properties of the DCP (Fig. 5-6I). The remainder of the screws are placed in the so-called neutral position using the neutral drill guide. The screws should avoid, at all costs, the articulation of the elbow joint. Shorter screws should be used in this region, or screws can be angled away from the joint (Fig. 5-6J). Intraoperative radiographs for this fracture are generally difficult as far as determining positioning, and the risk of breaking aseptic technique is increased. With preoperative planning and knowledge of where the elbow joint is in relationship to the fracture site, the surgeon can complete the operation without such an interruption. Because of the density of the bone in the proximal radius, the distal screws need only engage the caudal radial cortex (Fig. 5-6J). The blood vessels in the interosseous foramen should be avoided.[4] Cortical bone screws are used throughout the repair except when the bone of the proximal ulna is soft as may occur in foals or yearlings.

If a larger fracture gap exists, the tension device can be readily used, since additional distal exposure is easily obtained.[10] With this device a relatively large fracture gap can be closed and compressed. All the screws proximal to the fracture site are first inserted. The special drill guide for the compression device is secured to the plate and a 3.2-mm hole is drilled (Fig. 5-6K). The removable tension device is attached to the plate and secured to the bone with a 4.5-mm cortical bone screw. A socket wrench is used to slightly tighten the tension device and simultaneously provisionally reduce the fracture (Fig. 5-6L). The tension device is then tightened so as to produce compression at the fracture site. The distal screws are now inserted, and the compression device is removed (Fig. 5-6M).

The judicious use of power tapping and of the power screwdriver attachment will greatly speed up the operation and reduce the time the animal is anesthetized and the wound is exposed to room air. Reducing the pressure of the compressed nitrogen source to diminish the torque generated by the drill decreases the chances of instrument breakage.

In very young animals it is preferable that the ulna should not be attached to the radius with screws, as this procedure will cause abnormal development of the elbow joint as the proximal radial physis continues to grow. In such cases, the screws should be inserted *only* through the ulna if at all possible. If the ulna is so thin that screw fixation of the ulna alone would jeopardize the repair, the screws will have to be placed in the caudal cortex of the radius, but the plate needs to be removed before elbow dysplasia develops.

Suction drains should be used if excessive hematoma at the fracture site is anticipated. Pressure bandaging is difficult with the incision this far up the limb. Another option is to suture a stent bandage directly over the incision.

Postoperative Management

The postoperative management of olecranon fractures should consist of pressure bandaging while the animal is confined to a box stall. Casting or splinting is not only impossible but is probably detrimental because of placing unwanted forces on the fracture site.

If the fracture can be adequately stabilized at surgery, the prognosis for future soundness is generally good to excellent. Postoperatively, horses with olecranon fractures begin almost immediate weight bearing. Failure to bear weight within 7 to 10 days of surgery is usually indicative of continued instability at the fracture site or infection of the fixation.

It still has not been determined whether the plates should be removed from olecranon fractures in mature horses. Our tendency is to leave them in place unless there is a loose screw that could potentially migrate or there is infection around the implants. In this last situation the implants must not be removed until the fracture has healed. In young animals (less than 5 months) that still may have continued growth of the proximal radial physis, plate removal is necessary to avoid elbow dysplasia and subsequent lameness.

References

1. Brown, M.P., and Norrie, R.D.: Surgical repair of olecranon fractures in young horses. J. Equine Med. Surg. 2:545, 1978.
2. Colahan, P.T., and Meagher, D.M.: Repair of comminuted fractures of the proximal ulna and olecranon in young horses using tension band plating. Vet. Surg. 8:105, 1979.

3. Denny, H.R.: The surgical treatment of fractures of the olecranon in the horse. Equine Vet. J. 8:20, 1976.
4. Fackelman, G.E., and Nunamaker, D.M.: Manual of Internal Fixation in the Horse. New York, Springer-Verlag, 1982.
5. Fessler, J.F., and Amstutz, H.E.: Fractures. In Textbook of Large Animal Surgery. (E.W. Oehme and J.E. Prier, eds) Baltimore, Williams & Wilkins, 1974.
6. Fretz, P.B.: Fractured ulna in the horse. Can. Vet. J. 14:50, 1973.
7. Kopf, N., and Rettenbacher, G.: Die Zuggurtung der Olekranofractur Beim Pferd. Pract. Tierarzt. 7:598, 1981.
8. Levine, S.B., and Meagher, D.M.: Repair of an ulnar fracture with radial luxation in a horse. Vet. Surg. 9:58, 1980.
9. McGill, C.A., Hilbert, B.J., and Jacobs, K.V.: Internal fixation of fractures of the ulna in the horse. Aust. Vet. J. 58:101, 1982.
10. Milne, D.W., and Turner, A.S.: Atlas of Surgical Approaches to the Bones of the Horse. Philadelphia, W.B. Saunders, 1979.
11. Monin, T.: Repair of physeal fractures of the tuber olecranon in the horse using a tension band method. J. Am. Vet. Med. Assoc. 172:287, 1978.
12. Muller, M.E., Allgower, M., Schneider, R., and Willenegger, H.: Manual of Internal Fixation, 3rd ed. New York, Springer-Verlag, 1979.
13. Pettersson, H.: Die konservative und chirurgische Versorgung der Ulnafraktur. Pract. Tierarzt. 7:585, 1981.
14. Turner, A.S.: Fractures of the olecranon. In Symposium on Equine Orthopedics. Vet. Clin. North Am. (Large Anim. Pract.), 5:275, 1983.

Application of Fiberglass Cast

A cast is commonly an essential part of treatment of fractures and luxations. Frequently a cast is used to "protect" a fracture that has been repaired with plates and/or screws, especially during the recovery period from anesthesia when excessive forces may disrupt the repair. Casts are also useful for temporary immobilization of fractures distal to the distal third of the radius and tibia. Fractures proximal to this level are temporarily immobilized with a Robert-Jones bandage with a lateral splint to prevent abduction of the limb.[1] Casting is also used as a sole method of treating certain fractures that are too comminuted for repair by internal fixation with plates and/or screws.[3–5]

Some of the most frequent indications for cast application at Colorado State University Veterinary Teaching Hospital are distal limb lacerations, especially those involving the bulbs of the heels and coronet. Despite an initial higher expense, a cast provides superior immobilization of the wound edges to pressure bandaging alone. Pressure bandaging is sometimes useful in the initial stages of management when there is extensive suppuration or contamination, but a cast placed on the limb at the earliest opportunity is the best method to achieve rapid wound healing. Casts are also a vital adjunct to tendon lacerations in horses because of the inability of most commercially available suture materials to withstand the enormous tensile forces subjected to the repair by large animals. Certain cases of so-called "contracted" tendons or flexure deformities in foals require casts either as a sole method of treatment or as an adjunct to surgery.

One variation in the casting method that has become popular in recent years is the so-called "tube" or "sleeve" cast. This cast extends from the proximal end of the radius to just below the fetlock joint, the foot being exposed. In foals, the most common indication for a tube cast is the condition referred to as "hypoplasia" or delayed ossification of the carpal bones. We have also used it as a support to repair comminuted fractures of the carpus.

The greatest advantage of the tube cast is that normal weight bearing can occur, and the flexor tendons are under normal physiologic tension while the axial alignment of the limb is maintained. The limb will not adopt the hyperextension conformation due to tendon flaccidity seen if the entire limb, including the foot, is placed in the cast. In addition, the animal has better footing while in the cast.

Casting is by no means a benign procedure, and it does take experience and some practice to become confident in the technique. It is hoped that this section will aid the reader in becoming confident in the technique. Once perfected, fiberglass casting will become a useful method of therapy that will yield rewarding results.

Additional Instrumentation

Many different materials for cast application in horses have been available over the years. With recent advances in the fiberglass and plastic industry, strong lightweight materials are now in routine use.[4]

The fiberglass products used for boats and cars are widely available, but they are exothermic in the curing process and therefore a layer of plaster must be provided to protect the limb from excessive heat. A variety of knitted fiberglass fabrics, impregnated with a polyurethane resin that is activated upon exposure to water, are now the accepted norm for cast application on large animals (Fig. 5-7A). The material is lightweight and therefore ideal for use on foals, unlike the heavier plaster-based products that were previously used. The material is also durable and is unaffected by moisture once it has hardened. Most materials available rapidly harden to maximum strength, enabling the horse to stand and bear weight after approximately 20 minutes of curing. No longer is an awkward ultraviolet lamp (used for some of the earlier fiberglass products) required for the curing process.[2]

Manufacturers claim that fiberglass products are radiotransparent, enabling fracture healing to be evaluated under the cast. We find this method of evaluation somewhat inaccurate and prefer to change the cast under general anesthesia, radiograph the fracture without the cast on, and reapply the cast. It is possible, however, to check *fracture alignment* with reasonable accuracy after the cast has been applied.[5]

The fiberglass products are more expensive than the traditional plaster- and resin-impregnated plaster products. However, *less* material will be used, and with the greater durability of the fiberglass products, the cost is virtually the same. All fiberglass casting products have an expiration date stamped on the package, and this should be observed. The rolls are stored in sealed foil pouches that, if punctured, result in premature hardening. It has been recommended that the pouches be kept in a cool, dry atmosphere and the stock rotated. The pouches should remain in the original shipping boxes to avoid excess handling and the possibility of puncturing the pouches. Refrigeration will increase shelf life. During the actual casting procedure, one pouch should be opened at a time to minimize exposure to air. The roll of

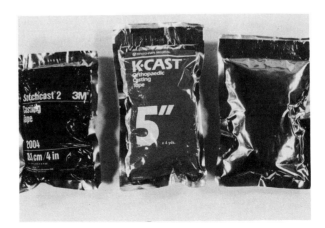

Fig. 5-7A. Types of fiberglass cast material available for large animals: Left, Scotchcast (3M Company); center, K-Cast (Kirschner Medical); right, Delta lite (Johnson and Johnson).

fiberglass tape and its resin should feel soft and pliable. If curing has occurred within the pouch, the roll will feel firm and be difficult or impossible to unravel. Disposable gloves should be worn during the casting procedure because the resin will adhere to the skin and allergic skin reactions are a possibility.

One of the disadvantages of the fiberglass products currently available is the relative difficulty in shaping the product to the contours of the limb. This seems especially true in foals where sharper corners have to be turned during the application process. We currently use "combination" casts, which consist of a very thin layer of resin-impregnated plaster (e.g., Specialist Cast®*), and then apply fiberglass over the plaster. Hopefully fiberglass products will become much softer and more supple, resembling the conforming characteristics of plaster, and the use of the initial plaster layer will become obsolete.

Veterinarians have been frequently confused as to *how much* padding to use under a cast. A good rule to follow, stated simply, is: "as little as possible." Through years of trial and error it has become customary to use no more than two layers of orthopedic stockinette. Some stockinette products are waterproof synthetic fiber, enabling hydrotherapy to be carried out *while the cast is on*. This is not a common method of therapy, and we do not insist that the stockinette be waterproof. The only bit of padding other than stockinette that is "permitted" is a strip of orthopedic felt placed at the top of the cast or an annulus or ring of felt to protect the prominence over the accessory carpal bone if the cast extends above the carpal joint.

One final word of advice prior to application of the cast: The operator should always assemble *all* the equipment needed to apply the cast and attend to the wound *before the general anesthesia is induced*.

The equipment necessary to apply the cast is listed in Appendix III and illustrated in Figures 5-7B and C.

* Specialist Cast, Johnson and Johnson Health Care Division, New Brunswick, N.J.

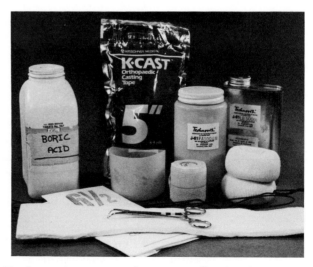

FIG. 5-7B. Equipment necessary for cast application (see Appendix I).

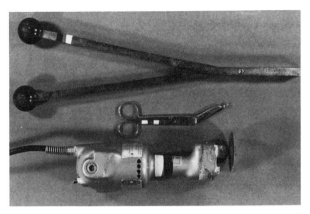

FIG. 5-7C. Equipment necessary for cast removal (see Appendix I).

Technique of Cast Application

METHOD OF RESTRAINT. Cast application is extremely difficult in the standing horse, and an optimal job is impossible unless the animal is motionless and relaxed. Nevertheless, cast application is occasionally indicated in standing horses for various reasons. Fractures of the long bones in yearlings and adults of such a size that physical restraint is out of the question are a real dilemma to manage on an emergency basis. Temporary immobilization is an important adjunct to treatment if the animal is to be transported to a facility where further treatment is undertaken. If the attending veterinarian is confident with intravenous anesthesia techniques, then a temporary bandage is applied, anesthesia is induced, and a cast is applied. However, a fiberglass cast is much easier to use in the standing horse than a plaster cast and is appropriate in many situations. Some fractures will be better handled using a Robert Jones dressing, with a lateral splint to prevent abduction, if the fracture is in the proximal two thirds of the radius or tibia.[2]

The horse should be positioned in lateral recumbency with the limb to be cast uppermost. The limb should be in "natural" position that will permit normal ambulation. Very slight flexion of the carpal joint will reduce the torsional forces at the fracture site.[4] Because of the reciprocal apparatus, the hindlimb will be more difficult to work with. Some slight flexion is desirable; but extension in the hindlimb will make the limb considerably longer than the opposite member, and the horse will tend to drag it as this leg attempts to ambulate.

With the exception of tube casts, the cast should encase the *entire* foot and end proximally at one of four points: the proximal end of the radius/axillary region and the proximal end of the tibia/tibial crest region or immediately distal to the carpus or tarsus, where cannon bones start to flare. A cast should never end in the mid-metacarpus (mid-metatarsus), as this causes intense stress and severe rub sores. Ending the cast in the midtibia, midradius region will result in a loose cast when the animal stands and the muscles are under tension. This will be accentuated when muscle atrophy occurs if cast immobilization is prolonged.

The golden rule for fracture treatment that states "the joint above the fracture and the joint below the fracture must be immobilized" for the most part is applicable to the horse. The notable exception to this would be management of a *very* distal fracture of the tibia or radius. A full limb cast does provide *some* immobilization of fractures in this region despite the inability to extend the cast above the elbow or stifle joint. Some of these fractures would obviously be supplemented with internal fixation.

Traction on the limb in some form or another is desirable in various instances. Traction will aid in positioning the limb as well as reducing and aligning the fracture fragments, especially comminuted fractures of the proximal and middle phalanges, and the cannon bones. The method we prefer to provide traction is widely accepted and not new. Holes are drilled in the hoof wall at the same angle as one would drive a horseshoe nail. Through these holes is looped a length of bailing wire, twisted on itself and wrapped around some sort of object that will allow an assistant to provide steady sustained traction during the casting procedure (Fig. 5-7D). A strong, well-trained assistant is indispensable during cast application in both foals and adult horses. Another assistant must diligently maintain alignment during the curing process. It is not uncommon for assistants to become so involved in the application of the cast that they neglect the posture of the limb. A common end result is a bow in the limb due to inadequate support under the carpus or tarsus. The assistant must support these areas with a *flattened* hand, so as not to indent the curing cast with the fingers.

PREPARATION OF THE LIMB. The wound or surgical site must be appropriately dressed and covered before application of the stockinette. This may entail clipping, shaving, debriding, and suturing or any combination of these procedures. A nonadhering dressing held in position with some cotton gauze (e.g., Kling) is now applied. If a cast is being applied to reduce formation of granulation tissue, then it is

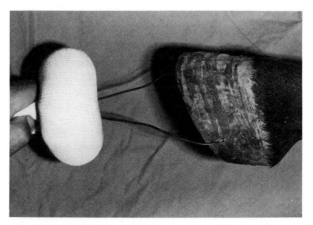

FIG. 5-7D. Baling wire used to provide traction. The stockinette is threaded over the wire in preparation to be rolled up the limb.

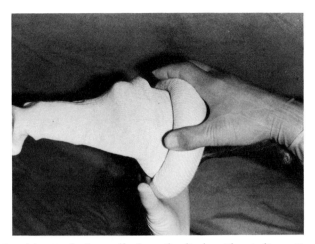

Fig. 5-7E. Stockinette being rolled up the limb without disrupting dressings or disturbing the flattened hair.

prudent to have trimmed the granulation tissue *before* the cast is applied, preferably the day before casting. We prefer to trim granulation tissue as generously as possible, apply a pressure bandage to the wound to allow for hemostasis, and *then* apply the cast the following day. The skin under the cast should be dry and the hair flat.

APPLICATION OF STOCKINETTE AND FELT. One or two layers of stockinette are now rolled up the limb, rather than pulled up the limb, which would disrupt any dressings and disturb the flattened hair (Fig. 5-7E). The size of the stockinette is important. Excessively large stockinette will not conform to the limb and will be "baggy," especially below the carpus and tarsus. Excessively small stockinette will be impossible to stretch over the hoof or impossible to roll up over the more muscular parts of the limb in the case of a full limb cast.

After the stockinette is in place, a strip of felt is positioned at the top of the cast and secured with a towel clamp (Fig. 5-7F). This felt and

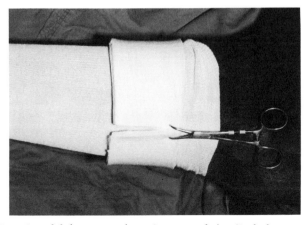

Fig. 5-7F. A strip of felt secured at the top of the limb by a towel clamp.

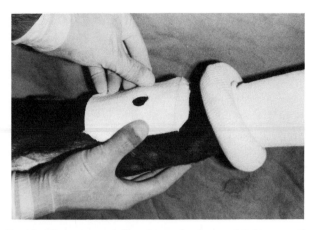

FIG. 5-7G. Positioning a specially shaped piece of felt over the accessory carpal bone region.

the stockinette are the *only* padding used in virtually all of our casts with one or two exceptions. For full limb casts above the carpus, an annulus or "doughnut" of felt must be positioned and secured over the accessory carpal bone region (Fig. 5-7G). Some surgeons will apply a thin strip of felt around the coronet to protect this region from the oscillating saw during cast removal. With a tube cast an additional strip of felt is necessary at the distal end of the cast.

APPLICATION OF FIBERGLASS TAPE. If available, a thin layer of resin-impregnated (or rapid-setting plaster) should be applied to the limb. This is an important step, especially in foals.

The fiberglass tape is available in various widths; 4-, 5- and 6-inch widths are suitable for all sizes of horse. We prefer to begin the cast with a few layers of the narrower tape (e.g., 4 inches), as it seems easier to conform it to the contours of the limb and then use wider tape for succeeding layers (e.g., 5 or 6 inches) to expedite the procedure.

The tape is removed from its foil pouch and immersed in water for 10 to 15 seconds. The recommended temperature for curing is 70 to 75° F (room temperature), but this can be varied accordingly to alter the speed of curing. Warmer temperatures will decrease the curing time and are recommended only when the operator has become familiar with the product and has had experience with the casting technique. The tape should not be wrung out.

The tape is applied in a spiral fashion, first encircling the felt at the top of the cast and proceeding distad (Fig. 5-7H). If plaster has already been applied, the fiberglass can be applied directly over the plaster. The tape should overlap the previous turn by about one half to one third the width of the tape. Slightly more tension should be applied than the operator has been used to with plaster products (Fig. 5-7I).

Exactly *how much* fiberglass to apply without compromising strength, yet avoiding a cumbersome overweight cast is a matter of

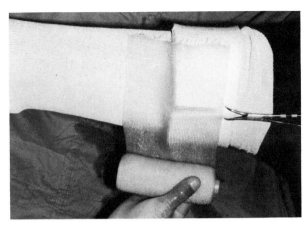

Fig. 5-7H. Application of the fiberglass tape, beginning at top of limb and proceeding distad.

judgment, and certainly there is no substitute for experience. At least 3 to 4 four layers are required for foals and 4 to 6 layers for adults. For the beginner, the first few casts may be a little heavier than desired, but subsequent ones can be made lighter when the properties of the fiberglass are discovered. A broken cast is not only expensive (time and materials), but it can spell disaster if the cast is intended to protect internal fixation of a fracture during recovery from the anesthesia. A broken cast will mean immediate anesthesia and reapplication of a new and stronger cast.

To produce a smooth cast, the tape must be folded, twisted, or pleated. Small pleats are advisable in the more contoured areas such as the articulations over the fetlock (Fig. 5-7J).

Longitudinal splints of casting material used in plaster casts are not necessary with fiberglass because of its inherent strength. Nevertheless, the cast should be reinforced around and immediately below the carpal and tarsal joints, which are regions where full limb casts frequently fail.

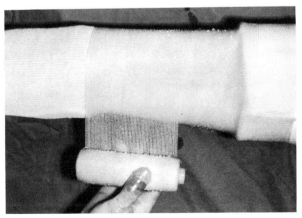

Fig. 5-7I. The tape should spiral distad, overlapping the previous turn by about one half to one third.

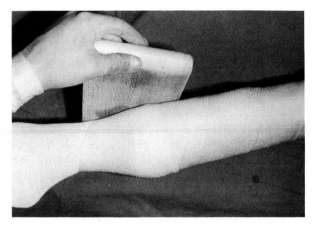

FIG. 5-7J. Folding or twisting tape in the more contoured areas such as fetlock joint.

As the cast is constructed, it will become obvious that eventually the traction device must be removed. If the device was necessary for fracture reduction and alignment, it is advisable to wait 10 minutes until some curing has occurred so that fracture reduction will not be compromised. Excess stockinette is then removed (Fig. 5-7K), followed by removal of the traction device by cutting the baling wire (Fig. 5-7L). The stockinette is folded up over the toe, and an additional roll of fiberglass tape is used to encase the entire toe (Fig. 5-7M). An important step at this point is the construction of some form of heel block to reduce the fulcrum effect that will occur if the horse bears weight purely on the toe and not the heel. The most expensive method is to place a roll of casting tape under the heel and secure this roll into position with the same roll of tape used to cover the toe (Fig. 5-7N). A cheaper method is to take a previously shaped block of wood that can be positioned and taped into place. At this point in the procedure an assistant should commence mixing the acrylic (Technovit, Kylzer & Co.) that will be used as a toe cap. An acrylic cap will

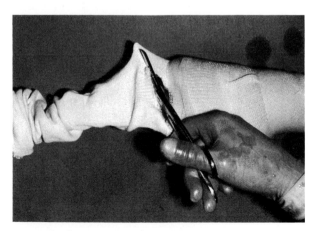

FIG. 5-7K. Removal of excess stockinette.

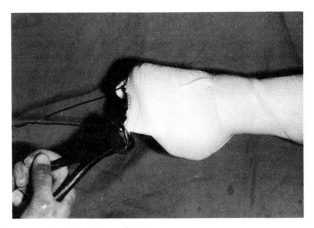

FIG. 5-7L. Removal of traction device.

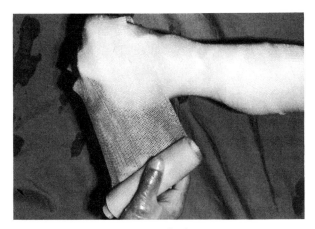

FIG. 5-7M. Encasing the entire foot with the cast.

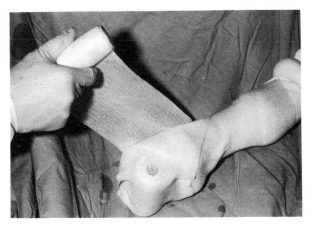

FIG. 5-7N. Roll of casting tape placed under the heel and secured in position with additional tape.

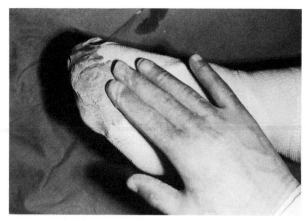

FIG. 5-7O. Acrylic cap placed on toe to reduce excessive wear on toe of the cast.

reduce a lot of wear on the toe of the cast (Fig. 5-7O). We have found that fiberglass tape is easily abraded on rough surfaces as the horse walks. Once the toe has been exposed, there will be an immediate reduction in the immobilizing effect of the cast and movement will produce rubbing sores on the coronet and heel bulbs. Sufficient stockinette and cast tape must be used to protect the toe from the exothermic reaction of the acrylic, but modern fiberglass tapes have a minimal exothermic reaction.

When the cast is complete and the toe cap (in the case of casts encasing the toe region) in place, silicone handcream is applied to the operator's gloved hands and then used to smooth out any sharp edges that may be remaining on the surface of the cast. The hand-cream should never be used until the completion of the cast, as it will interfere with the adherence of succeeding layers of casting tape.

Adhesive dressing such as Elasticon is applied to the top of the cast to secure the stockinette (Fig. 5-7P). It can be spiraled onto the bare limb to "seal" the top of the cast, preventing hay and debris from entering the cast.

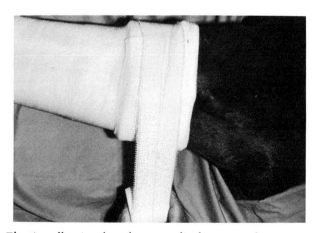

FIG. 5-7P. Elastic adhesive bandage applied to top of cast.

The currently quoted time required for the cast to harden to permit weight bearing in adult horses is 20 minutes. Certainly it is unwise to take shortcuts at this point just to expedite the procedure. As mentioned, a broken cast because of inadequate time to cure is not only costly in time and materials but could potentially mean the demise of the horse.

Tube or Sleeve Cast

A sleeve cast is used primarily for orthopedic conditions of the forelimb, such as collapsed or hypoplastic carpal bones in foals, and for this reason the description to follow will apply to the forelimb. The same principles apply to the hindlimb, as this cast is also used in early cases of collapsed tarsal bones. A sleeve cast extends from the proximal end of the radius to slightly distal to the fetlock joint. The stockinette is applied to the limb and the orthopedic felt is applied at the top of the cast in an identical fashion to that for the preceding cast. Then an additional piece of orthopedic felt about 6 cm in width is applied to the fetlock joint (Fig. 5-7Q).

The fiberglass tape is applied in a spiral fashion but ends at the fetlock joint articulation or slightly distal to it. Shortly into the curing process, the stockinette is cut at the tip of the toe and folded back on itself and taped onto the cast itself. This will cause the felt to curve around and produce a rounded edge of fiberglass tape that will be less likely to form a potentially dangerous sharp edge of fiberglass (Fig. 5-7R).

Convalescence

The equine patient with a limb in a cast must have diligent aftercare to ensure that minor problems do not develop into more serious ones. The patient should be hospitalized in a confined area with light bedding. We prefer straw. The bedding must be kept clean and dry. The cast should be closely inspected to see that it has not cracked. Frequently cracks are not obvious and may be nothing more than a

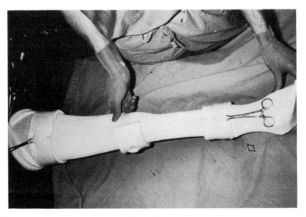

FIG. 5-7Q. Positioning of orthopedic felt for a tube or sleeve cast. Note additional piece of orthopedic felt at fetlock joint.

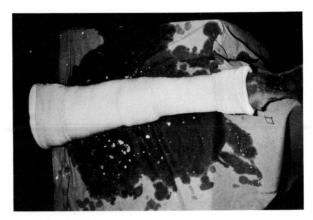

Fig. 5-7R. Completed tube or sleeve cast.

hairline fissure that will open up when the animal places an excessive amount of weight on the limb. If a cast breaks, its immobilizing effect is lost. Casts seem to break in certain areas, such as the proximal extremities of the cannon bones just distal to the carpus or tarsus, or in the pastern region.

A patient with a cracked cast should be scheduled for general anesthesia and replacement of the cast at the earliest opportunity. If the cast has become completely separated into two units, then it should be "patched up" with two or three rolls of fresh fiberglass tape immediately. If only a small hairline fissue has developed, it should be patched but the horse should be taken off feed and scheduled for general anesthesia and cast change the next day. No hard and fast rules can be established regarding the urgency of replacing a damaged cast, and each case has to be evaluated individually.

The value of daily grooming, adequate nutrition, and general tender loving care for orthopedic patients should never be underestimated.[4]

Pressure sores and rubbing sores should not be regarded as "occupational hazards" of casting the limbs of horses. All attempts must be made to minimize them, but occasionally they occur no matter how meticulously the cast is applied. The thin, fine skin in foals is particularly susceptible to pressure and rubbing sores. The most consistent sign of serious problems developing under a cast *is increased reluctance to use the limb.* We encourage that, at least daily, the horse be walked just a few paces out of its box stall and then returned to the stall so that the amount of weight bearing can be monitored from one day to the next. If the horse appears less agile and more reluctant to step out on the cast, then this should alert the clinician to a potential problem. When evaluating the use of the cast, one should always take into account if the horse is on analgesics such as nonsteroidal anti-inflammatory drugs. It is quite possible that such drugs are masking a serious problem under the cast. Swelling above the cast is cause for alarm, and in most cases it will warrant a cast change to investigate the problem. If the cast has been used for an extensive soft tissue injury, then swelling above the cast can be anticipated and can be remedied by pressure bandaging above the cast. If there is no apparent explanation for the swelling, then a cast change should be scheduled as early as practical.

Pressure sores under a cast occur more frequently in certain sites such as the accessory carpal bone, abaxial surface of the proximal sesamoid bones, and the proximal dorsal metacarpus/metatarsus in horses with casts that end in this region. Many pressure sores and rubbing sores will resolve merely by applying another cast. The next cast will often provide subtle alterations in fit that will allow the sores to resolve spontaneously. Rubbing and pressure sores should be cleaned of exudate and a nonadherent dressing applied and held in position with cotton gauze (e.g., Kling). Tetanus prophylaxis should be provided unless it was done previously.

Cast loosening is more likely to occur with the larger full length casts that end in the muscular regions of the proximal parts of the forearm and crus. This is caused by two factors, muscle atrophy due to disuse and sometimes swelling reduction due to the immobilizing effect of the cast. If the limb is severely swollen due to soft tissue injuries or cellulitis, then an attempt should be made to reduce the swelling with pressure bandaging, hydrotherapy, and antiinflammatory drugs before the cast is applied.

Localized osteoporosis is a loss of mineral content of the bones that are immobilized within the cast. The problem is most severe in growing animals because of the rapid bone turnover and is most noticeable in the proximal sesamoid bones and phalanges.[4] The process is reversible when the animal is free of the cast and some weight bearing is resumed. Despite its regular appearance, it is extremely rare for an animal with localized osteoporosis due to immobilization to sustain a pathologic fracture.

A more insidious problem associated with immobilization of the limbs is atrophy of articular cartilage. Immobilization impairs the diffusion of nutrients into the articular cartilage from the synovium because of the absence of the intermittent loading of the joint.

Joint laxity and flaccidity of the flexor tendons are also seen following cast application, especially in foals. Shoes with heel extensions are required if the condition is severe.

Joint stiffness, a problem that haunts human orthopedic surgeons, does not seem a problem in horses unless the joint itself has been injured.[4] Intraarticular fractures with accompanying joint capsule tearing are prone to this.

Cast Removal

In adult horses, the cast can be left in place for three to four weeks unless complications develop. Casts on the limbs of foals should be changed at least every 14 days because of limb growth within the cast. Casts used to immobilize extensive soft tissue injuries may require changing every 10 to 14 days, depending on the amount of wound drainage and suppuration

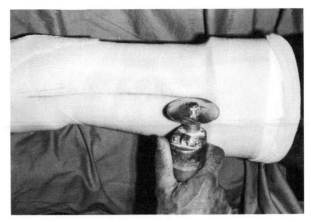

FIG. 5-7S. Cuts on the medial and lateral surfaces of the cast.

To remove a cast, an electric oscillating saw is the recommended instrument (Fig. 5-7C). Unfortunately, they are noisy and sedation is often necessary. These saws will cut skin if they are not used with care. Cuts are made on the medial and lateral surfaces of the cast, as well as under the hoof (Fig. 5-7S). Because of its strength, it is essential that complete full thickness cuts be made when removing a fiberglass cast. It is virtually impossible to remove a cast by cutting one side and merely scoring the other side in the hope it will fracture down the scored side.

It is usual to cut the last cast off with the horse standing so that anesthesia can be avoided. If anesthesia is necessary, the resultant two halves of the cast can be reapplied to the limb to protect the injury while the horse is recovering from anesthesia and then removed with the horse standing.

Following removal of the cast a "rebound" edema of the limb is common. Therefore, one should always anticipate pressure bandaging the limb for several weeks after cast application.

References

1. Bramlage, L.R.: Current concepts of emergency first aid treatment and transportation of equine fracture patients. Comp. Contin. Educ. 5:564, 1983.
2. Dingwall, J.S., Horney, F.D., McDonell, W., et. al.: A comparison of breaking strengths of various casting materials. Can. Vet. J. 14:62, 1973.
3. Edwards, G.B., and Clayton-Jones, D.G.: Use of Hexcelite for the immobilization of the limbs of large animals. Vet. Rec. 102:397, 1978.
4. Fessler, J.F., and Turner, A.S.: Methods of external coaptation. In Symposium on Equine Orthopedics, Philadelphia. Vet. Clin. North Am. (Large Anim. Pract.), 5:311, 1983.
5. Horney, F.D., and Dingwall, J.: The clinical use of light cast. Can. Vet. J. 16:201, 1975.

Cancellous Bone Graft Harvesting From the Tuber Coxae

Autogenous cancellous bone grafting is an important adjunctive procedure in the treatment of certain orthopedic problems in the horse. Cancellous bone grafting is used in the horse (1) as an aid in the ossification of defects accompanying primary internal fixation of fractures, (2) in the treatment of delayed or nonunions, (3) in the treatment of osteomyelitis, (4) in the promotion of surgical arthrodesis, (5) in the healing of midbody and basal sesamoid fractures, and (6) to promote healing in the treatment of subchondral cystic lesions.

The fate of autogenous cancellous bone grafting following transplantation has been the subject of many studies. It is generally believed that few cells survive the transplantation procedure, although both donor and recipient cells should be considered as contributing to the new cell population. More importantly, the graft stimulates the formation of new bone by osteoinduction and also provides a scaffold for ingrowth of blood vessels and multipotential mesenchymal cells (osteoconduction).[4] It is well recognized that autogenous cancellous bone revascularizes more quickly than homogenous cancellous bone with an earlier and greater production of new bone. In addition, autogenous cancellous bone is immunologically more desirable.[1] It is to be noted that a cancellous graft should be placed, ideally, in a region of rich blood supply.

Harvesting of cancellous bone graft is generally performed while surgery is being done on another part of the body (e.g., internal fixation of a long-bone fracture or surgical exposure of a sesamoid fracture). To minimize operating time, the use of two surgical teams is appropriate. If surgery time is delayed, the graft will suffer unnecessary exposure, thereby decreasing survival of graft cells.[3] The exposure of the cancellous bone is timed so that graft material can be transferred immediately from the donor site to the surgical region.

Harvesting of cancellous bone from the tuber coxae is described. This is the preferred technique of both authors, since we have experienced complications using the alternate sites of a rib or proximal tibia. More recently a technique of graft harvesting from the sternum has been also used and may achieve routine use.

Anesthesia and Surgical Preparation

The surgical procedure is performed with the horse under general anesthesia and in lateral recumbency. Generally, the tuber coxae that will be up when the horse is under surgery for the primary problem will be selected. A large area over the tuber coxae should be clipped prior to induction of anesthesia. Immediately before or after induction, the immediate area of the tuber coxae is shaved and surgical preparation is then made. The plastic adhesive drape is used.

Additional Instrumentation

It is convenient to have two sets of instruments, one for the primary procedure and the other for the bone graft because the surgeons are usually working on opposite sides of the horse.

Surgical Technique

There are two different approaches to the tuber coxae. The technique depicted utilizes a skin incision that passes in a perpendicular fashion over the tuber coxae as illustrated in Figure 5-8A. The length of the incision will vary according to the amount of bone graft needed (from 10 to 25 cm). If a small amount of graft is to be required such as with sesamoid bone grafting, a small incision is sufficient. If a major amount of cancellous bone is to be removed, as with an involved fracture, the incision needs to be larger to allow greater exposure of the tuber coxae. An alternative approach is to make a curvilinear incision over the caudal aspect of the tuber coxae and reflect the skin craniad.[2] The subcutaneous tissue and fascia are incised in the same plane as the skin to expose the tuber coxae (Fig. 5-8B). An incision is then made in the periosteum that outlines the area of the cortical window that will be made to expose the cancellous bone beneath (Fig. 5-8B). This incision passes through the lateral cortex of the tuber coxae and will be 5×2.5-cm if a large amount of bone is to be removed. An osteotome is used to cut a window through the bone (Fig. 5-8C). If a small amount of bone is required, a quarter-inch drill hole through the cortex is often sufficient. Once the osteotome has incised through the cortex into the cancellous bone space, the segment of corticocancellous bone is removed and discarded. Cancellous bone within the tuber coxae is then removed with a curette as required (Fig. 5-8C). Following completion of graft harvesting, the area is flushed with saline solution to remove all debris. The cortical bone is not replaced and only the soft tissue is closed. The fascia and subcutaneous tissue are closed with interrupted sutures of 2/0 synthetic absorbable material. The skin is closed with a row of simple interrupted or vertical mattress sutures using nonabsorbable monofilament material supported by vertical mattress tension sutures (Fig. 5-8D). A stent bandage using a roll of gauze (Kling) is sewn over the surgical site.

It is to be noted that in young animals, a thick layer of cartilage will be found over the end of the tuber coxae. The bone is soft enough that a curette can usually be used to create the window.

Postoperative Management

Phenylbutazone is administered postoperatively, since the pain from the graft site can be quite severe. The use of antibiotics is not necessary for the graft harvesting itself, but they may be used depending on the other primary surgical procedure being performed. If the graft is removed before the recipient site has been prepared, it should be placed on a sponge moistened with blood. The stent bandage is removed in a week, the tension sutures in 10 days, and the skin sutures closing the incision are removed in 14 days.

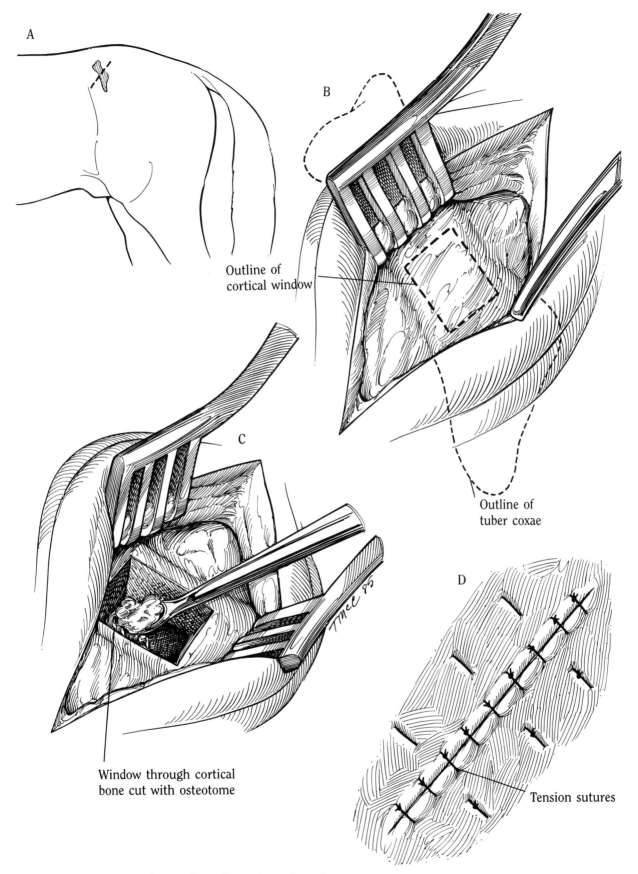

A

B

Outline of
cortical window

Outline of
tuber coxae

C

Window through cortical
bone cut with osteotome

D

Tension sutures

Fig. 5-8. Harvesting of cancellous bone from the tuber coxae.

Comments

Alternative approaches including the use of curvilinear incisions away from the prominence of the tuber coxae and a window in the gluteal cortex of the ileum have been described. However, the technique described here is simpler, and the authors have not experienced complications with it. It is important that the only cortex removed is from the end of the ilium, as damage to cortex on the sides could promote postoperative fracture.

References

1. Burchardt, H., and Enneking, W.F.: Transplantation of bone. Surg. Clin. North Am. 58:403, 1978.
2. Slocum, B., and Chalman, J.A.: Cancellous bone graft from the wing of the equine ilium: The surgical approach. Arch. Am. Coll. Vet. Surg. 4:39, 1975.
3. Stashak, T.S., and Adams, O.R.: Collection of bone grafts from the tuber coxae of the horse. J. Am. Vet. Med. Assoc. 167:397, 1975.
4. Turner, A.S.: Large animal orthopedics. In Practice of Large Animal Surgery. (P.B. Jennings, ed.) Philadelphia, W.B. Saunders, 1984.

Cancellous Bone Grafting of a Midbody or Basal Proximal Sesamoid Fracture

Fractures of the proximal sesamoid bones occur in fast-gaited horses such as Thoroughbreds, Standardbreds, and racing Quarterhorses.[1,3–6] The injury also is seen in western performance horses, such as barrel racing and cutting horses, and occasionally in hunters, jumpers, and eventing horses. Fractures of one or both of the sesamoid bones can involve any level of the bone. Fractures of the apex of the bone are operated on by removal of the fragment through an arthrotomy of the palmar or plantar recess (volar pouch) of the fetlock joint and have been discussed extensively elsewhere.[3,5,6]

A fracture of one proximal sesamoid bone in its midportion has been a dilemma for the equine surgeon with regard to surgical management. Treated conservatively, these fractures heal poorly because of poor blood supply and because the fragments are under continual tension of the suspensory apparatus. The resulting fibrous union lacks the strength to withstand strenuous exercise.[1] Resection of the proximal fragment necessitates transection of half of the suspensory ligament. It has been presumed that, following, such an operation, a fibrous tissue bridge would occur between the distal portion of the bone and the severed branch of the suspensory ligament. The end result would be of doubtful value to a fast-gaited horse. For this reason, alternative methods of management have been devised for the fracture of one sesamoid bone in its midportion. At the present time, there is no method that can be recommended because there has not been a sufficiently large series of cases that have been treated in different ways to compare the results, but the method we prefer is to insert an autologous bone graft between the fragments, using a modification of the method first described by Medina and coworkers.[4] Earlier attempts to reestablish the continuity of the suspensory apparatus included the use of bone screws inserted into the bone from its base.[2] This is technically difficult and results have been disappointing.

The bone grafting technique described is relatively quick and simple and can be done without the large array of ASIF equipment necessary for screw fixation. The technique involves insertion of the graft through the tendon sheath and the intersesamoidean ligament. Alternatively, the graft can be inserted through the lateral aspect of the bone without entering the tendon sheath, using a more abaxial approach, or through a routine arthrotomy of the plantar or palmar recess of the fetlock joint.[1]

Anesthesia and Surgical Preparation

The surgical procedure is performed with the horse under general anesthesia in lateral recumbency with the affected sesamoid bone uppermost. Prior to anesthetic induction, the limb is clipped from the coronet proximad to the proximal end of the cannon bone, around the limb's entire circumference. Following induction of the anesthetic, the area of the surgical incision is shaved. An Esmarch's bandage is applied to the limb, and a pneumatic tourniquet is applied just distal to the carpal joint. The surgical site is prepared for aseptic surgery in a routine manner.

Simultaneously the uppermost tuber coxae is clipped and prepared for harvesting an autogenous cancellous bone graft. The technique is described elsewhere in this book (pages 111–114).

Ideally, two surgical teams are needed for this procedure, one exposing the fracture site while the other harvests the bone graft. If this is not possible, then the surgeon must have a "scrubbed-in" assistant who can close the graft site as the surgeon does the operation on the limb; otherwise anesthetic time will be excessively prolonged.

Additional Instrumentation

Cancellous bone grafting requires bone curettes, a Weitlaner retractor, and casting material.

Surgical Technique

The approach to the fracture site is identical to that for severing the palmar (plantar) annular ligament.[6] A skin incision is made over the lateral edge of the superficial digital flexor tendon behind the palmar or plantar blood vessels and nerves. The incision is about 8 cm long and extends from above to below the proximal and distal limits of the annular ligament (Fig. 5-9A). Once the skin incision has been made, the lateral palmar or plantar nerve needs to be identified and the sparse subcutaneous tissue behind this structure separated. The incision is continued carefully through the annular ligament and digital tendon sheath to avoid incising the flexor tendons. The incision needs to pass immediately behind the palmar or plantar border of the sesamoid bone. The incision in the annular ligament is extended to complete sectioning of the entire ligament, and the flexor tendons are then retracted to reveal the intersesamoidean ligament and the fracture site. At this point in the operation the surgeon should go to the bone graft site and commence harvesting the cancellous bone from the tuber coxae. If two surgical teams are available, the approach to the tuber coxae is made simultaneously with the approach to the fracture site.

The fracture gap between the two portions of the sesamoid bone is usually evident visually and can be confirmed by probing with a sterile disposable needle. In the meantime the assistant has obtained a small amount of autologous cancellous bone from the wing of the ilium (about a teaspoonful is all that is needed). The intersesamoidean ligament is incised over the fracture, and the bone is carefully packed into the fracture gap so as *not to overfill the gap* and allow bone to fall into the palmar (plantar) region of the fetlock joint (Fig. 5-9B). The cut edges of the intersesamoidean ligaments are reapposed with simple interrupted sutures of a 2/0 synthetic absorbable suture material of the surgeon's choice (Fig. 5-9C).

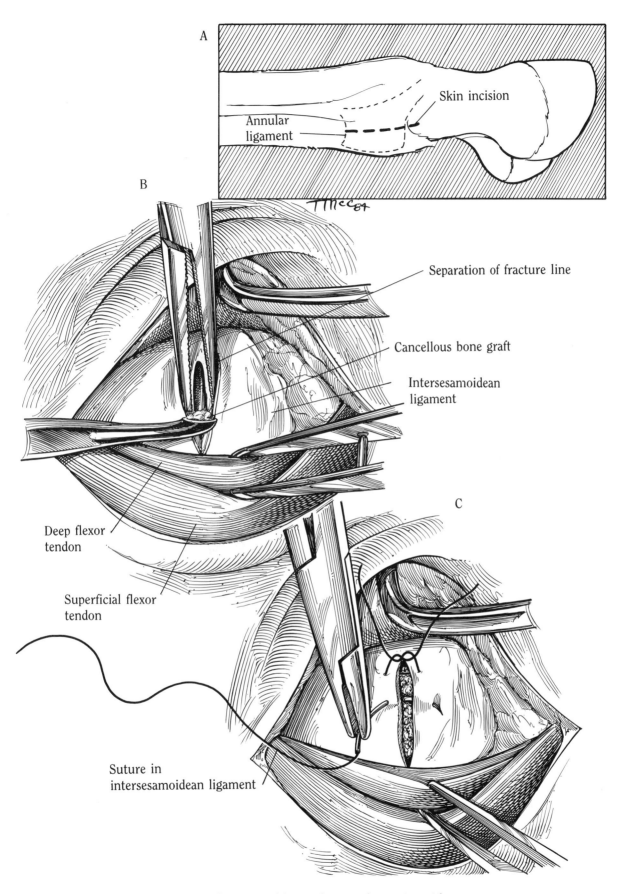

A

Skin incision

Annular ligament

B

Separation of fracture line

Cancellous bone graft

Intersesamoidean ligament

Deep flexor tendon

Superficial flexor tendon

C

Suture in intersesamoidean ligament

FIG. 5-9. Bone grafting of a proximal sesamoid bone, fractured near its midportion.

117

Neither the tendon sheath nor the annular ligament is sutured. The subcutaneous tissues are sutured closed with simple interrupted sutures of synthetic, absorbable material. It is important that this closure be tight to prevent leakage of synovial fluid from the tendon sheath and the subsequent development of synovial fistulae. The skin is closed with nonabsorbable sutures. A sterile dressing is placed over the incision, and a fiberglass cast that extends to the proximal extremity of the metacarpus (metatarsus).

Postoperative Management

Perioperative antibiotics are optional, and tetanus prophylaxis should be provided. The cast should be removed at 10 to 14 days, with the horse standing, and a pressure bandage applied. The limb should remain bandaged for two to three additional weeks during which time the bandage should be changed as required.

The healing of the fracture should be monitored periodically with radiographs of the affected bone. Care must be taken to use the same radiographic technique each time.

Although no definitive studies have shown just how long (if ever) the fractured bone takes to regain its original strength, we advise that racing not be resumed for at least 10 or 12 months. Naturally this decision will depend on what is revealed on the postoperative radiographs.

Comments

Patients with injuries to the sesamoid bones always should be carefully evaluated for concurrent injuries, such as suspensory desmitis, intraarticular chip fractures, and degenerative joint disease of the fetlock joint. Poor candidates for surgery of any description should be scheduled for breeding purposes if practical. Occasionally the distal fragment of a basal sesamoid fracture will have a sagittal fracture within it. Clearly this fracture is not a candidate for screw fixation, but it is a potential candidate for the bone grafting technique. In our opinion the injury does have a poor prognosis regardless of how this injury is managed, but we feel that bone grafting offers somewhat of an alternative procedure for what is otherwise a hopeless case with regard to future athletic performance.

We have not used a combination of lag screw fixation and bone grafting. This method should be given consideration, especially if the surgeon has experience at lag screw fixation of these fractures. If both techniques are used, then the lag screw must be placed first but not tightened, the bone graft then inserted, and then the lag screw tightened when the graft is in place.[1] It is hoped that in the future a more consistently predictable method for repairing midbody or basal sesamoid fractures will become evident.

References

1. Bukowiecki, C.F., Bramlage, L.R., and Gabel, A.A.: Proximal sesamoid bone fractures in the horse. A review, current treatments and prognosis. Compend. Contin. Educ. 7:S684, 1985.

2. Fackelman, G.E., and Nunamaker, D.M.: Manual of Internal Fixation in the Horse. New York, Springer-Verlag, 1982.
3. Fretz, P.B., and Barber, S.M., Bailey, J.V., et al.: Management of proximal sesamoid bone fractures in the horse. J. Am. Vet. Med. Assoc. 185:282, 1984.
4. Medina, L.E., Wheat, J.D., Morgan, J.P., et. al.: Treatment of basal fractures of the proximal sesamoid bones in the horse using an autogenous bone graft. *In* Proceedings of 26th Annual Conv. Am. Assoc. Equine Practitioners, 1980:1981, p. 345.
5. Spurlock, G.H., and Gabel, A.A.: Apical fractures of the proximal sesamoid bones in 109 Standardbred horses. J. Am. Vet. Med. Assoc. 183:76, 1983.
6. Turner, A.S., and McIlwraith, C.W.: Techniques in Large Animal Surgery. Philadelphia, Lea & Febiger, 1982.

Transphyseal Bridging With Screws and Wire

Angular limb deformities in foals are frequently caused by an imbalance of physeal growth. For various reasons, endochondral ossification is proceeding faster on one side of the growth plate than the other. The clinical appearance is a valgus or varus deformity. A *valgus* deformity is defined as a deviation of the line away from the midline distal to the joint in which the deviation originates.[5] A *varus* deformity is a deviation of the limb toward the midline distal to the joint in which the deviation originates. The most common location of angular limb deformities is the carpal joint where valgus deformities predominate.[4,8,9] In our experience the next most common location is the fetlock varus deformity with carpus varus and tarsus valgus being less common. Other deformities (e.g., tarsus varus) are extremely rare.

Conservative therapy is adequate for the management of most angular limb deformities seen in equine clinical practice. This would include trimming of the hooves to remove the fulcrum effect caused by a long toe, and confinement to reduce concussive forces that would occur if unrestricted exercise was permitted.

As part of the clinical examination of a foal with an angular limb deformity, a radiograph of the affected joint is indicated. This is particularly important in the carpal joint where the radiograph may reveal abnormalities within the bones of the carpus or at the level of the proximal ends of the metacarpal bones. If these abnormalities are severe, then surgery is not indicated as it will not be directed at the primary abnormality. Such foals may be candidates for other methods of therapy such as "tube" casting.[9]

Before attempting surgery that relies on active growth of a physis, it is vital that the surgeon appreciate how much *growth potential* remains in that physis. Although it is useful to know from radiographs when a growth plate has closed, it is of greater importance to the surgeon to know when the physis has completed most of its growth. For example, although radiographic evidence of closure of the distal metacarpal and metatarsal physes is seen at approximately 9 months, it is well known by surgeons who have attempted to correct angular deformities of the fetlock joint that most of the growth in this region is complete by 3 months of age. Therefore, it is our belief that deformities of the fetlock joint should be operated upon as soon as they are noticed, rather than adopting a wait-and-see policy that may work in certain deformities of the carpus and tarsus. Certain angular deformities of the distal metacarpus and metatarsus, as well as diaphyseal angular deformities can be corrected only by a wedge osteotomy and internal fixation using compression plating techniques.[6,10] These techniques are beyond the scope of this book, and the reader is encouraged to consult the bibliography.

Although the radiographic closure of the distal radial physis occurs between 24 and 30 months, most of the longitudinal growth has occurred by 9 to 10 months. Surgery is not advocated at this late stage either, as continual asymmetrical loading of the carpal or tarsal joints for this condition can lead to osteoarthritic changes. For this reason, surgery on the carpal and tarsal joints should be done when the foal is between 6 weeks of age and 4 months of age. One other factor that is operational in making such a decision is the severity of the deviation. If a relatively mild deformity has been steadily correcting itself following hoof trimming and confinement, then the surgeon may elect to delay surgery for a few weeks. This approach is not applicable to the fetlock joint.

Metallic implants to cause temporary physeal arrest have been used to correct certain angular limb deformities in man and animals. The aim of such surgical procedures is to temporarily bridge the metaphysis to the epiphysis, causing retardation of maturation and calcification of endochondral ossification on the metaphyseal side of the growth plate that will decrease longitudinal bone growth on that side. Metal staples have been used to bridge physes in both foals and children. The technique was modified in 1972 and now utilizes an ASIF bone screw placed on each side of the physis, with two figure-8 wires connecting the heads.[2] This is, in our opinion, the preferred method because the implants are easier to remove and the screws can be inserted independently at convenient sites on either side of the physis. In addition, it is felt that immediate compression is applied across the growth plate, thereby hastening correction, and the implants are stronger than staples.[4,8] Even though they are placed extraperiosteally, less soft tissue blemish is associated with the use of screws and wire than with staples.[4]

The procedure can be used alone or in combination with the technique of hemicircumferential transection of the periosteum and periosteal stripping for certain deformities, particularly in the fetlock joint, and is described in the next section of this book. The procedure of transphyseal bridging using screws and wire also has been performed in calves and llamas.[1,7]

Anesthesia and Surgical Preparation

The surgery is performed under general anesthesia. Inhalation anesthesia such as Halothane is preferable. In most foals that are candidates for this surgery, anesthesia can be induced by administration of the gas by mask. Anesthesia in older foals can be induced by intravenous techniques and maintained by an inhalation anesthetic. The foal is then placed in lateral recumbency with the side of the metaphysis/epiphysis that is to be bridged uppermost.

If the screws and wire are to be combined with the periosteal stripping procedure then the screws and wire should be inserted first because the risk of wound infection is higher and demand for asepsis greater when implants such as these are used. If both procedures are being performed on the same growth plate, then both surgical sites must be clipped, shaved, and prepared for surgery in a routine manner. A sterile plastic adhesive drape is applied to the limb so that it is tightly adherent to both surgical sites and stuck to itself in a seam at the cranial or caudal surface of the limb.

Additional Instrumentation

Transphyseal bridging requires a 3.2-mm drill bit (if ASIF cortical bone screws are to be used) or a 3.6-mm drill bit (if ASIF cancellous bone screws are to be used). An assortment of cortical or fully threaded cancellous bone screws, ranging from 32 to 40 mm in length is required. Also needed are the corresponding 4.5-mm or 6.5-mm cancellous bone tap, 4.5- or 6.5-mm ASIF tap sleeves, a power or hand-held drill, 18 gauge (1 to 2 mm) stainless steel wire, a wire twister of the surgeon's preference, and wire cutters. Equipment for taking intraoperative radiographs (without compromising sterile technique) is necessary. This includes a portable x-ray machine, sterile cassette covers, and cassettes.

Surgical Techniques

DISTAL END OF THE RADIUS (CARPUS VALGUS DEFORMITY). An 8 to 9-cm semielliptical incision is made with the apex facing caudally, centered over the medial radial epicondyle. The incision should end distally, at the level of the antebrachiocarpal joint (Fig. 5-10A). The skin and subcutaneous flap that has been created is reflected craniad, and its apex is grasped carefully with a Backhaus towel clamp. The distal radial physis is then located by probing the most prominent area in the surgical field with an 18- or 20-gauge sterile disposable hypodermic needle. Probing is best done by "walking" the needle along the metaphysis distad toward the epiphysis, exerting firm pressure by the index finger placed over the hub of the needle (Fig. 5-10B). Small hematomas may result from this procedure, but they are of no consequence. If the surgeon is unsure of where the needle is located, then an intraoperative radiograph is indicated at this point. As an additional aid, another needle can be placed in the antebrachiocarpal joint and then a radiograph taken.

To facilitate placement of the screw in the distal radial epiphysis, a small stab incision is made in the collateral ligament that invests the epiphysis of the distal extremity of the radius. A 3.6-mm or 3.2-mm hole is drilled to a depth of about 40 mm in the distal radial epiphysis, attempting to go parallel to the plane of the growth plate and antebrachiocarpal (radiocarpal) joint space. If a cortical bone screw is to be used, then a 3.2-mm drill bit will be used; if a cancellous bone screw is being used, then either a 3.6-mm or a 3.2-mm drill can be used. It is once again stressed that if the operation is being performed by the surgeon for the first time, we recommend that the surgeon take an intraoperative radiograph at this point to check to see if the drill, and subsequently the screw, is likely to endanger the physis or, more importantly, to invade the antebrachiocarpal joint. The soft tissues should be protected during drilling (and tapping) of these holes by using the appropriate tap sleeve. Once the surgeon feels confident with this operation, then insertion of the first screw hole can be done "freehand" without intraoperative radiographs. The hole is then tapped, using the 4.5-mm tap (cortical screws) or 6.5-mm tap (cancel-

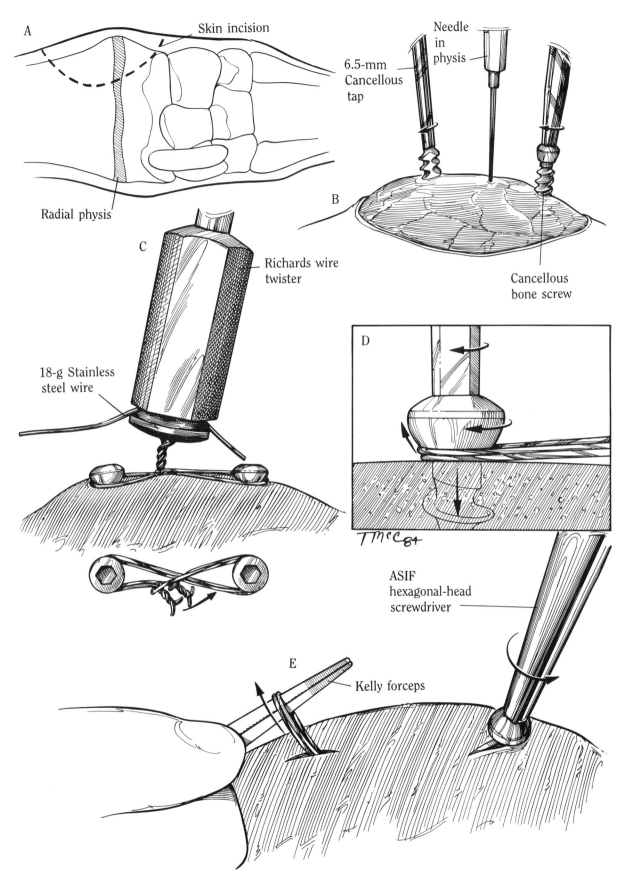

A
Skin incision
Radial physis

B
6.5-mm Cancellous tap
Needle in physis
Cancellous bone screw

C
Richards wire twister
18-g Stainless steel wire

D

ASIF hexagonal-head screwdriver

E
Kelly forceps

FIG. 5-10. Transphyseal bridging using screws and wire.

lous screws) and protecting the soft tissue with the appropriate tap sleeve (Fig. 5-10B). Tapping is an optional step, and it has been recommended that the screw in the epiphysis be placed in a self-tapping manner because the bone is relatively soft.[3]

A 4.5-mm cortical or 6.5-mm fully threaded cancellous bone screw of 32 to 38 mm in length is inserted. The screw should not be tightened to a point that the head disappears below the level of the collateral ligament. After this step we advise obtaining an intraoperative radiograph regardless of how experienced the surgeon is, as placement of this screw is one of the most critical steps of the whole operation. While the radiograph is being developed, the second remaining screw can be inserted in the metaphyseal region in a similar manner to the first. The hole should be placed in one cortex only. Because the bone is denser in this region, threads should be cut in the hole using the appropriate tap. The location of this screw is much less critical than the one located in the distal radial epiphysis; however, it must be located so that neither it nor the wire lies directly under the skin incision. If this occurs, infection may enter through the skin incision and establish itself around the implants during the convalescence. A chronically draining wound or even localized osteomyelitis and screw loosening may occur. The screw should not be seated so deeply that the head is buried in the bone.

Two independently placed figure-8 wires should be placed around the heads of the screws. The wire should be twisted to produce a symmetrical even twist in the wire (Fig. 5-10C). The wire is then cut, and the protruding twisted piece of wire bent down so as to lie alongside the figure-8 wire. A second similarly placed piece of wire is applied directly over the first, and the twisted ends are folded down beside the wire loops pointing distally so no sharp pieces of wire protrude from the surgical site (Fig. 5-10C). This is also important to facilitate removal. Any sharp protruding pieces of wire may cause pressure necrosis of the skin during the convalescence.

There are numerous ways to joint or twist wire to prevent it from loosening. Some texts advocate the ASIF cerclage wire tightener that uses a hook-in-eye configuration to hold the wire.[3] Specially prepared ASIF 1.2-mm cerclage wire with a loop twisted on the end by the manufacturer is required. We prefer the wire twister manufactured by Richards* but feel that surgeons should use whatever they feel comfortable with. When the surgeon is satisfied with the security of both wires, additional tension is then brought about in the wires by alternately tightening the screws. The wire will slide along the inclined plane of the spherical screw heads (Fig. 5-10D). The screws should not be tightened so much as to make them disappear from sight, or the wire may slip off the heads.[3] The surgeon should palpate the implants with the index finger to check that these implants are not protruding excessively.

---

* Richards Manufacturing Company.

The subcutaneous tissues are very thin in this area, but we strongly recommend that they be apposed over the implants during closure. A simple continuous suture of synthetic absorbable suture material should be used. Catgut is not recommended in this region because of its inflammatory properties. The skin edges are apposed using a simple interrupted pattern with the appropriate synthetic monofilament suture material. At this point an intraoperative radiograph is taken to check for correct placement of implants and for documentation in case postoperative problems arise.

DISTAL ENDS OF THE THIRD METACARPAL AND METATARSAL BONES. Angular limb deformities due to an imbalance of growth of the distal metacarpal or metatarsal physis are not as common as those occurring in the carpus. Because the distal metacarpal and metatarsal growth plates close much sooner, surgery for angular limb deformities of this region should be attempted as soon as the deformity is noticed, provided the foal is under 2½ months old. We also recommend that these deformities be treated by hemicircumferential transection of the periosteum and periosteal stripping on the opposite metaphysis of that bone *as well* as the transphyseal bridging described here.

Varus deformities in this region are the usual situation. In this case, transphyseal bridging is done on the lateral aspect of the physeal region, and the periosteal stripping is performed on the medial side. The surgical procedure is essentially the same as described for bridging of the distal radial physis. A semielliptical skin incision is made, making sure to stay dorsal to the palmar (plantar) vein artery and nerve in the region of the fetlock joint and at the same time ensuring there is no potential for implants to be situated directly under the skin incision. Because the epiphysis of these bones is relatively larger compared with the distal radial or tibial epiphyses, there is a little more room for error during the placement of the distal bone screw. Nevertheless, an intraoperative radiograph is indicated to be absolutely sure the metacarpophalangeal joint space or the physis has not been invaded and relocation of the screw is not indicated. Closure of the skin and subcutaneous layers should be performed meticulously in this area.

DISTAL END OF THE TIBIA. Deformities due to an imbalance of growth of the distal tibial physis are less common. Screw and wire insertion can be performed, but it requires meticulous placement of the distal bone screw because of the irregular shape of the distal tibial epiphysis. Intraoperative radiographs are mandatory for this surgery because it is relatively easy to inadvertently place the screw into the tarsocrural joint space. The screw in the epiphysis must therefore be angled upward to prevent this. We recommend taking an intraoperative radiograph following the placement of a sterile disposable hypodermic needle in both the physes and the tarsocrural joint. Another intraoperative radiograph is recommended to check the direction of the drill bit. Placement of the screw in the metaphysis is relatively straightforward. The end result will be two screws placed in different directions, something that cannot be achieved readily with staples.

Postoperative Management

A sterile nonadhesive dressing is placed over the incision, and then the affected joint is bandaged with materials of the surgeon's choice. A full-limb bandage using cotton may be indicated, but we feel that a light gauze and elastic adhesive bandage covering only the affected joint may be all that is required if it is carefully applied.

We feel perioperative antibiotics are indicated because implants such as screws have been shown to increase the likelihood of infection.[10] Nonsteroidal antiinflammatory drugs are not generally indicated. If the foal becomes lame during the convalescence, the causes of the lameness should be identified quickly and treated aggressively.

The foal should be confined during the convalescence to reduce concussion on the growth plates. The hooves should receive the appropriate trimming. Frequently foals are fed mineral supplements or given injections of various vitamins. We feel these are unnecessary in most situations unless a true deficiency can be identified. Certainly older animals undergoing this surgery (e.g., weanlings) should be fed a ration that has the appropriate calcium/phosphorus ratio. Analysis of the diet of older foals frequently reveals a mineral imbalance. The status of other trace minerals as an adjunct to the treatment of angular limb deformities in foals should also be determined; for example, a zinc excess or copper deficiency may exist in individual instances.

Removal of Implants

When the axis of the limb is straight, the implants must be removed to prevent *overcorrection* of the deformity. Owners must be alerted to this and good client education and communication are essential in this regard.

Removal of the screws and wire with the foal standing and under local anesthesia (around the screw heads) should not be considered because an uncooperative foal can easily cause a break in aseptic technique, especially if difficulty arises in locating the distal screw.

To remove the screws, a stab incision is made over the more readily palpable proximal (metaphyseal) screw head. Subcutaneous tissues are parted, using a mosquito hemostat, and then the hexagonally shaped "well" in the head of the screw is located. The hexagonal-tipped screw driver is carefully manipulated into the head of the screw to remove the screw (Fig. 5-10E). A second stab incision is then made in the vicinity of the head of the distal screw, and the hexagonal well in the screw head is located. Typically, more fibrous tissue will be covering the screw head of the distal screw. This screw is now removed (Fig. 5-10E). A pair of curved Kelly forceps is used to retrieve the two pieces of wire that formed a loop around the proximal screw head by hooking the tip of the forceps through this loop and bending the two bits of wire out the proximal stab incision. When the forceps are securely anchored through both pieces of wire, the wire is pulled out the *proximal* incision with a sharp tug. An assistant will be required to hold the limb during this maneuver (Fig. 5-10E).

One or two simple interrupted skin sutures are placed in each stab incision, and a light pressure bandage is applied to the affected joint for 7 to 10 days. Skin sutures are removed in 10 days.

References

1. Adams, S.B., and Amstutz, H.E.: Surgical correction of angular limb deformity of the forelimbs of a 7-month-old calf. Vet. Surg. 12:58, 1983.
2. Fackelman, G.E., and Frolich D.: The Current Status of ASIF Technique in Large Animals. In Proceedings of the 18th Annual Meeting of the American Association of Equine Practitioners, 1973, p. 325.
3. Fackelman, G.E., and Nunamaker, D.M.: Manual of Internal Fixation in the Horse. Berlin, Springer-Verlag, 1982, p. 91.
4. Fretz, P.B., Turner, A.S., and Pharr, J.: Retrospective comparison of two surgical techniques for correction of angular limb deformities in foals. J. Am. Vet. Med. Assoc. 172:281, 1975.
5. Fretz, P.B., Pharr, J.W., McIlwraith, C.W., et. al.: Varus vs. valgus. In Letters. J. Am. Vet. Med. Assoc. 181:636, 1982.
6. Fretz, P.B., and McIlwraith, C.W.: Wedge osteotomy for angular limb deformities in foals. J. Am. Vet. Med. Assoc. 182:245, 1983.
7. Fowler, M.E.: Angular limb deformities in young llamas. J. Am. Vet. Med. Assoc. 181:1338, 1982.
8. Leitch, M.: Angular limb deformities arising in the carpal region in foals. Compend. Contin. Educ. Pract. Vet. 1:539, 1979.
9. Leitch, M.: Musculoskeletal disorders in neonatal foals. In Symposium on Neonatal Equine Disease. Vet. Clin. North Am. (Equine Practice) 1:189, 1985.
10. Petty, W., Spanier, S., Shuster, J.J., et. al.: The influence of skeletal implants on incidence of infection. J. Bone Joint Surg. 67-A:1236, 1985.

Hemicircumferential Transection and Periosteal Stripping

The technique of horizontal transection of the periosteum and periosteal stripping has been used to achieve physiologic leg lengthening in man.[3,7] Two mechanisms explain this phenomenon. Earlier theories hypothesized that the periosteal stripping induced local vascular changes that subsequently affected bone growth. More recently, experiments have shown that periosteal transection allows a *mechanical release* of fibroelastic periosteal tension.[6] The technique of hemicircumferential transection of the periosteum and periosteal stripping (hereafter called simply periosteal stripping) was first successfully applied to correct angular limb deformities in foals by Auer et al. in 1982.[1]

We currently use periosteal stripping as the primary surgical technique for angular limb deformities caused by imbalance of physeal growth of the distal radius and tibia. For angular limb deformities of the fetlock joint (usually a varus deformity) we use periosteal stripping in combination with transphyseal bridging with screws and wire (discussed in the preceding section).

Because periosteal stripping is a "stimulation" procedure, i.e., it increases bone growth, it should be obvious to the reader that the procedure is performed on the opposite site of the metaphysis from that for the retardation procedure of transphyseal bridging. For a valgus deformity of the carpus, therefore, the periosteum is transected on the lateral aspect of the distal radial metaphysis.[1,2,8]

Anesthesia and Surgical Preparation

The surgical procedures must be done under general anesthesia with the side of the bone to be operated on uppermost. Alternatively, if both sides are to be operated on, the foal can be placed in lateral recumbency to avoid having to change position. If both periosteal stripping and transphyseal bridging are to be performed (e.g., on the distal metacarpal or metatarsal physis), then the procedure involving the implants (screws and wire) would logically be performed first. When implants are being used, the risk of wound infection is greater because of the "foreign body effect" of the implants; therefore, the demand for asepsis during surgery is more critical. Once the screws and wire have been inserted and the wound closed (see "Surgical Technique"), the animal can be rolled over, and the periosteal stripping performed on the opposite metaphysis. Care must be taken not to break aseptic technique as the foal is rolled over. Consequently, if both procedures are contemplated, then both surgical sites must be clipped, shaved, and prepared for surgery in a routine manner. A sterile plastic adhesive drape is applied to the limb so that it adheres tightly over both surgical sites and is stuck to itself in a seam at the cranial or caudal surface of the limb.

Additional Instrumentation

Periosteal stripping requires a periosteal elevator and a no. 12 Bard-Parker scalpel blade and a periosteal elevator.

Surgical Technique

The technique described herein is slightly modified from the one first described by Auer et al.[1] A 6-cm vertical straight skin incision is made on the most lateral (or medial) aspect of the metaphysis of the affected bone. The skin incision should extend distad to about the middle of the adjacent epiphysis (Fig. 5-11A). The subcutaneous tissue and areolar tissue also are incised carefully. Care must be taken to avoid nearby tendons and their tendon sheaths. In the carpus valgus deformity there is a natural depression between the common and lateral digital extensor tendons. The incision is located in this depression. In a varus deformity of the carpus the medial aspect of the distal end of the radius is relatively free of such structures. The approach for the lateral aspect of the distal tibial metaphysis is slightly different because of the lateral location of the lateral digital extensor tendon. Two vertical incisions through the skin and subcutaneous tissues (cranial and caudal to the lateral digital extensor tendon) are made to enable sufficient exposure of the metaphysis.

With the skin edges carefully held apart with two Backhaus towel clamps placed on the skin edges, an 18-gauge or 20-gauge sterile disposable needle is used to locate the physis. The distal radial physis is located close to the most prominent part of the bone in the surgical field. It can be found by "walking" the needle along the metaphysis distad toward the epiphysis, exerting firm pressure by the index finger placed over the hub of the needle (Fig. 5-11B). Small hematomas may result from this procedure, but they are of no consequence. An inverted T-shaped incision is made in the periosteum, using a bold stroke of a no. 20 scalpel blade (Fig. 5-11C). The horizontal component of the T should be about 1 cm proximal to the growth plate; however, the exact distance is apparently not critical (Fig. 5-11C). To ensure that the maximum amount of hemicircumference is transected, the surgeon can use the "hooked" blade of a no. 12 scalpel blade. The inverted T incision through the periosteum creates two triangular flaps that will be stripped from the underlying metaphysis (Fig. 5-11D). We have found that elevation of the periosteum by a periosteal elevator before using the no. 12 scalpel blade will facilitate further transection of the periosteum. The tendon sheaths of the extensor tendons are occasionally entered during this maneuver, but we have seen no untoward effects if this happens, and suturing should not be attempted. The periosteum is allowed to lie in its slightly retracted position and is not sutured.

In foals with valgus deformities of the carpus, as discussed, periosteal transection will be made laterally. An adjunctive surgical procedure that we now recommend is to palpate and transect the remnant of the distal extremity of the ulna with a no. 11 scalpel blade or a

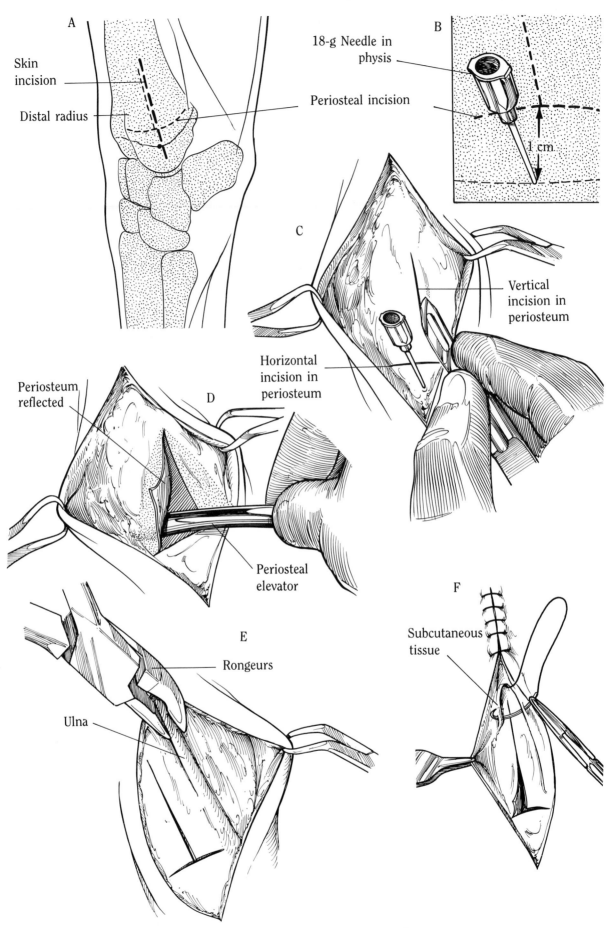

FIG. 5-11. Steps in correction of carpal valgus deformity by hemicircumferential transection of the periosteum and periosteal stripping.

rongeur forceps. This will eliminate any restraining (tethering) effect this bone may have on the lateral side of the bone[2] (Fig. 5-11E).

The subcutaneous tissues are apposed with a simple continuous pattern using a coated synthetic absorbable suture (e.g., 2/0 polyglactin 910 or polyglycolic acid) (Fig. 5-11F). Prior to finishing this layer of closure, we have found it useful to squeeze out any remaining hematoma, using several cotton gauzes rolled into a cylindrical shape. Skin edges are apposed using a nonabsorbable monofilament suture such as nylon or polypropylene (Fig. 5-11F). The hematoma can again be removed by squeezing it out one end of the incision with gauzes, just prior to placing the last two or three remaining skin sutures.

Postoperative Management

The skin incision is covered with a nonadhesive dressing and held in place with a gauze bandage. A light elastic bandage is then applied over the entire joint so that it adheres to the bare skin, thereby minimizing the chance of its slipping.

Preoperative antibiotics are administered only if the periosteal stripping procedure is combined with insertion of implants on the other side of the bone or in another location in the horse. They are not used for a routine uncomplicated case where periosteal stripping is the sole procedure.

The wound is kept under a sterile wrap for at least 10 days to minimize swelling at the surgical site. We change a bandage at day 3 to 5, with the second bandage being identical to the first. Skin sutures are removed at 10 to 14 days. Nonsteroidal antiinflammatory drugs are not necessary.

During the convalescence while the limb straightens, the foal must remain relatively confined to minimize concussion of the growth plate that would be caused by excessive activity. Although complete confinement of the mare and her foal to a box stall is desirable and recommended, this often meets with resistance from the owners. They frequently prefer the mare to be out in sunlight to help induce regular ovulation. As a compromise we recommend that they both be placed in a stall that has a small run attached to it. Under no circumstances, however, should the foal be running free with the mare in a large pasture.

Comments

The advantages of periosteal stripping are that it is a relatively straightforward procedure. It does not require implants nor does it require the mandatory second operation in transphyseal bridging for removal of screws and wire. Hospitalization is considerably shorter and the overall operation is therefore cheaper for the client. It is also cosmetically appealing, and the procedure can be repeated if further correction is needed.[1] Interestingly, the technique, if used as a sole procedure, has not in our experience resulted in overcorrection of an angular limb deformity.[2]

Failure to correct the angular limb deformity seems to be the only complication and occurs in only a small percentage of cases.[1,2] If this happens the surgeon is faced with a decision to either repeat the periosteal stripping or perform the more complicated and expensive transphyseal bridging on the opposite side of the metaphysis.

References

1. Auer, J.A., Martens, R.J., and Williams, E.H.: Periosteal transection for correction of angular limb deformities in foals. J. Am. Vet. Med. Assoc. 181:459, 1982.
2. Bertone, A.L., Turner, A.S., and Park, R.D.: Further observations of the use of periosteal transection and stripping for the treatment of angular limb deformities in foals. J. Am. Vet. Med. Assoc. 187:145, 1985.
3. Chan, K.P., and Hodgson, A.R.: Physiologic leg lengthening. Clin. Orthop. 68:55, 1970.
4. Crilly, G.R.: Longitudinal overgrowth of chicken radius. J. Anat. 112:11, 972.
5. Fretz, P.B., Pharr, J.W., McIlwraith, C.W., et al.: Varus vs valgus. In Letters, J. Am. Vet. Med. Assoc. 181:636, 1982.
6. Houghton, G.R., and Dekel, S.: The periosteal control of long bone growth. Acta Orthp. Scand. 50:635, 1979.
7. Jenkins, D.H.R., Cheng, D.H.F., and Hodgson, A.R.: Stimulations of bone by periosteal stripping. J. Bone Joint Surg. 57B:482, 1975.
8. Leitch, M.: Musculoskeletal disorders in neonatal foals. In Equine Practice Symposium on Neonatal Equine Disease. Vet. Clin. North Am. 1:189, 1985.

Arthrotomy of the
Dorsal Aspect of Fetlock Joint

The potential indications for dorsal arthrotomy of the fetlock joint include removal of osteochondral chip fragments from the dorsal proximal aspect of the proximal (first) phalanx, removal of osteochondritis dissecans fragments from the sagittal ridge of the distal articular surface of the third metacarpal bone and removal of chronic proliferative synovitis (villonodular synovitis) masses from the dorsal aspect of the fetlock joint.[1,3,4,6,7] The use of arthrotomy for removal of fragments from the dorsal aspect of the proximal end of the proximal first phalanx is controversial because of the finding that some fragments will heal with time and also that complications with periarticular new bone growth and a decreased range of motion have been reported following arthrotomy.[3,5] We believe that removal of these fragments by arthroscopy is the best means of maintaining soundness and providing the fastest resolution of the problem. For this reason, arthrotomy is considered virtually obsolete for the treatment of both proximal phalangeal chips and osteochondritis dissecans fragmentation from the distal metacarpus.[2,7] It is recognized, however, that removal of large fragments through arthrotomy may be indicated in a practice situation when arthroscopic surgery is not available. Arthrotomy still may be indicated for the removal of large masses of chronic proliferative synovitis,[4,6] since these are not always amenable to arthroscopic surgery.[2]

Anesthesia and Surgical Preparation

Dorsal arthrotomy is performed with the horse under general anesthesia and, depending on the surgeon's preference, in lateral or dorsal recumbency. With dorsal recumbency and the limb suspended, natural hemostasis is achieved. If the procedure is performed in lateral recumbency, an Esmarch's bandage and a pneumatic tourniquet are generally used. Prior to induction of anesthesia, the patient's limb is clipped from the hoof to just below the carpus all the way around the limb. Following anesthetic induction, the area of the surgical incision is shaved, and a routine surgical preparation is performed. Draping should include the use of a plastic adhesive drape. Some surgeons do the surgical preparation prior to induction of anesthesia. Radiographs should always include oblique views to ascertain the exact location of the lesion. Depending on the location of the lesion, the approach may be medial or lateral to the common digital extensor tendon.

Surgical Technique

A skin incision approximately 5-cm long is made 1-cm medial or lateral to the common digital extensor tendon over the fetlock joint. Figure 5-12A illustrates a medial approach to the metacarpophalangeal joint for removal of a fragment of the proximal phalanx. The subcutaneous fascia is incised along the same line as the skin incision.

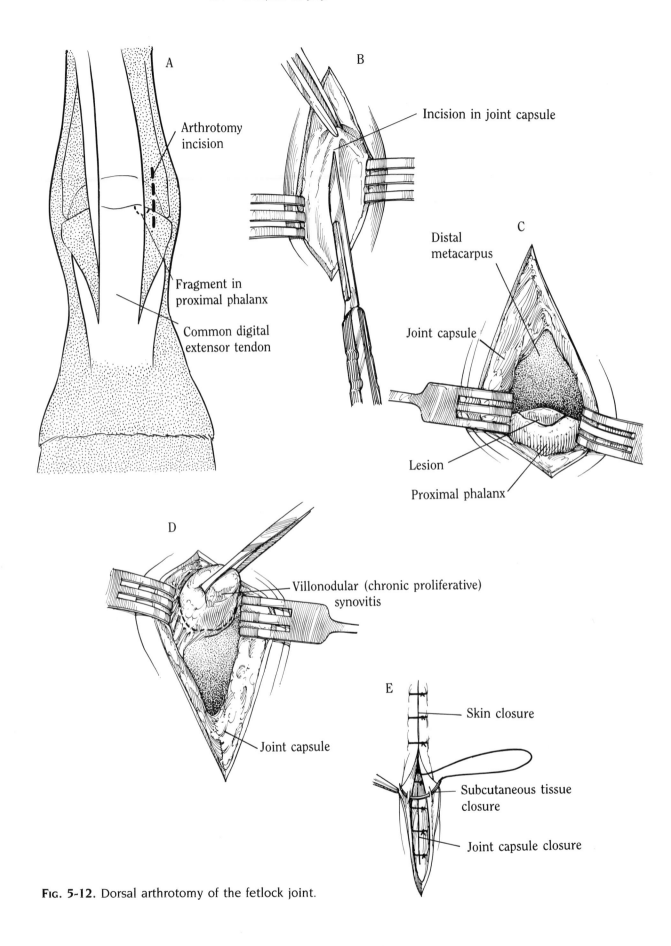

Arthrotomy
incision

Fragment in
proximal phalanx

Common digital
extensor tendon

Incision in joint capsule

Distal
metacarpus

Joint capsule

Lesion

Proximal phalanx

Villonodular (chronic proliferative)
synovitis

Joint capsule

Skin closure

Subcutaneous tissue
closure

Joint capsule closure

Fig. 5-12. Dorsal arthrotomy of the fetlock joint.

The incision is continued through the fibrous joint capsule (Fig. 5-12B). The dorsal branch of the palmar metacarpal artery and dorsal branch of the artery of the proximal phalanx are ligated or cauterized if encountered. The incision is completed through the synovial membrane. The fetlock joint is flexed slightly, and the edges of the incision are retracted to expose the articular cartilage of the distal metacarpus and the proximal rim of the proximal phalanx (Fig. 5-12C).

When a chip fracture off the proximal phalanx is being removed (Fig. 5-12C), it is elevated from the bone with a periosteal elevator and the soft tissue attachments are severed with a scalpel blade.

With villonodular (chronic proliferative) synovitis, the arthrotomy incision is in a slightly more proximal position centered over the synovial reflection of the distal metacarpus. The mass is removed after grasping it with Allis forceps and severing the base with a scalpel (Fig. 5-12D). With large lesions the mass can extend across the entire side of the joint, and in some situations two arthrotomy incisions, one on each side of the common digital extensor tendon, may be necessary. Sagittal sectioning of the mass before severing the base may also facilitate removal.

Following any procedure in the joint, it is flushed with saline solution or balanced electrolyte solution, and suction is used to remove fluid. The fibrous joint capsule is closed, using interrupted sutures of 2/0 synthetic nonabsorbable or absorbable material. The sutures in the joint capsule do not penetrate synovial membrane, and preplacement of the sutures in the joint capsule ensures that penetration does not occur and that there is ideal approximation of the incision edges (Fig. 5-12E). The subcutaneous fascia is closed in a continuous pattern using 2/0 synthetic absorbable suture material. (Fig. 5-12E). The skin is closed in an interrupted pattern using 2/0 nonabsorbable monofilament suture material (Fig. 5-12E). The tourniquet is removed (if one has been used), a sterile dressing is placed over the incision, and a firm pressure bandage is placed immediately on the leg from just below the carpal joint to the foot.

Postoperative Management

The use of antibiotics is optional. The skin sutures are removed in 10 to 12 days, but the bandage is maintained on the limb for another 10 days. Postoperative radiographs are taken within 24 hours of surgery; these films are of value for comparative purposes when follow-up progressive radiographs are made at a later date. The horse is stall-rested with hand-walking for six weeks and then can be turned out in a small area. At least four months' rest before training is recommended.

References

1. Haynes, P.F.: Disease of the metacarpophalangeal joint and metacarpus. Vet. Clin. North Am. (Large Anim. Pract.) 2:49: 1980.
2. McIlwraith, C.W.: Diagnostic and Surgical Arthroscopy in the Horse. Edwardsville, KS, Veterinary Medical Publishing Co., 1984.

3. Meagher, D.M.: Joint surgery in the horse: The selection of surgical cases and the consideration of alternatives. In Proceedings of the Annual Meeting of the American Association of Equine Practitioners, 1973, p 81, 1974.
4. Nichols, F.A., Grant, B.D., and Lincoln, S.D.: Villonodular synovitis of the equine metacarpophalangeal joint. J. Am. Vet. Med. Assoc. 168:1043, 1976.
5. Raker, C.W.: Calcification of the equine metacarpophalangeal joint following removal of chip fractures. Arch. Am. Coll. Vet. Surg. 4:66, 1975.
6. Van Veenendaal, J.C., and Moffatt, R.E.: Soft tissue masses in the fetlock joint of horses. Aust. Vet. J. 56:533, 1980.
7. Yovich, J.V., McIlwraith, C.W., Stashak, T.S.: Osteochondritis dissecans of the sagittal ridge of the third metacarpal and metatarsal bones in horses. J. Am. Vet. Med. Assoc. 186:1186, 1985.

Arthrotomy of the Tarsocrural (Tibiotarsal) Joint

Arthrotomy of the tarsocrural joint is indicated for the surgical treatment of osteochondritis dissecans lesions and removal of fragments associated with trauma when the alternative technique of arthroscopic surgery is not available. Such lesions occur in the distal intermediate ridge and malleoli of the tibia and the trochlear ridges of the talus.[1] Arthroscopic surgery is the preferred technique for the treatment of such lesions,[3] but the technique is not always conveniently available and may not be feasible in occasional cases when a large fragment off the distal aspect of the lateral trochlear ridge of the talus may be embedded in the soft tissue. In addition, fragments from the lateral malleolus are seldom operable by arthroscopic techniques.

The exact location and extent of the lesions should be ascertained with preoperative radiographs. Lesions of the distal intermediate ridge of the tibia, lateral trochlear ridge of the talus, and lateral malleolus of the tibia are operated on through a dorsolateral arthrotomy approach. This technique is presented sequentially below. The indications for a dorsomedial arthrotomy approach are fewer but include lesions on the medial trochlear ridge of the talus and the medial malleolus of the tibia.

Anesthesia and Surgical Preparation

The dorsolateral arthrotomy is performed under general anesthesia either with the horse placed in lateral recumbency with the affected limb up or in dorsal recumbency with the limb extended. Prior to induction of anesthesia, the patient's limb is clipped from the middle of the crus to the fetlock joint all the way around the leg. Following induction of anesthesia, the immediate surgical area is shaved and the limb prepared. The use of a tourniquet is optional.

Additional Instrumentation

The procedure requires retractors, curettes, periosteal elevators, and a bulb syringe.

Surgical Technique

The limb is draped with a draping system of the surgeon's choice, which should include plastic adherent drapes. A 3-cm vertical skin incision is made lateral to the long digital extensor tendon from the lateral malleolus distad to the level of the middle extensor retinaculum (Fig. 5-13A). The incision is continued through the subcutaneous tissue, avoiding the cranial tibial artery and deep peroneal nerve that lie plantar to the long digital extensor tendon. Synovial distention of the joint, which is usually present in these cases, facilitates identification of the dorsolateral pouch of the tarsocrural joint. If synovial distention is not obvious, the joint pouch can be made more obvious by intraarticular injection of fluid. The joint capsule is incised in the cen-

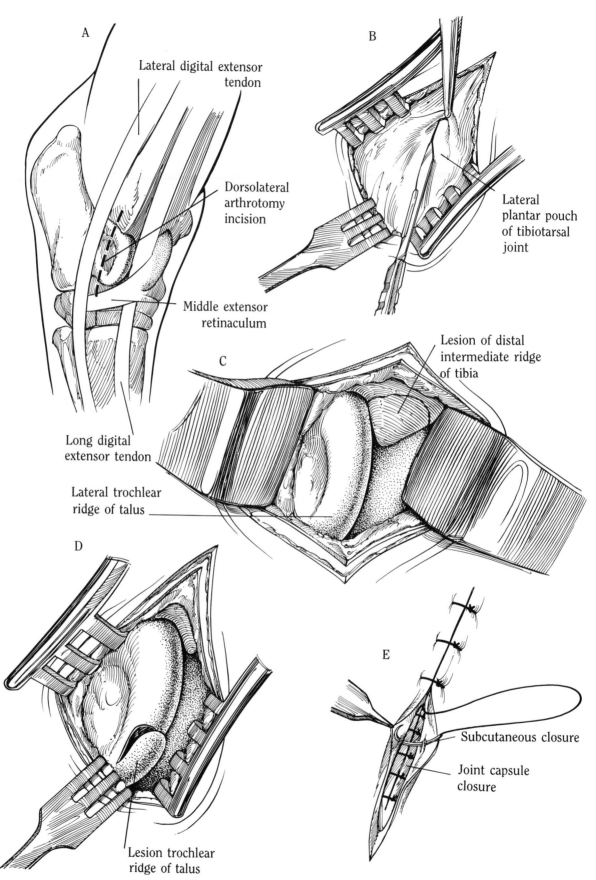

A

Lateral digital extensor tendon

Dorsolateral arthrotomy incision

Middle extensor retinaculum

B

Lateral plantar pouch of tibiotarsal joint

C

Lesion of distal intermediate ridge of tibia

Long digital extensor tendon

Lateral trochlear ridge of talus

D

Lesion trochlear ridge of talus

E

Subcutaneous closure

Joint capsule closure

FIG. 5-13A–E. Arthrotomy of the tarsocrural joint.

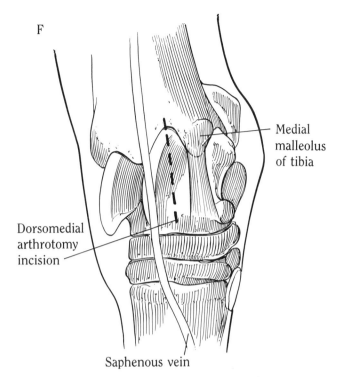

F

Medial
malleolus
of tibia

Dorsomedial
arthrotomy
incision

Saphenous vein

FIG. 5-13 (*Continued*). **F.** Arthrotomy of the tarsocrural joint.

ter of this pouch (Fig. 5-13B). Hand-held retractors will facilitate exposure of the lesion, particularly those of the intermediate ridge of the tibia proximally (Fig. 5-13C).

Lesions of the distal intermediate ridge of the tibia are operated on by retracting the incision proximad and reaching over the lateral trochlear ridge to the lesion. The fragments may be loose (and can be simply lifted out), or separation of the fragment from the parent bone with an elevator or osteotome may be required. Following removal of the fragment, any loose tags of bone and cartilage are removed.

With lesions of the lateral trochlear ridge of the talus a flap is generally present, and this is elevated and removed (Fig. 5-13D). In some instances, a large osteochondral fragment requiring dissection from the joint capsule is present. Any loose or undermined articular cartilage is removed, and the subchondral bone in the base of the defect is curetted. Some surgeons will also elect to drill holes in the healthy subchondral bone to facilitate vascularization and subsequent healing of the defect (forage).[1] In some cases of lateral trochlear ridge osteochondritis dissecans, an osteochondral fragment will have already completely separated from the defect and be located in the dorsomedial joint pouch. It may be possible to grasp this lesion through the dorsolateral arthrotomy, but in some situations an additional dorsomedial arthrotomy may be necessary. The removal of these loose bodies is important, since these separated fragments continue "to grow" and may become very large.

A lesion of the lateral malleolus will require some additional dissection of the fragment from the fibrous capsule (most of these should not be operated on).

Once all intraarticular lesions have been attended to, the joint is flushed and the arthrotomy is closed. The fibrous joint capsule and retinaculum are closed with simple interrupted sutures of absorbable synthetic material or monofilament nonabsorbable material (Fig. 5-13E). The sutures should not penetrate the synovial membrane. Preplacement of the sutures in the joint capsule and retinaculum ensures accurate apposition and a tight seal. The subcutaneous tissue is closed with a simple continuous suture of absorbable synthetic material and the skin closed with interrupted sutures using monofilament nonabsorbable material (Fig. 5-13E). The immediate surgical site is covered with a nonadherent pad and gauze bandage, and the limb is wrapped with a tight pressure bandage up to the middle of the crus.

If dorsomedial arthrotomy is necessary, it also is performed through the large dorsomedial joint pouch, with care being taken to avoid the cranial branch of the medial saphenous vein (Fig. 5-13F).

Some cases of osteochondritis dissecans necessitate two arthrotomies to manage both the original defect and the loose body or bodies. If arthroscopic surgery is available, double arthrotomies are not necessary.

Postoperative Management

The limb is maintained in a firm pressure bandage for two weeks, during which time the bandage is changed on several occasions. Skin sutures are removed at 10 to 12 days. During convalescence the horse is kept in a stall and walked in hand. Training is not resumed for at least four months after surgery.

References

1. Ficat, R.P., Ficat, C., Gedeon, P., et al.: Spongialization: A new treatment for diseased patellae. Clin. Orthop. 144:74, 1979.
2. McIlwraith, C.W.: Surgery of the hock, stifle and shoulder. Symposium on Equine Orthopedics. Vet. Clin. North Am. 5:333, 1983.
3. McIlwraith, C.W.: Diagnostic and Surgical Arthroscopy in the Horse. Edwardsville, KS, Veterinary Medicine Publishing Company, 1984.

Arthrotomy of the Femoropatellar Joint

Arthrotomy of the femoropatellar joint is indicated for the surgical treatment of osteochondritis dissecans of the femoropatellar joint. These lesions may be located on the lateral or medial trochlear ridge of the femur or the articular surface of the patella, but the lateral trochlear ridge of the femur is the most common site. The technique of arthrotomy of the femoropatellar joint for the treatment of the lesions has been commonly replaced by arthroscopic surgery. Arthrotomy is still, however, used when arthroscopic surgery is not available or the surgeon feels inadequately experienced at the technique.

As with other joint operations, the exact location of the lesions should be ascertained as much as possible with preoperative radiographs, but it is now known that the correlation between radiographic findings and findings at surgery are often poor.[1] Two techniques of femoropatellar arthrotomy have been developed and compared,[2,3] and both are illustrated here. The location of the lesion is the main criterion for selecting the surgical approach.

Anesthesia and Surgical Preparation

Prior to induction of anesthesia the area of the stifle joint is clipped. The immediate surgical area is shaved immediately before or immediately after induction of anesthesia.

Additional Instrumentation

Arthrotomy of the femoropatellar joint requires retractors, curettes, periosteal elevators, and a bulb syringe.

Surgical Technique

The locations for the two different approaches to the femoropatellar joint are illustrated in Figure 5-14A.

For the craniolateral approach the patient is positioned in dorsal recumbency with the limb extended. A 12-cm linear skin incision is made between the lateral and middle patellar ligaments (Fig. 5-14A). The thin, superficial fascia is incised in a similar fashion to expose the thick deep fascia of the stifle. This layer is incised to expose the underlying fat pad (Fig. 5-14B). Sufficient fat pad is removed with Metzenbaum scissors to expose the thin femoropatellar joint capsule deep to the fat pad. The joint capsule is then elevated and incised over the lateral trochlear ridge (Fig. 5-14C). Retractors are used to improve exposure, and the limb is flexed and extended to position the lesion satisfactorily within the incision (Fig. 5-14D). The craniolateral approach provides good exposure to the distal two thirds of the lateral trochlear ridge. Visualization of other areas of the joint are limited with this approach.

The joint capsule is closed with single interrupted sutures of 2-0 absorbable synthetic suture material. The deep fascia is closed with simple interrupted sutures of 0 or 1-0 synthetic absorbable suture (Fig. 5-14E). Closure of the superficial fascia is optional. Follow-up

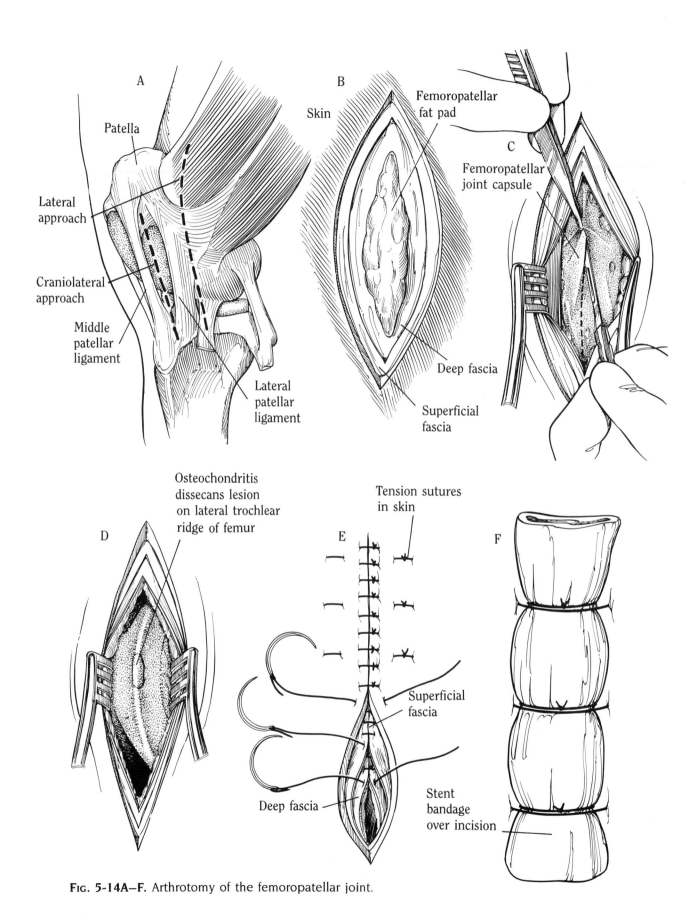

A

Patella

Lateral approach

Craniolateral approach

Middle patellar ligament

Lateral patellar ligament

B

Skin

Femoropatellar fat pad

Deep fascia

Superficial fascia

C

Femoropatellar joint capsule

D

Osteochondritis dissecans lesion on lateral trochlear ridge of femur

E

Tension sutures in skin

Superficial fascia

Deep fascia

Stent bandage over incision

F

Fig. 5-14A–F. Arthrotomy of the femoropatellar joint.

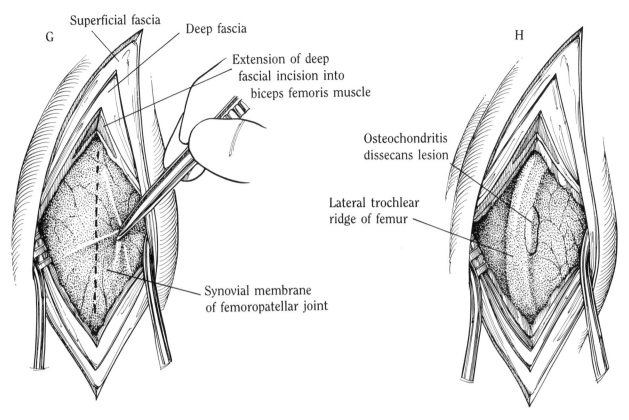

FIG. 5-14 (*Continued*). **G, H.**

data suggest this layer will commonly dehisce[3]. The skin is closed with nonabsorbable sutures; tension sutures are also used (Fig. 5-14E). A stent bandage (either a sterile 4-inch gauze bandage or rolled up 4 × 4-inch sponges are used) is sutured over the incision (Fig. 5-14F).

The lateral surgical approach provides exposure of the entire lateral trochlear ridge, the distal articular surface of the patella, the middle trochlear ridge and trochlear groove, and the synovial membrane at the cranial aspect of the joint. Because of this versatility it is the more common method of arthrotomy despite slightly increased requirements for closure.

For the lateral approach the patient is positioned in lateral recumbency, and the limb is supported horizontally in a limb stand. A 15-cm skin incision is made parallel and lateral to the lateral patellar ligament (Fig. 5-14A). The incision curves caudad in its proximal position to be lateral to the patella. The superficial fascia is similarly incised. The deep fascia is incised parallel to the lateral patellar ligament, and in the proximal aspect, this incision enters the biceps femoris muscle (Fig. 5-14G). The incision through the deep fascia exposes the femoropatellar joint capsule over the lateral aspect of the lateral trochlear ridge, and this thin joint capsule is then incised. Retractors are again used to facilitate exposure (Fig. 5-14H).

The lesions of osteochondritis dissecans in the femoropatellar joint will vary from wrinkling and cracking of the articular cartilage to flaps or loosely attached osteochondral fragments within an obvious defect. Also, osteochondral fragments may be free floating or attached to synovial membrane distant from the site of the lesion, and in some cases subchondral defects will be located beneath intact, normal-appearing articular cartilage. The surgical manipulations performed within the joint vary, therefore, depending on the lesion but will include removal of loose bodies as well as elevation of flaps and fragments and their removal followed by debridement of pathologic tissue. The joint is flushed copiously with sterile electrolyte solution before closure of the arthrotomy.

The joint capsule is closed in the same fashion as with the craniolateral approach. The deep fascia does need to be closed in two layers proximally where the fascia divides and lies superficial and deep to the biceps femoris muscle. The superficial fascia, as well as the skin, is closed in this approach. The superficial fascia is closed with 0 synthetic absorbable suture material and the skin is closed with 2-0 monofilament nonabsorbable material supported with vertical mattress tension sutures of 0 monofilament nonabsorbable material. Again, a stent bandage is placed over the incision.

Postoperative Management

Antibiotic (Procaine penicillin) is administered prior to surgery and continued for 5 days postoperatively. Phenylbutazone is also administered for 5 to 7 days to minimize swelling in the surgical region and decrease the chance of fasciitis, which can be a complication in this region. It is the authors' feeling that edema and inflammation between the fascial layers of the stifle can progress to cellulitis. This is a problem unique to the stifle. Another important part of the postoperative management is the maintenance of the horse in a standing position for two to three weeks postoperatively. This is achieved in our Clinic by placing a wire across the stall and having the lead shank attached to the wire with a ring. The skin sutures are removed two weeks following surgery. The horse is confined to a stall for at least six weeks postoperatively (with daily hand-walking) and then can be turned out into a small lot. Training should not be commenced within 4 months of surgery.

References

1. Pascoe, J., Wheat, J.D., and Jones, K.: A lateral surgical approach to the equine femoropatellar joint. Vet. Surg. 9:141, 1980.
2. Pascoe, J.R., Pool, R.R., Wheat, J.D., and O'Brien, T.R.: Osteochondral defects of the lateral trochlear ridge of the distal femur of the horse: Clinical, radiographic and pathological examination and results of surgical treatment. Vet. Surg. 13:99, 1984.
3. Trotter, G.W., McIlwraith, C.W., and Norrdin, R.W.: A comparison of two surgical approaches to the equine femoropatellar joint for the treatment of ostechondritis dissecans. Vet. Surg. 12:33, 1983.

Arthrotomy of the Femorotibial Joint

Arthrotomy of the femorotibial joint is indicated for the surgical treatment of subchondral cystic lesions of the medial condyle of the femur.[2,5,8] This technique has been developed because our results with conservative management of femoral cystic lesions have been poor at Colorado State University despite some reports of a reasonable return to clinical soundness with conservative treatment.[6] It has been noted that horses with cystic lesions may perform well up to a certain level and then become lame with harder work. Some horses can perform satisfactorily within a certain range of work. With more athletic pursuits, problems may be anticipated.

Surgical techniques that have been investigated include an extraarticular approach to the cyst with curetting and packing of the defect with a cancellous bone graft,[4] open curettage of the cyst through a femorotibial arthrotomy with[3] or without[5,8] cancellous bone grafting, or replacement of the defect with a polymer carbon fiber and fluorocarbon (Proplast, Dow Corning Corp., Midland, Michigan).[7] The first technique has been abandoned because of poor results and, at present, we recommend open arthrotomy, curettage of the cyst, and forage of the subchondral periphery of the cyst without cancellous bone grafting.

Anesthesia and Surgical Preparation

The arthrotomy is performed under general anesthesia with the horse placed in dorsal recumbency and the stifle joint flexed. Prior to induction of anesthesia the patient's limb is clipped in the area of the stifle, and the immediate surgical site is shaved directly after induction of anesthesia and positioning of the patient.

Additional Instrumentation

This arthrotomy procedure requires retractors and curettes as well as a flushing and vacuuming system.

Surgical Technique

Following surgical preparation the site is draped. With the limb in a flexed position, the femorotibial joint can be directly approached between the middle and medial patellar ligaments (Fig. 5-15A). A 5-cm vertical skin incision is made from below the patella distad to the tibial tuberosity, over the medial condyle that can be palpated. The incision is extended through superficial and deep stifle fascial layers into the femoropatellar fat pad (Fig. 5-15B), and the femoropatellar fat pad is dissected away at this location to expose the femorotibial joint capsule. This latter dissection should be conducted with care in the more proximal part of the incision to avoid penetration of the femoropatellar joint capsule. Using this approach, the femorotibial joint is reached and is identified by palpating the medial femoral condyle beneath it. After the joint capsule has been cleared of fat and elevated away from the condyle with forceps, a 2-cm inci-

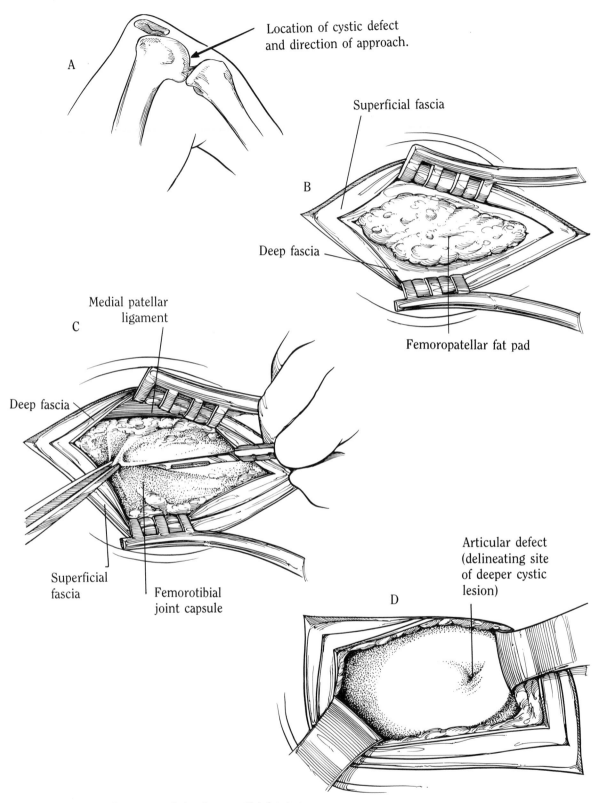

Location of cystic defect and direction of approach.

A

Superficial fascia

B

Deep fascia

Femoropatellar fat pad

Medial patellar ligament

C

Deep fascia

Superficial fascia

Femorotibial joint capsule

Articular defect (delineating site of deeper cystic lesion)

D

Fig. 5-15A–D. Arthrotomy of the femorotibial joint.

sion is made through the joint capsule (Fig. 5-15C). With the aid of hand-held retractors and limb manipulation (slight flexion or extension) the articular component of the lesion can be exposed (Fig. 5-15D).

The articular defect serves as identification for the deeper cystic lesion. It will vary from a small dimple or crack to a more widely eroded area. The latter situation tends to occur in horses that have been worked while under antiinflammatory medication because of lameness. The articular cartilage and bone are then penetrated to enter the cyst for curettage (Fig. 5-15E). Curettage of the cystic lesion should be thorough with careful debriding of the entire wall of the cyst and eliminating sclerotic bone, which is commonly present at the periphery. Once the cystic lesion is completely debrided, forage in the bone is performed to enhance revascularization of the defect (three or four holes of 2-mm diameter are drilled from the cystic cavity out into the bone of the femoral condyle in various directions).

Prior to closure, the femorotibial joint is irrigated thoroughly. The femorotibial joint capsule is closed with simple interrupted sutures of 2-0 synthetic absorbable suture material (Fig. 5-15F). The deep fascia is closed with simple interrupted sutures of 0 or 1 synthetic absorbable material (Fig. 5-15G), and the superficial fascia and subcutaneous tissues are closed with a continuous suture using 0 synthetic absorbable suture material. The skin incision is closed with simple interrupted sutures using 2-0 nonabsorbable monofilament material, supported by vertical mattress tension sutures of 0 nonabsorbable monofilament material (Fig. 5-15G, H). The incision is covered with a stent bandage as previously illustrated in the femoropatellar arthrotomy technique.

Postoperative Management

Postoperative management is the same as for femoropatellar arthrotomy. Skin sutures are removed at two weeks. The horse is maintained standing, using an overhead wire, for three weeks. The horse is maintained in a stall for six weeks (with daily hand-walking) and then can be turned out into a small area. The horse is not put into training for six months and then is brought back into training gradually.

Postoperative radiographs will show variable degrees of osseous healing of the defect.[8] However, continued lucency of the cystic defect is not incompatible with functional soundness.[8] It is suggested that the degenerate tissue within the cystic lesion is replaced with fibrous tissue. Lack of osseous healing has also been reported following adjunctive cancellous bone grafting.[3]

Femorotibial arthrotomy through an approach between the medial patellar ligament and the medial femorotibial (collateral) ligament has worked well for other surgeons.[2,8] Based on personal experience, we feel the approach described is more convenient and has worked well for us. Follow-up results in over 60 cases of surgical treatment of subchondral cystic lesions have been excellent and include successful racing performances.[8] Although cancellous bone grafting is a logical

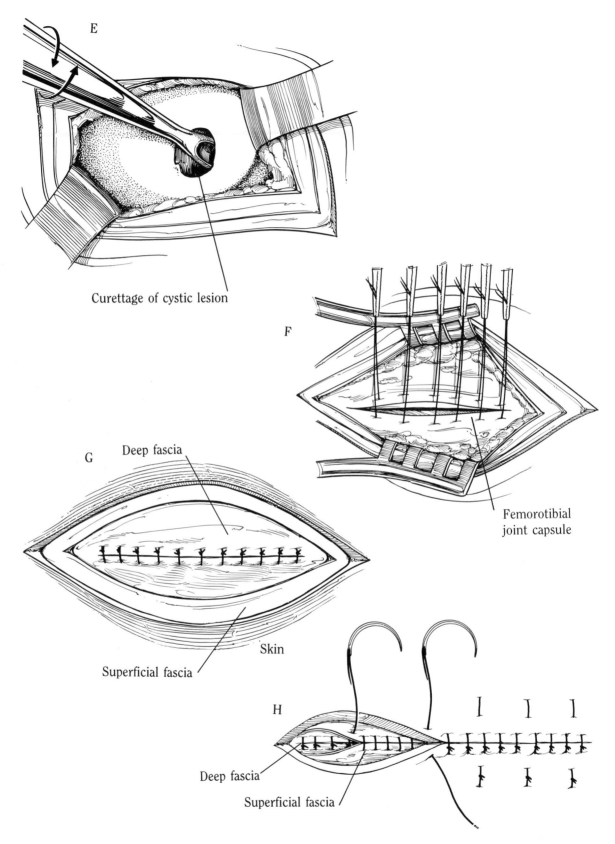

E

Curettage of cystic lesion

F

Femorotibial
joint capsule

G

Deep fascia

Skin

Superficial fascia

H

Deep fascia

Superficial fascia

FIG. 5-15 (Continued). E–H.

adjunct, we do not perform it because our results have been the same as those reported with grafting[3,8] thereby making the second surgical procedure unnecessary. Also, we are apprehensive about maintaining the cancellous bone in situ when there is an open communication distad from the cystic cavity to the joint.

References

1. Jeffcott, L.B., and Kold, S.E.: Clinical and radiological aspects of stifle bone cysts in the horse. Eq. Vet. J. 14:40, 1982.
2. Kold, S.E., and Hickman, J.: Use of an autogenous cancellous bone graft in the treatment of subchondral bone cysts in the medial femoral condyle of the horse. Eq. Vet. J. 15:312, 1983.
3. Kold, S.E., and Hickman, J.: Results of treatment of subchondral bone cysts in the medial condyle of the femur with an autogenous bone graft. Eq. Vet. J. 16:414, 1984.
4. McIlwraith, C.W.: Unpublished data, 1981.
5. McIlwraith, C.W.: Surgery of the hock stifle and shoulder. Vet. Clin. North Am. (Large Anim. Pract.) 5:333, 1983.
6. Stewart, B., and Reid, C.F.: Osseous cyst-like lesions of the medial femoral condyle of the horse. J. Am. Vet. Med. Soc. 180:254, 1982.
7. Valdez, H.: The use of carbon bio materials in repairing osteochondritic lesions in the horse. Proceedings of the 27th Annual Meeting, American Association of Equine Practitioners in 1981.
8. White, N.A., and McIlwraith, C.W.: Abstract, 1985 Meeting, American College of Veterinary Surgeons.

Arthrotomy of the Shoulder Joint

Arthrotomy of the shoulder joint is indicated for the treatment of osteochondritis dissecans (OCD).[6,7,9] There are few reports in the literature of surgically treating OCD in this joint, probably because of the difficulty in adequately exposing the humeral and glenoid surfaces of the shoulder joint and the knowledge that degenerative joint disease commonly occurs in association with OCD in the equine shoulder.[8]

Recent follow-up on operations for OCD using the technique about to be described is encouraging.[7] Not only was it possible to return horses to athletic soundness, but it was also possible to markedly improve function where extensive degenerative change was present. The surgical approach described has been reported previously[7] and is modified from one described for the dog.[2]

Anesthesia and Surgical Preparation

Accurate identification of the problem prior to the operation is important. Intraarticular analgesia is usually induced to localize the lameness problem to the shoulder joint, and radiographs are made under general anesthesia. Radiographs with the horse standing are often inadequate and may not demonstrate lesions. An arthrogram can be performed by introducing 7 ml of diatrizoate methylglucamine (Renografin, E.R. Squibb & Sons, Inc., Princeton, NJ, 08540) into the affected joint, but the authors do not consider this to be necessary routinely.

The shoulder is clipped prior to surgery, and the horse is placed on a regimen of perioperative antibiotics and given tetanus toxoid. Phenylbutazone is also administered perioperatively.

Surgical Technique

After draping, a 20-cm skin incision is made, beginning 2.5 cm caudal to the spine of the scapula and curving over the shoulder joint caudal to the infraspinatus tendon (which can be palpated) (Fig. 5-16A). The deep fascia is incised to expose the caudal border of the brachiocephalicus muscle. This is elevated and retracted craniad to expose the underlying aponeurosis of the deltoideus muscle, which is located over the infraspinatus muscle. The dense aponeurotic portion at the cranial aspect of the deltoid muscle is severed, and the deltoideus muscle retracted caudad to reveal the teres minor muscle below (Fig. 5-16B). This exposure is also facilitated by cranial retraction of the infraspinatus muscle (Fig. 5-16B). The insertion of the teres minor on the humerus is transected, leaving enough of the attachment to be sutured, and the muscle belly is retracted caudad, using Gelpi retractors to expose the joint capsule beneath. Care must be taken to avoid the caudal circumflex humeral artery and vein and axillary nerve, which are positioned caudad to the surgical region. The joint capsule may sometimes be distended. The joint capsule is incised parallel to the palpable rim of the glenoid cavity (Fig. 5-16C).

Accessibility to lesions will vary with access tending to be easier

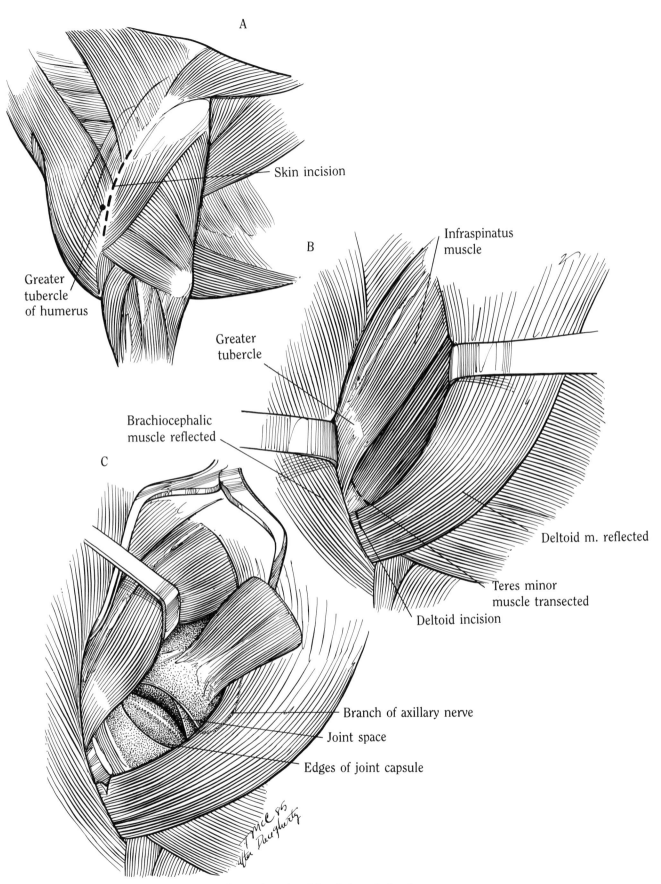

A

Skin incision

Greater
tubercle
of humerus

B

Infraspinatus
muscle

Greater
tubercle

Brachiocephalic
muscle reflected

C

Deltoid m. reflected

Teres minor
muscle transected

Deltoid incision

Branch of axillary nerve

Joint space

Edges of joint capsule

FIG. 5-16. Muscle-separating approach to the shoulder joint of the horse.

when bone remodeling is extensive. In other situations the careful insertion of a curved instrument into the glenoid notch to distract the humeral head from the glenoid cavity is important. Extreme adduction of the distal limb will expose additional portions of the caudal humeral head, and this maneuver needs to be performed rather forcibly. As with other cases of OCD, detached or loose cartilage flaps are removed and the subchondral bone is debrided of all abnormal tissue with a curette. The use of a fiberoptic lighting source to expose deeper regions of the joint is also advantageous. Cystic lesions in the glenoid cavity are identified by cartilagenous dimpling or cracking and curetted. An angled curette is useful. After debridement and removal of fragments, the joint is flushed thoroughly to remove loose pieces of bone and cartilage.

The joint capsule is closed with interrupted sutures of 2-0 polyglactin 910. The teres minor muscle is reattached to the humerus with simple interrupted sutures of 1 polyglactin 910 and the severed aponeurotic origin of the deltoid muscle is similarly sutured. The free caudal border of the brachiocephalic muscle is replaced over the deltoid muscle and sutured with a simple continuous pattern using 1 polyglactin 910. The subcutaneous tissue is also apposed using a simple continuous suture of 0 polyglactin 910, and the skin is apposed with simple interrupted sutures of monofilament nonabsorbable suture material, or with skin staples. A stent bandage is secured over the wound.

Postoperative Management

Antibiotics and phenylbutazone are administered for 5 days following surgery. The horse is stall rested with hand-walking for one month and then can be turned out into a small area with a gradual increase in exercise. A total of six months' rest is allowed before resuming training.

Comments

This surgical approach to the shoulder joint differs from two previous techniques for arthrotomy in the horse that have involved longitudinal or transverse tenotomy of the infraspinatus tendon.[3,9] The approach described maintains the stability of the joint afforded by the infraspinatus tendon and allows better exposure of the caudal humeral head than we have been able to achieve by longitudinal tenotomy.

Adequate surgical access does require manipulation and traction. Arthroscopic techniques have now been developed that allow superior visualization to the shoulder.[1] Surgical manipulations with arthroscopy are difficult, however, and do not yet fit into the description of routine arthroscopic surgery. Arthrotomy does not require the specialized experience of the arthroscopic technique, and no healing problems have been observed. On the other hand, the visualization within the joint is superior with arthroscopy.

References

1. Bertone, A.L., McIlwraith, C.W.: Arthroscopic anatomy of the equine shoulder joint and approaches for the surgical treatment of osteochondrosis. Vet. Surg. In press.
2. Birkeland, R.: Osteochondritis dissecans in the humeral head of the dog: Comparison of results achieved with conservative and surgical treatment. Nord. Vet. Med. 19:294, 1967.
3. De Bowes, R.M., Wagner, P.C., and Grant, B.D.: Surgical approach to the equine scapulohumeral joint through a longitudinal infraspinatus tenotomy. Vet. Surg. 11:125, 1982.
4. McIlwraith, C.W.: Subchondral cystic lesions (osteochondrosis) in the horse. Comp. Cont. Educ. Pract. Vet. 4:394, 1982.
5. McIlwraith, C.W.: Diagnostic and Surgical Arthroscopy in the Horse. Edwardsville, KS, Veterinary Medicine Publishing Company, 1984.
6. Mason, T.A., and MacLean, A.A.: Osteochondrosis dissecans of the head of the humerus in two foals. Eq. Vet. J. 9:189, 1977.
7. Nixon, A.N., Stashak, T.S., McIlwraith, C.W., et al.: A muscle separating approach to the equine shoulder joint for the treatment of osteochondritis dissecans. Vet. Surg. 13:247, 1984.
8. Nyack, B., Morgan, J.P., Poole, R.R., and Meagher, D.M.: Osteochondritis of the shoulder joint of the horse. Cornell Vet. 71:149, 1981.
9. Schmidt, G.R., Dueland, D.R., and Vaughan, J.T.: Osteochondrosis dissecans of the equine shoulder joint. Vet. Med. Small Anim. Clin. 70:542, 1975.

Arthroscopic Surgery of the Carpal Joints

Arthroscopic surgery in the carpal joints is indicated for the removal of osteochondral chip fractures from these joints. The advantages of arthroscopic surgery over conventional arthrotomy for the treatment of these problems has been documented.[1-3] It is our opinion that these advantages are sufficient to make the use of arthrotomy for the removal of such fragments obsolete. The equine carpal joints have been the most frequently operated on by arthroscopic surgery and have served somewhat as the showpiece for the procedure. Basic principles of arthroscopic surgery for the removal of small fragments will be described. For more details the reader is referred to another textbook.[3]

Arthroscopic surgery is also used by the authors to operate on carpal slab fractures. However arthrotomy is still considered an appropriate technique in the management of this condition, because the advantages of using arthroscopic surgery are less defined at this stage.

Anesthesia and Surgical Preparation

This surgical procedure is performed with the horse under general anesthesia. The horse may be placed in lateral or dorsal recumbency, but we prefer dorsal recumbency with the limb suspended. This facilitates operation on the horse from both sides (this is commonly necessary when multiple fragments are present). Prior to induction of anesthesia, the patient's limb is clipped from the midradius to the distal cannon area. The immediate surgical site on the dorsal aspect of the joint is shaved immediately before or after induction of the anesthesia. Draping will include a plastic adhesive drape as well as a special impervious drape (General Econopak Inc.).

Additional Instrumentation

Appropriate arthroscopic instrumentation is required (see Appendix IV).[3]

Surgical Technique

Arthroscopic surgery uses the principle of triangulation. Preoperative radiographs will have ascertained the site of the chip fractures. It is to be noted, however, that arthroscopic examination frequently finds additional pathologic change that was not identified on the radiographs. As a general principle, the arthroscope is inserted on the side opposite the lesion, and surgical instruments are inserted over the lesion. When lesions are present on both sides, the positions of instrument and arthroscope will be reversed appropriately.

A chip fracture off the distal aspect of the radial carpal bone will be used as an example. Two skin incisions are made prior to distention of the joint. The incision for the arthroscope is placed laterally, between the extensor carpi radialis and the common digital extensor tendons. The portal for the instrument is located medially, medial to the extensor carpi radialis tendon. These incisions are made before joint distention in order that the surgeon can be sure they are located away from the tendon sheaths. The intercarpal (midcarpal) joint is then distended with saline or polyionic electrolyte solution, and the arthroscopic cannula is inserted through the joint capsule using the sharp trocar. The sharp trocar is then exchanged for a blunt obturator to complete placement of the arthroscopic sheath within the joint. The arthroscope is then inserted, and the ingress fluid line and light cable are attached. The joint can then be examined. The pathologic changes at various sites within the joint are ascertained. This examination is facilitated by the placement of an egress cannula through the site of the instrument portal (Fig. 5-17A). The egress cannula is used to allow flushing of fluid through the joint to clear it of any debris or blood. When the view is clear, the stopcock on the egress cannula is closed and the egress cannula can be used as a palpating instrument to ascertain the mobility of chips and the size and nature of other lesions. Once the diagnostic arthroscopy is completed, the chip can be removed.

An instrument portal through the joint capsule is then made, using a trocar or no. 15 scalpel blade (Fig. 5-17B). Carpal chips can be divided into four categories, and the techniques for their removal vary accordingly. If the chip is fresh and mobile, forceps are inserted through the instrument portal, and the chip is removed. When there are strong fibrous attachments at the fracture line or to the fibrous joint capsule, the fragment is loosened with a periosteal elevator inserted through the instrument portal (Fig. 5-17C). When bony reattachment is developing or has occurred, an osteotome is used to free the fragment from the parent bone. The osteotome is held in correct position by the surgeon who is visualizing its position, and an assistant taps the osteotome on command. When there is extensive bony reattachment, a motorized burr can be used to remove the protruding lesion.

After removal of the separated chip fragment using forceps (Fig. 5-17 D, E), the defect is then debrided with a curette (Fig. 5-17 F, G). (The selection of forceps to remove fragments depends on both the preference of the surgeon and the size of the fragment). Debridement of the defect includes the removal of defective bone as well as elevated, fragmented or loose articular cartilage. Partial thickness defects of articular cartilage (where there is firm attachment of the remaining cartilage to the bone) are not debrided. These principles are based partly on knowledge of cartilage healing in the horse and partly on subjective feeling.[3] When debridement of the defect is completed, the joint is irrigated, using a large bore (4.5 mm) egress cannula.

Chip fragments at different locations vary in their ease of removal, the degree of associated joint damage, and also the prognosis. Chip fractures off the distal intermediate carpal bone are removed using a medial arthroscopic approach and a lateral instrument approach (it is

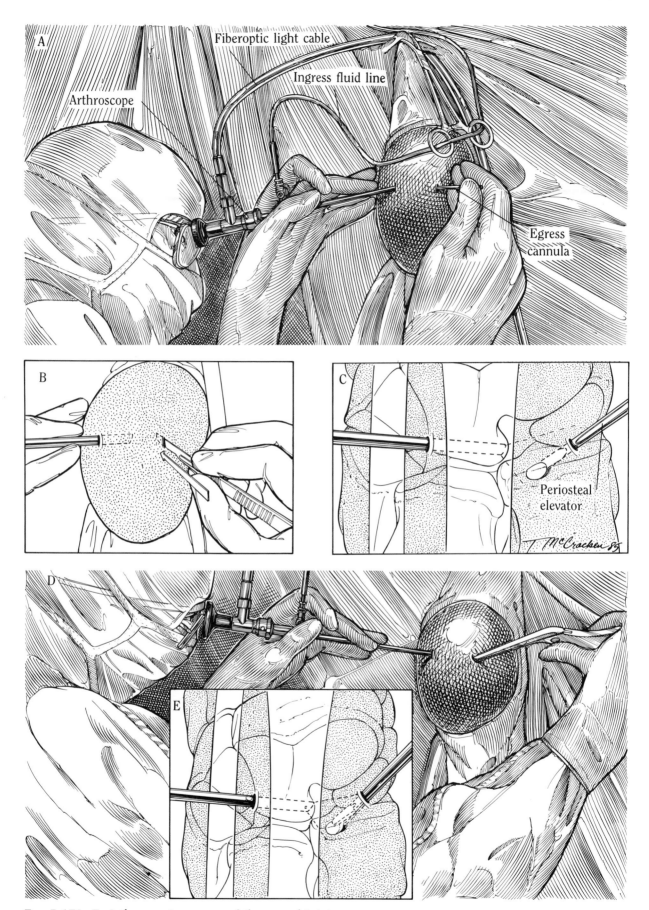

Labels in figure: Fiberoptic light cable, Ingress fluid line, Arthroscope, Egress cannula, Periosteal elevator

Fig. 5-17A–E. Arthroscopic surgery of the carpal joint.

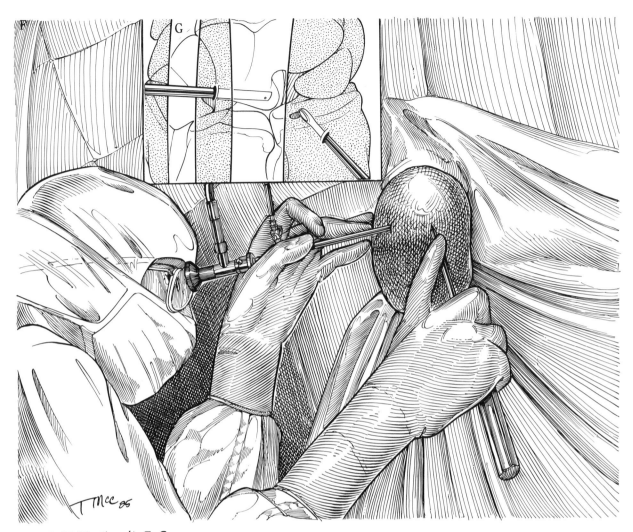

Fig. 5-17 (Continued). **F, G.**

to be noted that the actual site of these lateral and medial portals is always the same with any chip in the carpal joint). Chip fragments off the proximal aspect of the third carpal bone are removed with a lateral arthroscopic approach and a medial instrument approach. Generally, lesions in the radiocarpal (antebrachiocarpal) joint are more difficult to operate on because the joint capsule is drawn more tightly against the dorsal surface of the bones in this joint, thus allowing less room for manipulation of the instruments. Surgery in this joint is facilitated if the limb being operated on is in about 30 degrees of flexion in contrast to 90 degrees of flexion in the intercarpal joint. With lesions of the proximal radial and proximal intermediate carpal bone, the forceps have to approach the lesion end on, and the distance from the synovial membrane to the lesion is small. For lesions of the proximal radiocarpal bone, the arthroscope is placed through the lateral portal and the instrument through the medial portal. These positions are switched for operating on the proximal aspect of the intermediate carpal bone. Fractures off the distal lateral aspect of the radius are operated on with the arthroscope placed medially and the instrument placed laterally. These fragments are generally of a larger size. Similarly, fragments off the medial aspect of the distal radius are operated on with the arthroscope placed laterally and the instrument placed medially. Further detail on surgery at each of these locations is presented elsewhere.[3]

Carpal fragments of all sizes are amenable to arthroscopic surgery, and suturing of portals in the joint capsule is unnecessary even with large fragments. Multiple fragments in multiple joints can be conveniently operated on with arthroscopic surgery, whereas multiple arthrotomies in such situations would not be appropriate. Spurs or osteophytes are removed only if they are broken off or if their interposition into the joint makes them likely candidates for later fracture or if they will preclude normal joint closure. Most spurs visible on preoperative radiographs are *not* candidates for removal, and the best example of these are ones that commonly occur on the proximal aspect of the intermediate carpal bone.

Intraoperative and/or postoperative radiographs are important to ensure that no fragments are left within the joint. While the arthroscopic surgeon must be careful to ensure that all interarticular fragments are removed, at the same time it is important that he realize that osseous densities within the joint capsule are not candidates for removal.

Postoperative Management

While patients are recovering from anesthesia, full-length padded bandages are applied to the operated limbs to avoid trauma to the carpal joints. After recovery from anesthesia, small bandages consisting of a nonadhesive pad, a sterile gauze (Kling), and an elastic adhesive (Elastikon) are applied. These bandages facilitate early exercise and passive flexion of the joint. Hand-walking is commenced at 7 to 10 days. Swimming is commonly used during the convalescent period of many horses. With simple fractures, horses can be put into training at six weeks, and some horses are started considerably earlier than this without any problems. Horses with associated cartilage and bone damage have appropriately longer periods of convalescence.

Comments

The advantages of arthroscopic surgery can be listed as follows:

1. Less trauma to the soft tissues with resultant benefits both in the cosmetic appearance of the carpus as well as decreased functional compromise.
2. Better visualization of lesions.
3. Earlier return to racing or other athletic activity. This advantage is considered to be related to maintenance of normal joint function, particularly in the soft tissues, rather than differences in cartilage healing.
4. Improved racing performance after surgery.[2]

5. Treatment of more cases possible (multiple lesions).
6. Correction of the problem rather than treatment with medication. Many trainers who were not satisfied with the results from arthrotomy and therefore would rely on rest, retirement, or continued work with medication, now request arthroscopic surgery.
7. Considerably decreased convalescent costs for arthroscopy compared to arthrotomy. Not only is the time from surgery to commencement of training decreased, but training time will be decreased also because of less loss of fitness.[2]

Although these advantages have made arthroscopic surgery the technique that should be used for the removal of carpal chip fractures, it is also to be recognized that the technique requires skill and experience. The technique requires careful learning. Without these qualifications the advantages of arthroscopic surgery are quickly lost.

References

1. McIlwraith, C.W.: Experiences in diagnostic and surgical arthroscopy in the horse. Equine Vet. J. 16:11, 1984.
2. McIlwraith, C.W.: Arthroscopy in retrospect. Proceedings of the 30th Annual Convention of the American Association of Equine Practitioners in 1983.
3. McIlwraith, C.W.: Diagnostic and Surgical Arthroscopy in the Horse. Edwardsville, KS, Veterinary Medicine Publishing Company, 1984.

Arthroscopic Surgery of the Dorsal Aspect of the Fetlock Joint

Arthroscopic surgery in the fetlock joint is indicated for the following conditions:

1. Proximal dorsal chip fractures of the proximal phalanx.[1-3]
2. Proximal palmar/plantar fractures off the proximal phalanx.[1-3]
3. Villonodular (chronic proliferative synovitis) of appropriate size.[1-3]
4. Osteochondritis dissecans of sagittal ridge of distal metacarpus or metatarsus.[3,6]

The removal of osteochondral chip fragments from the proximal dorsal aspect of the proximal phalanx is the most common indication for arthroscopic surgery in this joint. The use of arthrotomy in such conditions is now generally considered inappropriate unless there are special circumstances. The technique for removing these chip fractures will be illustrated. Arthroscopic surgery for the removal of avulsion fragments of the proximal palmar or proximal plantar rim of the proximal phalanx is difficult, but a technique has been developed. Whether it has advantages over the arthrotomy for these fractures is still uncertain. It is also a particularly difficult arthroscopic technique and is not described in this atlas. For additional details, the reader is referred to another textbook.[3] Arthroscopic surgery is appropriate for less extensive villonodular synovitis cases, but arthrotomy may still be necessary when large masses fill the entire dorsal joint space. This procedure is described elsewhere in the preceding section. With osteochondritis dissecans of the distal sagittal ridge of the distal articular surface of the third metacarpal or metatarsal bone, we recommend arthroscopic surgery.[3]

At the present time the authors do not use arthroscopic surgery to remove apical chip fragments from the proximal sesamoid bones (the arthrotomy technique has been described in our previous textbook*). Midbody and basal sesamoid fractures are currently treated using cancellous bone grafting (also described in a preceding section of this chapter).

Anesthesia and Surgical Preparation

For arthroscopic surgery in the dorsal aspect of the fetlock joint, the horse is placed under general anesthesia in dorsal recumbency. The limb is suspended for surgical preparation, and it may be suspended or rested on the horse's forearm during the operation. The limb is clipped prior to surgery from below the carpus to the foot and shaved immediately before or after induction of anesthesia.

---

*Techniques in Large Animal Surgery. Philadelphia, Lea & Febiger, 1982.

Additional Instrumentation

These arthroscopic procedures require arthroscopic instrumentation (see Appendix IV).

Surgical Technique

A chip fracture off the medial aspect of the proximal phalanx within the fetlock joint will be used as an example. The joint is distended with saline or electrolyte solution prior to making any incisions (Fig. 5-18A). The general principles of triangulation and arthroscopic surgery have been previously described in the section on carpal arthroscopy. The skin incision for the arthroscopic portal is made over the bulge lateral to the common digital extensor tendon created by joint distention. The arthroscopic sleeve is inserted using the sharp trocar, and after passing through the joint capsule, it is angled proximad to avoid creating iatrogenic damage to the sagittal ridge of the distal metacarpus. After placement of the arthroscopic sheath, the arthroscope is inserted and the fluid line and light cable are attached.

For surgical procedure on a chip fracture off the medial proximal aspect of the proximal phalanx, the instrument portal is made in the lower half of the medial bulge created by joint distention. The portal through the joint capsule is made with a trocar or scalpel blade as previously described in the procedure on carpal arthroscopic surgery. If there is a question regarding the correct site for placement of the instrument portal, it can be ascertained by inserting an 18-gauge needle through the proposed site to check for positioning. The external and internal positioning of the arthroscope and instrument is illustrated in Figures 5-18B and 5-18C. As in the carpus, fragments can be removed with forceps if they are loose or may require separation with a periosteal elevator. Following removal of the fragment, loose tags are removed from the defect, but debridement is kept to a minimum in an attempt to avoid any potential periosteal proliferation at the surgical site due to capsular trauma.[5] The joint is irrigated with polyionic solution and the skin incisions are closed.

For surgery on villonodular synovitis or osteochondritis dissecans lesions, the arthroscopic approach is the same, but the instrument is inserted more proximad than it is for proximal phalanx chips (Fig. 5-18D, E). These techniques are detailed elsewhere.[3]

Postoperative Management

A sterile dressing is placed over the incisions, and a firm leg bandage is applied to the lower leg. This wrap is maintained with changes for 10 days, at which time the sutures are removed and no further bandaging is necessary. Hand-walking is begun 7 to 10 days after surgery. Swimming is used during the canvalescence of some of these cases. For horses with uncomplicated chip fractures of the proximal dorsal aspect of the proximal phalanx, training can be resumed two months after surgery.[6] A longer lay-up time of four months is recommended for horses with chronic proliferative synovitis and larger fractures off the proximal aspect of the proximal phalanx.

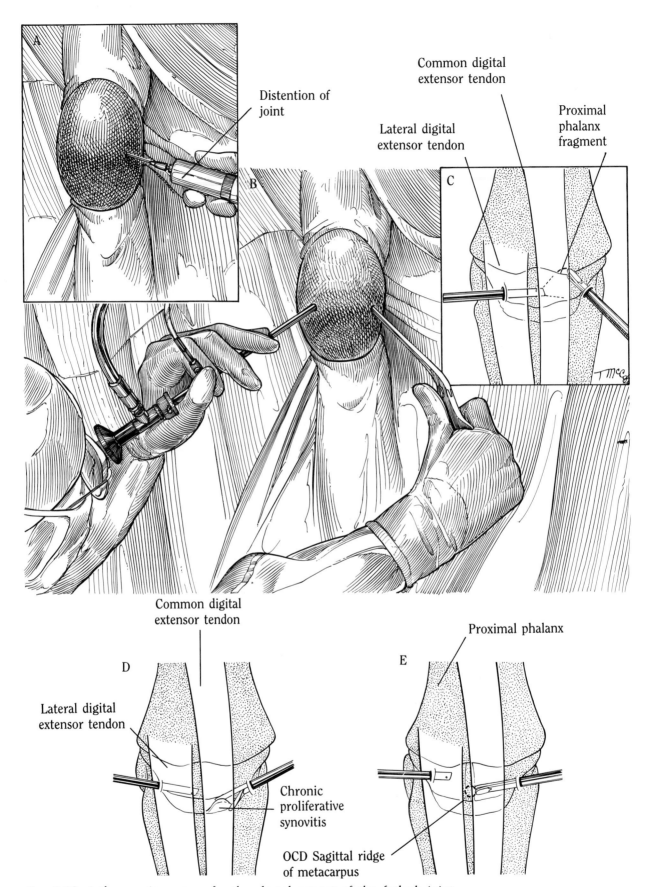

A Distention of joint

B

C Common digital extensor tendon

Lateral digital extensor tendon

Proximal phalanx fragment

D Common digital extensor tendon

Lateral digital extensor tendon

Chronic proliferative synovitis

E Proximal phalanx

OCD Sagittal ridge of metacarpus

FIG. 5-18. Arthroscopic surgery for the dorsal aspect of the fetlock joint.

Comments

The advantages of arthroscopic surgery over arthrotomy have been described elsewhere in this textbook and are well documented in the literature.[2,3] As mentioned before, caution is needed in that these advantages apply only when sufficient skill and experience in the technique have been developed.

References

1. McIlwraith, C.W.: Experiences in diagnostic and surgical arthroscopy in the horse. Eq. Vet. J. 16:11, 1984.
2. McIlwraith, C.W.: Arthroscopy in retrospect. Proceedings American Association of Equine Practitioners AAEP Meeting, 1984, pp. 57–66.
3. McIlwraith, C.W.: Diagnostic and Surgical Arthroscopy in the Horse. Edwardsville, KS. Veterinary Medicine Publishing Company, 1984.
4. Petterson, H., and Ryden, G.: Avulsion fractures of the caudoproximal extremity of the first phalanx. Eq. Vet. J. 14:333, 1982.
5. Raker, C.W.: Calcification of the equine metacarpophalangeal joint following removal of chip fractures. Arch. Am. Coll. Vet. Surg. 4:66, 1975.
6. Yovich, J.V., McIlwraith, C.W., and Stashak, T.S.: Osteochondritis dissecans of the sagittal ridge of the third metacarpal and metatarsal bones in horses. J. Am. Vet. Med. Assoc. 186:1186, 1985.
7. Yovich, J.V., McIlwraith, C.W.: Arthroscopic surgery for removal of chip fragments of the first phalanx. J. Am. Vet. Med. Assoc. 188:273, 1986.

Arthroscopic Surgery of the Tarsocrural (Tibiotarsal) Joint

Arthroscopic surgery is the preferred method of treatment for cases of osteochondritis dissecans or traumatically created fragments involving the tarsocrural joint.[1] The sites of such lesions include the distal intermediate ridge and medial malleolus of the tibia and the trochlear ridges of the talus. Traumatically induced fragments off the lateral malleolus generally require arthrotomy if they are considered suitable for surgical treatment.

The exact location of the lesions should be ascertained as well as possible with preoperative radiographs. Experience with arthroscopy has taught us, however, that the surgeon must be prepared to find lesions that were not demonstrable on preoperative radiographs. In addition to decreasing the trauma associated with removal of these fragments, compared to arthrotomy, arthroscopic surgery has improved the surgeon's diagnostic capabilities in this joint and ability to identify "new" lesions.

Anesthesia and Surgical Preparation

The surgical procedure is performed under general anesthesia with the horse in dorsal recumbency. Frequently, bilateral lesions are present, and both joints are operated at the same time. Prior to induction of anesthesia, the patient's limb(s) is(are) clipped from the middle of the crus to the middle of the metatarsus. Following induction of anesthesia the areas over the dorsolateral and dorsomedial pouches of the tarsocrural joint are shaved, and a routine surgical preparation of the hock is performed.

Additional Instrumentation

This procedure requires arthroscopic instrumentation (see Appendix IV).

Surgical Technique

An impervious draping system is used, as well as sterile plastic adherent drapes in the immediate area. The general technique of arthroscope and instrument insertion and triangulation has been discussed under arthroscopic surgery of the carpal joint. One difference with the tarsocrural joint is that the joint is distended with sterile fluid *prior* to making any skin incisions. This joint distention is effected through the dorsomedial pouch and 50 to 100 ml of fluid are injected. This distention enables identification of both the dorsolateral and the dorsomedial outpouching of the tarsocrural joint. To operate on lesions of the distal intermediate ridge of the tibia, or the lateral trochlear ridge of the talus, a medial approach with the arthroscope is made. The lateral approach with the arthroscope is made if the primary area of concern includes the medial trochlear ridge of the talus.

For lesions of the medial malleolus of the tibia, lateral and medial arthroscopic approaches have been used.

To insert the arthroscope through the medial pouch, an 8-mm skin incision is made slightly dorsal to the center of the outpouching but lateral to the cranial branch of the medial saphenous vein. This incision will be approximately 1 cm lateral to the complex of extensor tendons over the dorsal aspect of the joint. The arthroscopic sheath and sharp trocar are then pushed through the subcutaneous tissue and joint capsule with the limb maintained in extension. When the bone on the medial nonarticular portion of the talus is contacted, the sharp trocar is replaced with the blunt obturator, and the limb is flexed to enable passage of the arthroscopic sheath across the joint. The arthroscope, the fiberoptic cable, and the ingress fluid system are then connected, and visualization can begin.

If the arthroscope is to be placed from the lateral side, it is inserted through the dorsolateral pouch. The skin incision is made in the center of the dorsolateral pouch with the limb in extension. Flexion is again used to facilitate passage of the sheath and obturator over the dorsal aspect of the trochlear ridges of the talus.

The placement of the instrument and arthroscope to operate on a lesion off the distal intermediate ridge of the tibia is illustrated in Figure 5-19A. The instrument is placed through the distal part of the bulge of the dorsolateral pouch. Such a placement is necessary to enable passage of the instrument over the lateral trochlear ridge and onto the intermediate ridge lesion. This approach is also represented diagramatically in Figure 5-19B. The technique for operating on a lesion on the lateral trochlear ridge is illustrated in Figure 5-19C. Alternatively, the arthroscope may also be placed laterally. Lesions of the medial malleolus are operated on using a triangulating approach from the same side or the opposite side, depending on the surgeon's preference. Unless fragments of the lateral malleolus are small, their embedment in other soft tissues of the joint is too extensive for arthroscopic surgery to be carried out conveniently. Further details on the arthroscopic techniques in the tarsocrural joint are available elsewhere.[1]

Fragments and flaps are separated with an elevator or osteotome followed by removal with forceps. The area of the lesions is debrided with a curette. The joint is then flushed, and the arthroscope and sheath are removed from the joint. Each skin incision is closed with one or two simple interrupted sutures of nonabsorbable material. The tarsus is bandaged using a nonadhesive pad, gauze bandage, and elastic adhesive bandage. A full pressure wrap is not considered necessary.

Postoperative Management

The bandage is maintained with changes for ten days at which time the sutures are removed and bandaging is no longer necessary. The horse is maintained in a stall for one month and then can be

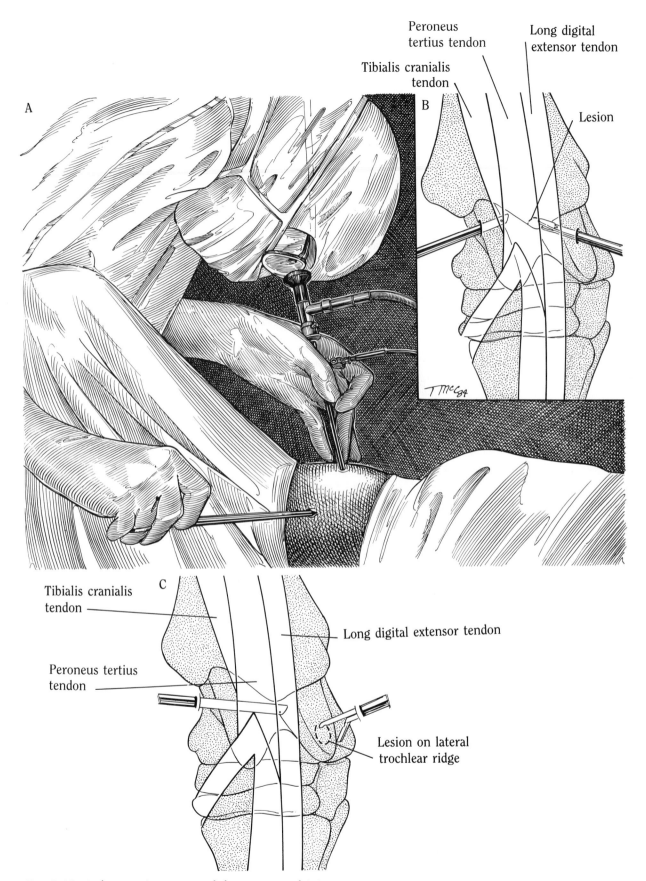

Peroneus
tertius tendon

Long digital
extensor tendon

Tibialis cranialis
tendon

Lesion

A

B

Tibialis cranialis
tendon

C

Long digital extensor tendon

Peroneus tertius
tendon

Lesion on lateral
trochlear ridge

Fig. 5-19. Arthroscopic surgery of the tarsocrural joint.

turned out into a small area. Athletic training (if the age of the animal is appropriate) can be resumed in six to eight weeks.

Reference

1. McIlwraith, C.W.: Diagnostic and Surgical Arthroscopy in the Horse. Edwardsville, KS, Veterinary Medicine Publishing Company, 1984.

Arthroscopic Surgery of the Femoropatellar Joint

Arthroscopic surgery of the femoropatellar joint is the preferred method of surgically treating osteochondritis dissecans of the lateral trochlear ridge, medial trochlear ridge, or the patella. The advantages include decreased tissue trauma, a less complicated convalescence, and good results in terms of return to athletic function.[1-3] There is rapid resolution of both synovial effusion and lameness following the surgery. Contraindications to surgery include marked loss of articular cartilage and bone on the trochlear ridges, lateral luxation of the patella, or remodeling change of the patella seen on radiographs. The use of arthroscopy has improved our diagnostic capabilities in this joint, as well as offering an improved method of surgical treatment.

Anesthesia and Surgical Preparation

The surgical procedure is performed with the horse under general anesthesia and in dorsal recumbency. The limbs are maintained in extension during surgical procedures, but the opposite limb is flexed when they are not being performed to minimize the risk of postoperative femoral nerve paresis. Prior to induction of anesthesia the area of the stifle is clipped, and the immediate surgical site is shaved either before or after induction. An impervious draping system is used.

Additional Instrumentation

Arthroscopic instrumentation including motorized abrading equipment is necessary (see Appendix IV).

Surgical Technique

Both limbs may be operated on at once. The affected limb is maintained in an extended position during surgical procedures while the other limb is kept in a flexed position. Prior distention of the femoropatellar joint is not usually necessary. An 8-mm skin incision is made midway between the distal border of the patella and the tibial crest between the lateral and middle patellar ligaments. This incision is continued through the superficial and deep fascia into the femoropatellar fat pad. The arthroscopic sleeve, containing a blunt obturator, is then inserted through this incision and directed at an angle of 45 degrees up under the patella. With pressure, the sheath and obturator will pass through the thin femoropatellar capsule and up the trochlear groove. If resistance is encountered, the sheath is moved lateral to pass up the gap between the patella and lateral trochlear ridge into the suprapatellar pouch. When the arthroscopic sleeve is inserted up into the suprapatellar pouch, the examination is begun in this position. Sequential examination of the femoropatellar joint is continued by withdrawing the scope down the trochlear groove and alternatively examining the lengths of the medial and lateral trochlear ridges. The entire examination of the joint can be completed with the arthroscope placed through this single portal.

The site of instrument portals will vary depending on the location of the lesion. The same principles of triangulation as described in the carpus are used, but the angles are more acute (Fig. 5-20A, B). The instruments and arthroscopic approaches used to operate on a lesion on the lateral trochlear ridge of the femur (the most common site) are illustrated in Figure 5-20A and B. The instrument portal is proximal and lateral to the arthroscopic portal and frequently passes through the lateral patellar ligament. If attempts are made to make the portal more lateral than the lateral patellar ligament, it is difficult to manipulate the instrument to operate effectively on lesions on the lateral trochlear ridge. Making an instrument portal through the lateral patellar ligament does not seem to be of any consequence. Lesions are operated on by elevating the flaps or fragments and removing them

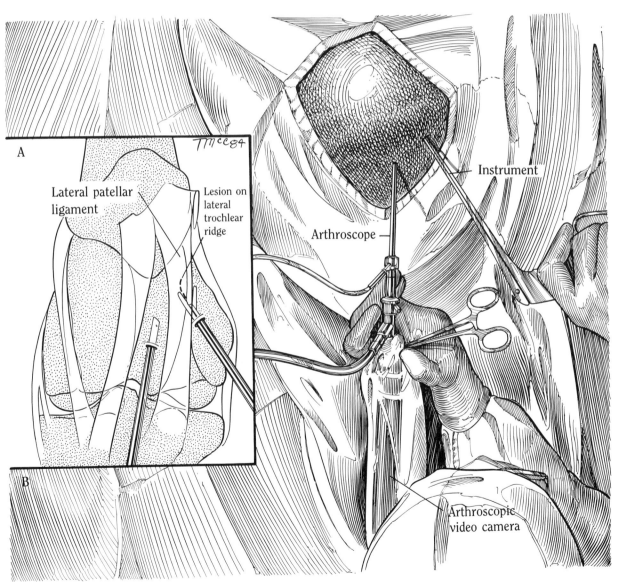

FIG. 5-20. Arthroscopic surgery of the femoropatellar joint.

with forceps. Loose bodies are similarly removed with forceps. The lesions are debrided with a combination of basket forceps, curettes, and mechanical abrading equipment. These maneuvers are presented in more detail elsewhere.[1]

For the lesions in less frequent locations, different instrument portals are necessary. A more distal portal is required for lesions of the distal lateral trochlear ridge. Similarly, proximal and distal portals between the middle and medial patellar ligament are used to operate on the medial trochlear ridge of the femur. If lesions are on the underside of the patella, a distal portal medial or lateral to the middle patellar ligament is necessary for the instrument to be effectively passed proximad under the patella and be manipulated on the articular surface of the patella.

Following debridement of lesions, the joint is flushed and the skin incisions are closed with nonabsorbable suture material. No bandaging is necessary.

Postoperative Management

The use of antibiotics is optional, but the horses are placed on phenylbutazone for 5 days following surgery. Skin sutures are removed in 12 to 14 days. The horse is maintained in a stall for one month and then can be turned out into a small area. Training exercise can be resumed in three months after the arthroscopic surgery. Synovial effusion generally resolves within one month of surgery.

References

1. McIlwraith, C.W.: Diagnostic and Surgical Arthroscopy in the Horse. Edwardsville, KS, Veterinary Medicine Publishing Company, 1984.
2. McIlwraith, C.W., and Martin, G.S.: Arthroscopic surgery for the treatment of osteochondritis dissecans in the equine femoropatellar joint. Vet. Surg. 14:105, 1985.
3. Martin, G.S., and McIlwraith, C.W.: Arthroscopic anatomy of the equine femoropatellar joint and approaches for treatment of osteochondritis dissecans. Vet. Surg. 14:99, 1985.

Surgical Treatment of Infectious (Septic) Arthritis

In addition to antibiotic therapy, the institution of some form of joint drainage and irrigation is usually appropriate in the treatment of infectious arthritis. The presence of a purulent effusion retards the action of many antibiotics by decreasing the metabolic rate of the bacteria. In addition, pH values drop in septic effusions, and the activity of aminoglycosides is reduced significantly with a decrease in pH.[6] The primary indication for joint drainage, however, is the removal of substances potentially deleterious (lysosomal enzymes, E group prostaglandins) to the articular cartilage.

Methods of joint drainage include needle aspiration, through-and-through lavage, distention irrigation, and arthrotomy with or without synovectomy. The selection of a particular technique depends on the individual case as well as the preference of the clinician. Techniques have been adapted from the human medical literature, but controlled data in the horse are necessary to assess relative efficacy of the different methods. Recent experiments have attempted to elucidate the situation.[2] It should not be implied that the use of any of these techniques will lead consistently to a successful result. In our experience there is still no panacea for the condition and there is marked variation in success.

Two drainage techniques will be described. In early cases of infectious arthritis through-and-through lavage of the joint is appropriate. When the inflammatory process becomes chronic, lavage and distention irrigation lose their effectiveness because fibrin clots become too large or too organized for aspiration. In these instances arthrotomy and joint debridement are indicated. In studies with induced septic arthritis in rabbits, it was found that by seven days postinfection, the exudate had organized to the extent that surgical debridement was the only means of effective removal.[3] More recent work in the human clinical literature emphasizes that arthrotomy needs to be performed at an early stage rather than being done as a last resort.[5] In analysis of results in the treatment of 28 cases of septic arthritis of the human wrist, of the 10 wrists with good or excellent results, all had had the arthrotomy within 10 hours of diagnosis. Of the 13 with a fair or poor result, surgery had been delayed for 16 hours or longer.[5] The long-term results deteriorated in direct proportion to increasing time until treatment and the number of procedures performed.[5] The tendency of the authors with cases of equine septic arthritis now is for earlier intervention or earlier arthrotomy.

The degree of increased surgical aggressiveness proposed for the treatment of equine septic arthritis and the timing are still a little uncertain. Recent work with an experimental model did document that arthrotomy more effectively removed fibrin from the joint than any one of three lavage regimes.[2] However, when horses were euthanized and the joints examined, most parameters were not significantly different. It is considered that the advantages of aggressive surgical debridement differ among clinical cases of diverse pathogenesis.

Through-and-Through Lavage

Through-and-through lavage is generally performed by placing two needles or catheters on opposite sides of the joint (Fig. 5-21A). One serves as an inflow tract and the other as an outflow tract, and periodic distention of the joint is achieved by occluding the outflow tract and applying pressure to the ingress line. This procedure is ideally performed under general anesthesia and aseptic conditions, but in some instances the lavage while the horse is standing is appropriate. Three to 6 liters of fluid are flushed through the joint. A balanced polyionic electrolyte solution is preferred, as this will more closely approximate the pH of normal synovial fluid. The addition of antibiotics to the irrigating solution is optional, but we do not do it. Some clinicians add providone-iodine solution (Betadine) to the irrigating solution. However, recent experimental work has shown that too concentrated a solution is deleterious to the joint. It has been shown that if concentration of providone-iodine in solution is 0.2% or less, no deleterious effects are experienced.[1] On the other hand, addition of chlorhexidine-surfactant (Novalsan) solution is definitely contraindicated.[1] Opinions among clinicians also vary on the timing for irrigation or lavage. The recent experimental work at Colorado State University did not show significant differences between one, two, and three lavage regimes.[2]

Arthrotomy with Implantation of an Ingress Flushing System

The site of the arthrotomy incision is usually the same as for an elective arthrotomy in the respective joint. Identification of landmarks will be more difficult, however, because of the periarticular swelling generally associated with septic arthritis. The technique is a simple one and is illustrated, using the tarsocrural joint as an example. In this case an arthrotomy incision is made through the dorsomedial pouch of the tarsocrural joint (Fig. 5-21B). After the skin incision is made distal to the medial malleolus of the tibia, a careful inspection is made to ensure that the cranial branch of the medial saphenous vein is not within the area. Because of the capsular and subcutaneous swelling, the location of the vein may be difficult to ascertain prior to making the skin incision. The incision is then continued through the subcutaneous tissue and fibrous joint capsule. Gray, hyperplastic synovial membrane will usually be encountered at this stage and it is similarly incised.

This arthrotomy will be left open to heal on its own. With resolution of infection, the synovial membrane will close over the defect and second intention healing will occur. Once arthrotomy has been performed, a quarter inch fenestrated drain (Orthopedic Equipment,

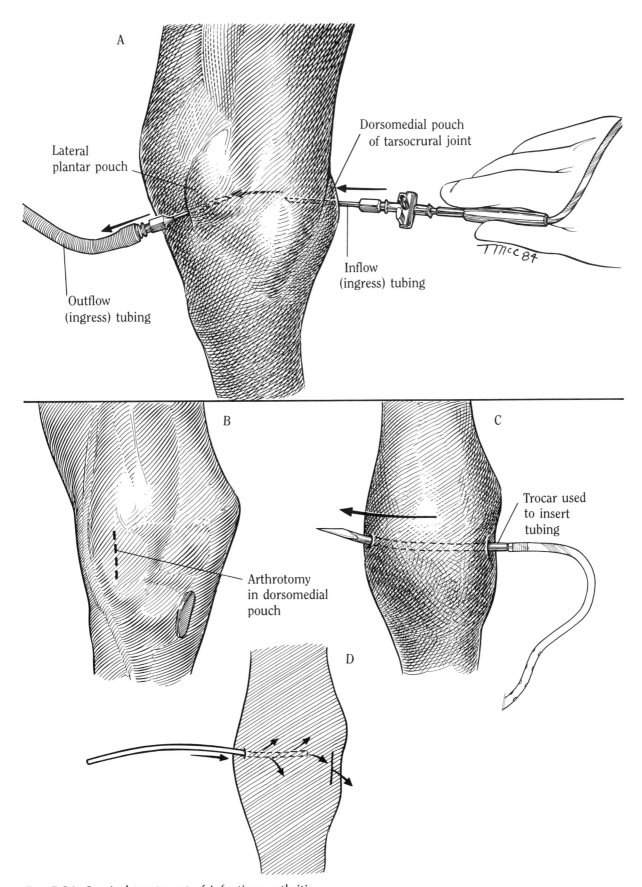

Lateral
plantar pouch

Dorsomedial pouch
of tarsocrural joint

Outflow
(ingress) tubing

Inflow
(ingress) tubing

A

B

Arthrotomy
in dorsomedial
pouch

C

Trocar used
to insert
tubing

D

FIG. 5-21. Surgical treatment of infectious arthritis.

Bourbon, Indiana) is inserted through the dorsolateral pouch using a trocar as illustrated in Figure 5-21C. Care must be taken to ensure that the fenestrations are within the joint rather than being in the subcutaneous tissue (Fig. 5-21D). A three-way stop cock is connected to the drain, the drain is sutured in an appropriate position, and the limb is bandaged. This technique is always performed under general anesthesia with aseptic conditions. At the time of surgery the joint is flushed thoroughly, and flushing is continued on a twice daily basis for 7 to 10 days. The length of the fenestrated portion and the number of fenestrations on the drain are recorded (a case of part of the drain being pinched off and left in the joint has been recorded[2]).

During arthrotomy as much pathologic synovial membrane as possible is removed. Fibrin is also debrided from the joint. However, synovectomy is very difficult because chronically affected joints have extensive thickening of the fibrous joint capsule, and multiple arthrotomy incisions will be required to remove the entire synovial membrane. Suction drains and closure of the arthrotomy are unsatisfactory due to clogging of the drain and rapid cessation of effective drainage. The Penrose drain is an alternative, but retrograde contamination of the joint is a risk. The leaving of an open arthrotomy has not been associated with untoward complications.

Postoperative Management

The joint is flushed twice daily through the ingress system and the bandage is changed daily. Broad-spectrum antibiotics are of course maintained systemically throughout the period of treatment. When the joint has closed, analysis of synovial fluid is one of the methods of gauging the effectiveness of treatment. Sequential follow-up radiographs are also recommended.

Other ancillary follow-up medications have been proposed. The use of systemic nonsteroidal antiinflammatory agents is logical both for comfort of the patient and to decrease prostaglandin levels within the inflamed joint. Although the use of intraarticular corticosteroids has been proposed once the actual sepsis is apparently resolved, we feel it is a hazardous practice. While it is acknowledged that they aid circulation and plasma membrane integrity, prevent intracellular water sequestration, stabilize lysosomes, inhibit capillary and fibroblast proliferation, and prevent kinin release, complement activation, and prostaglandin synthesis, we need to recognize that our experimental work has shown that 50% of joints still cultured positive at necropsy after apparent clinical resolution of the problem.[2] Sodium hyaluronate has been used by some clinicians with reportedly good results.

References

1. Bertone, A., McIlwraith, C.W., Powers, B., and Radin, J.: The effect and comparison of four antimicrobial joint lavage solutions on synovial membrane and articular cartilage in the horse. Vet. Surg. 15:305, 1986.

2. Bertone, A., McIlwraith, C.W., Jones, R., and Norrdin, R.: Comparison of treatments for induced equine infectious arthritis. AJVR. In press.
3. Daniel, D., Akeson, W., Amiel, D., et al.: Lavage of septic joints in rabbits: Effects of chondrolysis. J. Bone Joint Surg. (Am.) 58-A:393, 1976.
4. McIlwraith, C.W.: Treatment of infectious arthritis. Vet. Clin. North. Am. (Large Anim. Pract.) 5:363, 1983.
5. Rashkoff, E.V.: Septic arthritis of the wrist. J. Bone Joint Surg. 65-A:824, 1983.
6. Ward, T.T., and Steigbigel, R.T.: Acidosis of synovial fluid correlates with synovial fluid leukocytosis. Am. J. Med. 64:933, 1978.

Surgical Relief of Carpal Canal Syndrome

A condition somewhat related to annular ligament constriction of the fetlock occurs in the carpal canal of the horse.[3,6] It is also a well-recognized condition in the wrist joint of man known as "carpal tunnel syndrome."[3,4] Through the carpal canal of the horse run the deep and superficial flexor tendons as well as the medial palmar artery and vein, the lateral palmar artery and vein, and the medial palmar nerve[1] (Fig. 5-22A). The accessory carpal bone and the palmar carpal annular ligament contribute to the relatively nondistensible carpal canal. The carpal synovial sheath invests the tendons in this area.

Any enlargement of the contents of or narrowing of the carpal canal can cause pain and lameness in a fashion similar to that seen in the palmar or plantar tendon sheath of the fetlock joint. Infection and trauma in the region are also potential causes of the condition.[4] Pressure on the medial palmar nerve may also contribute to the lameness.[3] Any thickening of the flexor tendons, such as would occur in a case of very proximally located tendinitis of either the deep or superficial flexor tendon, can cause the condition. The most common cause of carpal canal syndrome in the horse is a fracture of the accessory carpal bone.[1,3,5,6] This fracture is more common in jumping and steeplechase horses, although all breeds are potentially susceptible. Following fracture, swelling at the fracture site with subsequent fibrosis and callus formation results in a relative narrowing of the canal with pressure on the flexor tendons, nerves, and blood vessels.

Carpal canal syndrome is manifested by a bulging of the carpal sheath adjacent to the digital extensor and ulnaris lateralis muscles. There may be reduced arterial pulse distal to the lesion.[5] There is pain on flexion or extension of the limb.[3] Radiographs may reveal a healing fracture of the accessory carpal bone. Nerve conduction studies used in man have not been performed in horses but would be of interest in this condition. The surgical technique is similar to that described previously.[3]

Anesthesia and Surgical Preparation

The operation is performed with the patient under general anesthesia in lateral recumbency with the affected limb down. The caudal aspect of the carpus is prepared for aseptic surgery in a routine manner.

Surgical Technique

A 15-cm long incision is made longitudinally from 3 cm above to 5 cm below the accessory carpal bone, parallel and caudal to the common digital vein (Fig. 5-22B). A longitudinal strip of the volar annular ligament up to 1-cm wide is removed parallel to the axis of the limb (Fig. 5-22C). Care must be taken not to lacerate the lateral palmar vein, which is close to the retinaculum[5] (Fig. 5-22A). The length of the strip should be a little greater than the zone of thickening, but rarely does it include the entire longitudinal length of the annular ligament (Fig. 5-22D).

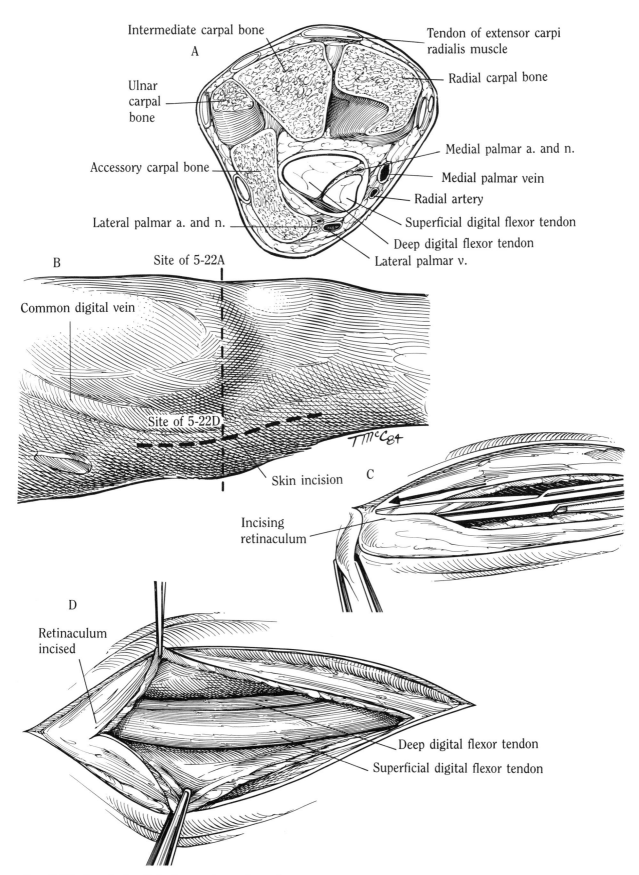

Intermediate carpal bone

A

Tendon of extensor carpi
radialis muscle

Ulnar
carpal
bone

Radial carpal bone

Accessory carpal bone

Medial palmar a. and n.

Medial palmar vein

Radial artery

Superficial digital flexor tendon

Lateral palmar a. and n.

Deep digital flexor tendon

Lateral palmar v.

B

Site of 5-22A

Common digital vein

Site of 5-22D

Skin incision

C

Incising
retinaculum

D

Retinaculum
incised

Deep digital flexor tendon

Superficial digital flexor tendon

FIG. 5-22. Surgical relief of carpal canal syndrome.

The subcutaneous tissues are closed using either continuous or simple interrupted sutures of synthetic absorbable material. These sutures should provide a good watertight seal to prevent the formation of synovial fistula. The skin is closed with nonabsorbable sutures in a suture pattern of the surgeon's choice.

Postoperative Management

A sterile dressing is placed over the incision, and the entire limb is placed in a protective bandage. Care must be taken to avoid a pressure sore over the prominence of the accessory carpal bone when a bandage is applied to this area. In our experience with limited numbers of cases we have observed an early favorable response following surgery.

Phenylbutazone is administered intravenously to reduce postoperative pain and facilitate early return of use of the limb. Antibiotics are not administered routinely. Sutures are removed at 12 to 14 days, and bandaging may be discontinued 3 to 4 days later.

Comments

Case selection is important in this condition. Ideally, a surgical candidate should be free of chip fractures within the carpus or associated degenerative joint disease. These conditions would affect the prognosis adversely. The most difficult decision that faces the surgeon is whether the cause of the lameness is instability at the fracture site of the accessory carpal bone or the carpal tunnel syndrome itself. Injecting local anesthesia into the carpal sheath may aid in the localization of the lameness. The dramatic response to surgery seen in selected cases is similar following treatment of carpal tunnel syndrome in human patients.[4]

References

1. Getty, R.: Heart and arteries. In Sisson and Grossman's The Anatomy of the Domestic Animal, 5th Ed. (R. Getty, ed.) Philadelphia, W.B. Saunders, 1975, p. 592.
2. Lieberman, J.S.: Neuromuscular electrodiagnosis. In Neurological Surgery, Vol. 1. (J.R. Youmans ed.) Philadelphia, W.B. Saunders, 1982, p. 630.
3. MacKay-Smith, M.P., Cushing, L.S., and Leslie, J.A.: "Carpal canal" syndrome in horses. J. Am. Vet. Med. Assoc. 160:993, 1972.
4. Milford, L.: The hand. In Campbell's Operative Orthopedics, 6th ed. A.S. Edmonson and A.H. Crenshaw, eds. St. Louis, C.V. Mosby, 1980, p. 361.
5. Radue, P.: Carpal tunnel syndrome due to fracture of the accessory carpal bone. Equine Pract. 3:8, 1981.
6. Turner, A.S.: Large animal orthopedic surgery. In Textbook of Large Animal Surgery. (P. Jennings, ed.) Philadelphia, W.B. Saunders, 1984, p. 934.

Arthrodesis of the Proximal Interphalangeal Joint

Arthrodesis of the proximal interphalangeal joint is used in treating degenerative joint disease (DJD) of the pastern joint, luxations of the pastern joint, and fractures involving the pastern joint. The proximal interphalangeal (pastern) joint is a common site for DJD in horses.[1,5,7] It can occur as a sequela to a severe sprain of the pastern or a deep wire cut in the pastern region.

In young horses, high ringbone is occasionally seen in the hindlimbs, secondary to subchondral cystic lesions.[1-7] These cysts are possible manifestations of osteochondrosis. The exact cause of the subchondral cyst is uncertain, but it appears to be unrelated to the smaller subchondral cysts seen in humans secondary to degenerative joint disease. The pastern joint of the opposite hindlimb should also be radiographed. There may be lesions in the opposite pastern joint as well as in other joints that are predisposed to the syndrome of osteochondritis dissecans and subchondral bone cyst formation.[1,7]

Arthrodesis is also indicated for certain fractures of the middle phalanx (P2) that do not involve the distal interphalangeal joint.[2-6,8] It has been our experience that, if such fractures are allowed to heal by external coaptation alone, the resulting callus enlarges the pastern area and may interfere with tendon function. Such fractures are usually so unstable that not only is healing protracted but the proximal phalanx becomes driven into the fracture site to produce severe hyperextension of that joint and a limb that may be even nonfunctional for pasture soundness.[2] Various techniques of arthrodesis of the equine pastern joint have been documented.[8] Earlier techniques used a joint drilling procedure that removed as much of the articular cartilage as possible. Other methods employ a more radical approach to the joint, utilizing a variably shaped skin incision and a transection of the dorsal joint capsule of the pastern joint. With these methods, a more thorough curettage of the joint surface is possible.

Arthrodesis for high ringbone usually entails removal of a variable amount of periosteal new bone from the dorsal region of the joint, which forms in response to the original disease. To gain access to the joint, some collateral ligament transection is necessary, although we recommend that these ligaments be preserved as much as possible because they contribute to the final stability of the joint. The use of internal fixation as part of the surgical procedure aids in the horse's convalescence. The method described here is a modification of the lag screw fixation as described by Schneider and co-workers.[5] The convalescent time and cost of hospitalization can be reduced because the cast can be removed earlier, since the lag screws make the joint inherently more stable.[5,8] This finding has also been substantiated by others.[6]

Clipping of the entire limb up to the level of the proximal end of the metatarsus or metacarpus is best done prior to induction of anesthesia to reduce the time under anesthesia.

Anesthesia and Surgical Preparation

The surgical procedure is performed with the horse under general anesthesia with the affected limb uppermost. The limb is positioned on a leg stand so that placement of a cassette for intraoperative radiographs will be possible without having to move the horse and risk a break in aseptic technique. We prefer to have the limb supported just below the hock or carpus with the rest of the limb free, approximately half a meter above the table surface.

The dorsal aspect of the affected pastern joint is shaved; then an Esmarch bandage and a pneumatic tourniquet are applied just below the carpal or tarsal joint as appropriate. The area of the surgical incision is prepared for aseptic surgery in a routine manner.

The use of a plastic adhesive drape is recommended. Since the foot region will be fairly close to the surgical site, it is advisable to place a separate plastic drape and a pair of sterile rubber surgical gloves over the foot prior to applying the drape over the surgical site.

Additional Instrumentation

ASIF equipment for lag screw fixation with 4.5-mm cortical bone screws (see appendix), includes curettes, chisel (1 to 2 cm wide), mallet, strong periosteal elevator, and equipment for intraoperative radiographs.

Surgical Technique

To obtain adequate exposure of the pastern joint thereby ensuring a more thorough removal of articular cartilage, the joint must be exposed through its dorsal aspect. An I-shaped incision is made over the dorsal surface of the proximal and middle phalanges. The proximal part of the incision extends across the middle of the proximal phalanx, and the distal part of the incision is placed approximately 0.5 cm above the coronet (Fig. 5-23A). The two incisions are connected by a sagittal incision down the dorsal aspect of the proximal and middle phalanges. The skin is reflected, exposing the common (or long) digital extensor tendon and the two branches of the interosseous (suspensory) ligaments. A Z-plasty is performed in the common (or long) extensor tendon and, if necessary, the branches of the suspensory ligament (Fig. 5-23B). The extensor tendon is carefully dissected away from the joint capsule of the pastern joint, and the pastern joint is identified by probing with sterile disposable hypodermic needles. Following identification of the joint, the joint capsule is transversely incised using sharp dissection. The collateral ligaments can be completely severed to allow exposure of the joint surfaces. In the authors' experience partial severance is usually adequate. If arthrodesis is performed for a proximal middle phalangeal fracture, then there is usually enough instability of the joint that even less collateral ligament need be severed to permit adequate exposure. However, in arthrodesis for the treatment of ringbone, severing a certain amount of collateral ligament is necessary.

Following the arthrotomy, a suitable instrument such as a heavy-duty periosteal elevator is used to pry the joint surfaces apart so that as much hyaline cartilage as possible can be visualized. A curette is then used to denude as much cartilage from the ends of the bone as possible. Access to the caudal aspects of the proximal and middle phalanges for curettage is facilitated by an assistant forcefully flexing the joint[5,8] (Fig. 5-23C).

Following removal of the articular cartilage, a shelf is made approximately 2.5 cm proximal to the joint and on the middle of the proximal phalanx. This shelf is used to seat the heads of the screws. Two or three lag screws (depending upon the size of the horse) are placed across the pastern joint, engaging as much of the middle phalanx as possible (Fig. 5-23D, E, F). Care must be taken not to drill the 3.2 mm pilot hole too far and damage the navicular bone when the drill emerges from the caudal cortex of the middle phalanx. A roughly parallel configuration of the lag screws is recommended[3] (Fig. 5-23G, H). With the avulsion fractures of the middle phalanx, care must be taken not to direct the screws into the fracture site.[2] Intraoperative radiographs are an essential part of this surgical procedure. We feel the best time to take one is following the placement of the first lag screw. Only a true lateral view need be taken. From the radiograph the surgeon will be able to note if the screw is (1) in the correct direction and engaging as much of P2 as possible and (2) of the correct length. The screw must not protrude beyond the palmar cortex of P2 and endanger the navicular bone; yet at the same time, it should engage this cortex to ensure maximum holding power. Following placement of the first screw, the remaining two or three screws are placed on either side of this screw, making the necessary adjustments in screw direction and length for them. A lateral and dorsopalmar/plantar radiograph is then taken as a final record of the arthrodesis.

We have found that it is virtually impossible to include any subcutaneous layer in the closure. For that reason, we proceed directly to closure of the skin when the joint capsule and extensor tendons have been apposed. Following closure of the wound and removal of the adhesive drapes, nonadherent dressings are applied and maintained in position with cotton gauze such as Kling. The tourniquet is released and a fiberglass/plastic combination cast is applied to the top of the proximal extremity of the metatarsus or metacarpus.

Postoperative Management

Prophylactic antibiotics are administered for 3 to 5 days. Horses usually require analgesics such as phenylbutazone for several days and sometimes for as long as 10 days. Preoperative administration of phenylbutazone is also recommended. The dose of phenylbutazone can be reduced gradually over the period of administration. If the horse begins to use his cast less well, it should be removed and the cast changed.

The horse should be kept in a clean, dry box stall, bedded with material that allows some ambulation without hindering forward mo-

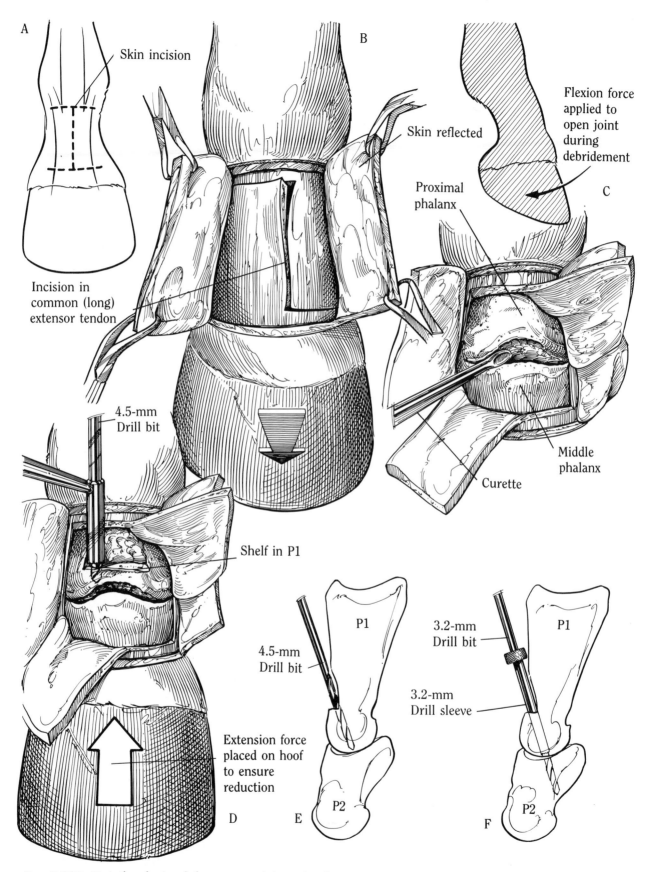

A — Skin incision

Incision in common (long) extensor tendon

B — Skin reflected

Flexion force applied to open joint during debridement

C

Proximal phalanx

Middle phalanx

Curette

4.5-mm Drill bit

Shelf in P1

Extension force placed on hoof to ensure reduction

D

E — 4.5-mm Drill bit — P1 — P2

F — 3.2-mm Drill bit — 3.2-mm Drill sleeve — P1 — P2

Fig. 5-23A–F. Arthrodesis of the pastern joint using lag screws.

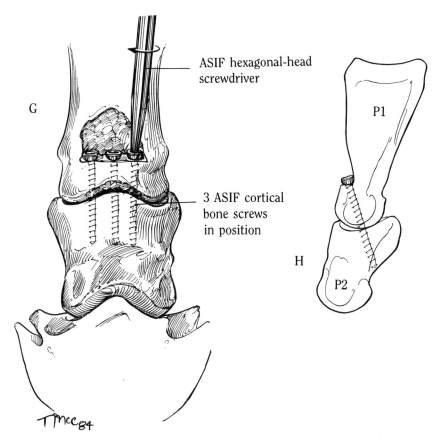

ASIF hexagonal-head
screwdriver

G

P1

3 ASIF cortical
bone screws
in position

H

P2

Fig. 5-23 (*Continued*). G, H. Arthrodesis of the pastern joint using lag screws.

tion of the cast limb. If straw is all that is available, it should be used sparingly for this reason. The limb should be kept in a cast for about six weeks. Young animals with ringbone secondary to osteochondrosis will generally show much earlier signs of fusion of the proximal phalanx to the middle phalanx than an adult horse. These cases may require less than six weeks in a cast during which time two or three changes of the cast can be anticipated. At each cast change, a radiograph will indicate the degree of fusion.

The last cast should be cut off with the horse standing and lightly tranquilized if necessary. The limb should be maintained in a pressure bandage for two to three weeks following cast removal to prevent the limb swelling that typically occurs at this time.

Comments

In our experience, the prognosis for complete return to athletic function following arthrodesis of the pastern in the hindlimb is slightly greater than 80%. Approximately 60% of horses will be sound if this joint in the forelimb is fused.[4]

Complications we have seen following this surgical procedure are distal interphalangeal degenerative joint disease (low ringbone) screw breakage, and excessive formation of callus, all of which produced continued lameness. A small number of horses exhibit toe elevation during weight bearing. We have also witnessed fracture of the small shelf created on the distal end of the proximal phalanx. The shelf must be made sufficiently high up P1 and be large enough to avoid this.[4]

The convalescence after this procedure is long, and it is unusual for the horse to become sound within one year after surgery.[4] It is also an expensive operation for most owners. It does, however, offer reasonable hope for horses that would otherwise be permanently lame or, at best, require years, if ever, for the joint to ankylose spontaneously.[2,4–6,8]

The convalescent period of certain middle phalangeal (P2) fractures can be shortened and greater stability can be achieved with the lag screw technique. This technique is limited to the middle phalangeal fracture that is not severely comminuted and has only one or both caudal eminences fractured off, as well as high ringbone. This technique essentially involves an approach similar to that described above. In some instances where the P2 fracture is severely comminuted, arthrodesis and internal fixation are performed using an ASIF T plate. Whenever possible, the lag screw technique is preferred for pastern arthrodesis because of less exposure to the coffin joint area.

References

1. Ellis, D.R., and Greenwood, R.E.S.: Six cases of degenerative joint disease of the proximal interphalangeal joint of young Thoroughbreds. Equine Vet. 17:66, 1985.
2. Gabel, A.A., and Bukowiecki, C.F.: Fractures of the phalanges. Vet. Clin. North Am. (Large Anim. Pract.), 5:233, 1983.
3. Genetzky, R.M., Schneider, E.J., Butler, H.C., and Guffey, M.M.: Comparison of two Surgical procedures for arthrodesis of the proximal interphalangeal joint in horses. J. Am. Vet. Med. Assoc. 179:464, 1981.
4. Martin, G.S., McIlwraith, C.W., Turner, A.S., et al.: Long term results and complications of arthrodesis of the proximal interphalangeal joint. J. Am. Vet. Med. Assoc. 184:1136, 1984.
5. Schneider, J.E., Carinine, B.L., and Guffy, M.M.: Arthrodesis of the proximal interphalangeal joint in the horse: A surgical treatment for high ringbone. J. Am. Vet. Med. Assoc. 173:1364, 1978.
6. Steenhaut, M., Verschooten, F., and De Moor, A.: Arthrodesis of the pastern joint in the horse. Equine Vet. J. 17:35, 1985.
7. Trotter, G.W., McIlwraith, C.W., Norrdin, R.W., and Turner, A.S.: Degenerative joint disease with osteochondrosis of the proximal interphalangeal joint in young horses. J. Am. Vet. Med. Assoc. 180:1312, 1980.
8. Turner, A.S.: Large animal orthopedic surgery. In Textbook of Large Animal Surgery (P. Jennings, ed). Philadelphia, W.B. Saunders, 1984, p. 858.

Arthrodesis of the Distal Tarsal Joints

Bone spavin is degenerative joint disease of the "low-motion joints" of the hock, usually involving the distal intertarsal and tarsometatarsal joints.[2] Occasionally the proximal intertarsal joints are involved. Typical radiographic evidence includes subchondral lysis with loss of joint space and periosteal proliferation, most commonly on the medial aspect of the hock. At Colorado State University it is a common cause of hindlimb lameness, with usually a progressive course finally rendering the horse unsuitable for its intended use. Currently, nonsurgical treatment has included rest, exercise with or without the use of nonsteroidal antiinflammatory drugs, intraarticular corticosteroids, and corrective shoeing. We are currently recommending the second option to clients who do not want surgery. We feel that continued exercise is more likely to result in spontaneous bony ankylosis of the joints and remission of lameness. This is unpredictable, however, and may take a long time (years).[2]

Arthrodesis of these joints is aimed at eliminating pain, presumably by improving joint stability. Numerous surgical techniques have been performed to achieve this in these joints, but the easiest and most practical entails destruction of the articular cartilage by means of a drill introduced on the medial side of the joints involved. Earlier reports of this technique revealed a mixed success rate. It was recommended that at least 60% of articular cartilage be destroyed.[1] Horses frequently suffered pain, lost weight, and continued to be lame. The author of a more recent report evaluating this technique encountered such a high incidence of complications that he could not recommend the procedure.[3]

We reevaluated the technique following the paper by Edwards[4] and a report on a modified technique in the United States.[6] It appears that if one is too radical in removing articular cartilage, then excessive instability occurs and results in the high morbidity observed with the previous technique. Early postoperative exercise also seems to help the convalescence.[6] We now recommend this procedure for the treatment of bone spavin, realizing that an attempt to remove all articular cartilage from these joints is not only contraindicated but is unnecessary for a successful outcome.[1]

Before surgery is attempted, a good clinical examination is indicated to rule out existing lameness. If possible, we like to see some response to intraarticular anesthesia of these joints. To place local anesthesia in this region, the most practical way is to place anesthesia into the tarsometatarsal joint, under pressure. The tarsometatarsal joint is most easily punctured plantar-laterally between the head of the 4th metatarsal and 4th tarsal bones. By forcing the anesthetic solution under pressure some may be forced into the distal intertarsal joint because of dissection of the anesthetic material through internal connective tissue spaces. This does not happen with consistency. Reliable anesthetization of the distal intertarsal joint therefore requires a separate injection. This joint is more difficult to enter and must be done from the medial side of the hock. The needle is placed through the gap between the fused first and second tarsal bone and the central tarsal bone. A 1-inch needle is placed as far proximally as possible and advanced almost to the hub so that the tip remains in the joint.

Both hocks should be radiographed, as frequently the condition is bilateral although worse in one. If both hocks are involved clinically, then we currently operate on both at the same time. Previously we felt that both hocks should be done a week apart because of the possibility that one or both of the operations will produce excessive postoperative pain, but this has not been the case. If there is radiographic evidence of disease in both hocks but the horse is lame in only one, then two options are available: both can be operated on or the lame leg can be operated or a "wait-and-see" policy adopted for the other limb.

Anesthesia and Surgical Preparation

The surgical procedure is performed under general anesthesia with the horse placed in lateral recumbency with the affected limb down or, alternatively, in dorsal recumbency. Prior to induction of anesthesia, the entire hock region of the horse is clipped if it will tolerate this; otherwise, clipping may be done when the horse is anesthetized. Following positioning of the horse on the appropriate padding (waterbed, innertubes, air mattress) the upper hindlimb is secured in such a way as to allow access to the medial side of the affected hock (when the surgery is performed in lateral recumbency). We use a leg stand and pull the uppermost limb slightly caudad to the one being operated on. Allowance also must be made for positioning of an x-ray cassette caudal to the hock, since one intraoperative radiograph will be necessary to ensure that the joints are located. We have found it useful to position the head of the x-ray machine in its approximate location to save time.

When the horse is positioned, the medial side of the hock dorsal to the chestnut is shaved and prepared for surgery in a routine manner.

An Esmarch's bandage and a tourniquet are not necessary for this operation.

Additional Instrumentation

Arthrodesis of the distal tarsal joint requires a power drill (e.g., ASIF compressed nitrogen drill, hand drill, or sterilized electric drill, 3.2-mm drill bits, and a drill guide).

Surgical Technique

After draping (sterile plastic adherent drapes are recommended for this procedure) the cunean tendon is identified by deep palpation. A 5-cm vertical skin incision is made slightly caudal to the cranial branch of the medial saphenous vein to expose the cunean tendon (Fig. 5-24A). The cunean bursa is entered, and forceps are directed under the tendon. The cunean tendon is severed, and a 1 to 2 cm

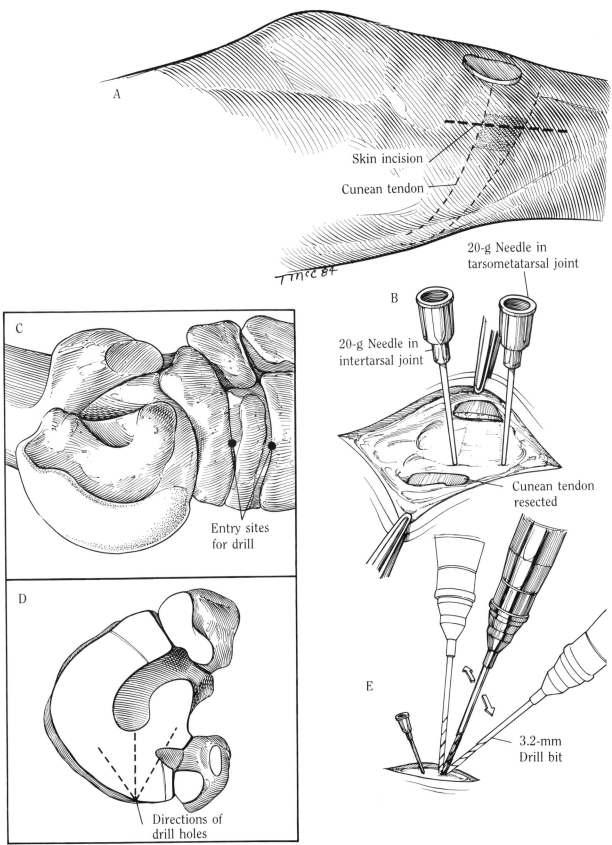

FIG. 5-24. Arthrodesis of the distal intertarsal joint and tarsometatarsal joint.

section of the tendon is removed to provide better access to the joints. The area under the tendon is probed with 20-gauge ½-inch needles to find the distal intertarsal and tarsometatarsal joints (Fig. 5-24B). With practice, the surgeon can locate the joints quickly, although if any bony exostosis exists, entry into these joints may be difficult or impossible. Even if the needle has not entered the joint, it can still function satisfactorily as a marker, especially if it is placed securely in soft tissue. A dorsopalmar radiograph is then made.

When the film has been developed, the surgeon may need to either reposition the needles and take another radiograph (if the needles had completely missed the joint) or proceed with the arthrodesis. From the radiographs not only the *location* of the needles can be checked but also their *direction*; this precaution will enable the drill to be directed *along the plane of the joint* (Fig. 5-24C).

Without disturbing the other needle, one needle is removed and the drill positioned and aligned so as to follow the plane of the joint. We currently use an ASIF 3.2-mm drill and make three drill tracks through each joint (Fig. 5-24D, E). The use of power equipment and a new sharp drill bit is strongly recommended. It is imperative that the drill remain in the joint space. Frequent cleaning of the drill bit is essential to ensure efficient cutting. If the drill hole becomes impacted with bone swarf, binding may occur and the drill bit may break. The risk of this happening is also enhanced when using old drill bits. We have broken several drill bits, but fortunately they all broke close to the skin edge and were easily retrieved with an autoclaved pair of vise grips. If the drill bit broke deep within the joint, its retrieval would be impossible. The first author (C.W.M.) has recently used a 4.5-mm drill bit; although it is more difficult to "feel" the joint space, breakage of the drill bit is less likely.

The length of each track is somewhat difficult to determine, and we feel that 2 to 3 cm depth is adequate. Again, frequent withdrawal of the drill bit and cleaning with mosquito forceps and cotton gauzes is essential. If the drill bit does emerge from outside the articular surface, a periosteal reaction may be stimulated, but no untoward sequelae have been observed.[4] The most dorsally located drill track that is directed obliquely across the cranial aspect of the joint is more likely to be overdrilled, because it is more difficult to ascertain the exact depth.[4]

The procedure is repeated on the other joint. The drill track for each joint enters through one medially located hole under the cunean tendon. Following drilling of both joints, the wound is flushed and bony debris removed. The subcutaneous tissues are closed with simple continuous sutures using a synthetic absorbable suture material of the surgeon's choice. The skin is closed with simple interrupted sutures using a synthetic monofilament nonabsorbable material. A subcuticular suture using an absorbable material can also be used,[4] but we would recommend this only if there were minimal to no tension on the skin edges at the time of closure. This latter technique obviates the need for suture removal.

A sterile nonadherent dressing is applied and held in position with cotton gauze. The entire hock is bandaged, using an elastic adhesive bandage that will adhere readily to the skin and, prevent slippage of the dressing during recovery from anesthesia. The remainder of the limb distal to the hock is wrapped with a firm pressure bandage to reduce limb swelling distal to the surgical site.

Postoperative Care

Postoperative pain is surprisingly minimal. We administer phenylbutazone immediately before and for several days after operating if the horse requires it. Most patients require 3 to 4 days of this medication. Antibiotics are not administered routinely. The limb is kept under a pressure bandage for 7 to 10 days, during which time one complete bandage change may be all that is required. Healing is typically uncomplicated despite the difficulty in maintaining constant, firm pressure over the incision.

The horse is discharged 10 to 12 days postoperatively with instructions to the owner to commence hand-walking immediately. Light riding can begin four weeks after the arthrodesis. Since no hard and fast rules can be laid down regarding exercise, we recommend a judicious approach. It is often possible to return the horse to full work at 12 days if postoperative pain is minimal. If a particular horse has more pain than usual, then we may delay the recommendation and begin handwalking by 1 to 2 weeks. Walking is begun despite a mild lameness, since it is felt that exercise hastens fusion of the joints.[1,2,4]

Comments

Arthrodesis of the tarsal joint is relatively simple, and the complications with the technique described have been low. During drilling, profuse hemorrhage has emerged occasionally from one of the drill holes. This is probably due to trauma to the proximal perforating branch of the cranial tibial artery. Although the bleeding is alarming at first glance, we have proceeded with the operation by placing a finger over the drill hole when the drill is removed for cleaning. At the end of the operation the bleeding usually subsides, and in all cases the bleeding has been inconsequential following skin closure.

Theoretically, to hasten fusion, any arthrodesis technique should involve removal of as much articular cartilage as possible to ensure maximum bony contact.[8] In the initially described technique, efforts were directed at maximum joint destruction, even to the point of "fanning" the drill bit.[3] In our opinion this is contraindicated because it appears to create severe postoperative pain. Although we have no biomechanical evidence of this, we suspect that the more radical techniques produce a greater instability to the joint. It seems that three carefully placed 3.2-mm drill holes through each joint are all that are required.

Our results agree with those of Edwards,[4] demonstrating that approximately 80% of cases will return to full function after the surgery. The time from surgery to full working soundness varies from a few weeks to a year. Surprisingly, horses have shown improvement quite soon after surgery even though it has been too early to expect bony union. Our recommendation to owners has been not to make a decision on the outcome of the surgery before 12 months.

Several modifications of this surgery do exist. These include packing the holes with cancellous bone, the use of lag screws, ASIF T plates and Steinnman pins. These are all designed to either speed fusion or provide quicker stability. From a practical standpoint the method described is simple and less expensive to the owner. If more radical drilling and removal of tissue is required, then we agree that some form of fixation (e.g., plate) is appropriate.

References

1. Adams, O.R.: Surgical arthrodesis for the treatment of bone spavin. J. Am. Vet. Med. Assoc. 157:480, 1970.
2. Adams, O.R.: Lameness in Horses, 3rd ed. Philadelphia, Lea & Febiger, 1974, p. 326.
3. Barber, S.M.: Arthrodesis of the distal intertarsal and tarsometatarsal joints in the horse: J. Vet. Surg., 13:227: 1984.
4. Edwards, G.B.: Surgical arthrodesis for the treatment of bone spavin in 20 horses. Equine Vet. J. 14:117, 1982.
5. Mackay, R.C.J., and Liddell, W.A.: Arthrodesis in the treatment of bone spavin. Equine Vet. J. 4:34, 1982.
6. Murray, E.S.: Personal communication. 1983.
7. Sack, W.O., and Orsini, P.G.: Distal intertarsal and tarsometatarsal joints in the horse: Communication and injection sites. J. Am. Vet. Med. Assoc. 179:355, 1981.
8. Turek, S.L.: Orthopedics, Principles and Their Application. Philadelphia, J.B. Lippincott, 1984.

Decompression of the Suprascapular Nerve

Paralysis of the suprascapular nerve (sweeny) results in atrophy of the supraspinatus and infraspinatus muscles. It is usually caused by direct trauma to the nerve and was frequent in draft horses with poorly fitting collars.[1] It has also been seen when there is overstretching of the nerve as may occur when the shoulder is thrust caudad when an animal slips.[1,5]

In the *acute* stage, the gait of a horse with sweeny is almost unmistakable. During the support phase of the stride there is a rapid outward excursion of the shoulder, observed best when the horse is walked toward the examiner.[1,2,8] This occurs because the infraspinatus muscle and, to a lesser degree, the supraspinatus muscle contribute to the lateral support of the shoulder. The abnormal gait is frequently seen shortly after injury. Eventually the muscles atrophy and the spine of the scapula becomes obvious. The onset of muscle atrophy is usually evident within 7 to 14 days following trauma.[2]

The outward movement of the scapula during weight bearing is believed to cause intermittent *overstretching* of the suprascapular nerve resulting in continued trauma. Additionally, scar tissue around the nerve can be responsible for the paralysis, because as the collagen in the scar tissue matures, nerve conduction is constricted and impaired.[3]

The diagnosis of suprascapular nerve paralysis should be made only after a thorough physical and radiographic examination to rule out fractures and arthritis of the shoulder region and osteochondritis dissecans (OCD) in young horses. When available, electromyography of the infraspinatus and supraspinatus muscles is helpful, particularly in the early case (before muscle atrophy) to identify denervation.

Surgical treatment is aimed at decompression of the suprascapular nerve as it passes over the cranial edge of the scapula[3] and at removal of the surrounding organizing hematoma or scar tissue (neurolysis). Reduction of the tension being exerted on the nerve is achieved by removing a piece of scapula that underlies the nerve. This procedure reduces tension on the nerve created by the abrupt change of its dissection over the cranial edge of the scapula and removes the potential for intermittent tension on the nerve during full weight bearing.[1,8]

Anesthesia and Surgical Preparation

The operation is performed with the horse in lateral recumbency with the affected limb uppermost. Prior to anesthesia, the shoulder region is clipped to reduce anesthetic time. Following induction of anesthesia the area of surgical incision (Fig. 5-25A) is shaved and routine surgical preparation is performed.

Additional Instrumentation

Decompression of the suprascapular nerve requires a wire bone saw or osteotome, a chisel, and a mallet, curettes, rongeurs, Penrose drain, tubing (e.g., ¼-inch). An air drill is helpful if available.

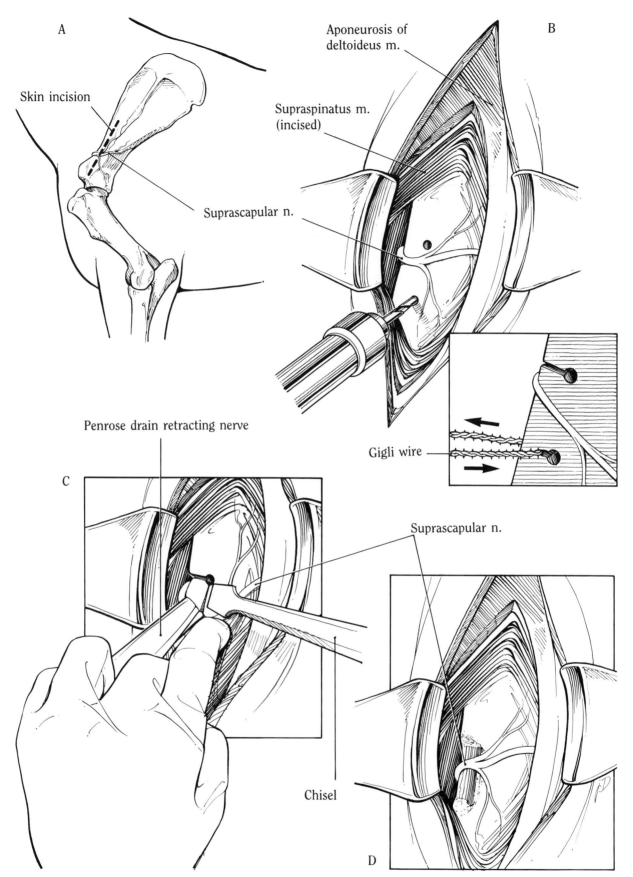

FIG. 5-25. Decompression of the suprascapular nerve for the treatment of sweeny.

192

When an osteotome is used, the ventral osteotomy should be made first to reduce the chances of creating a fracture of the supraglenoid tuberosity that could extend into the shoulder joint.[7]

Surgical Technique

After draping (the use of sterile plastic adherent drapes is recommended for this procedure), the spine of the scapula is identified. A 15-cm skin incision is made 4 cm proximal to the end of the scapular spine and 1 cm cranial to it. The dissection plane continues down to the origin of the supraspinatus muscle on the scapular spine (Fig. 5-25A). This origin is then incised 1 cm cranial to the scapular spine, and the supraspinatus muscle is reflected craniad to expose the suprascapular nerve.

Organizing hematoma or scar tissue surrounding the nerve is dissected free from the nerve as atraumatically as possible (this procedure is called external neurolysis). Hemostasis should be attended to as hemorrhage arises. All attempts should be made to reduce the inflammatory response and resultant scar tissue that will arise from healing at the surgical site.

When the external neurolysis is complete, the nerve is gently retracted by an encircling Penrose drain, and a piece of bone 1.2 × 2.5 cm lying directly under the nerve is removed using a wire saw, an osteotome, a chisel, or an air drill. If a wire saw is used, then holes should be drilled into the neck of the scapula to initiate the path for the saw cuts (Fig. 5-25B, C). The vertical component of the saw cuts can be connected by chiseling the fragment of bone away from the parent structure (Fig. 5-25C). If an osteotome is used, the vertical osteotomy should be made first to reduce the chances of creating a fracture of the supraglenoid tuberosity that could extend into the shoulder joint.[7] The defect created will have sharp edges that must be smoothed or removed with the selected use of bone curettes, rongeurs, or a burr and air drill (Fig. 5-25D). When available, an air drill with a medium fluted burr facilitates the removal of a curved piece of bone underlying the suprascapular nerve. The advantages of the burr air drill technique is that it is quicker and, with practice, safer. Since a curved piece of bone is removed instead of a rectangular piece, there is less risk of the ventral aspect of the osteotomy site fracturing into the shoulder joint.[9]

During the closure, a Penrose drain may be inserted under the supraspinatus muscle and anchored by a long horizontal mattress suture that exits near the proximal end of the incision. Subcutaneous tissues and skin are apposed in a routine manner. A stent bandage is sutured over the incision line.[1,5]

Postoperative Management

The Penrose drain is removed in 24 to 48 hours, depending on its rate of decline of exudate productivity. Hand-walking is commenced one week following surgery and increased depending on the degree of improvement shown by the horse. The stent bandage is removed 4 to 5 days after the operation. If the surgical procedure has been successful, the horse can be turned out to pasture in six weeks.

Comments

It is obvious to any student of wound healing that the surgical manipulation involved in removal of the organizing hematoma or scar tissue from around the nerve, especially dissections of the epineurium, results in re-formation of scar tissue. Theoretically, this could result in a secondary reentrapment of the nerve.[2] To avoid this, the nerve should be dissected meticulously, beginning in normal tissue, both proximally and distally if possible, so that all branches of the nerve can be identified and preserved. Dissection then progresses centripetally, exposing the region of nerve damage.[3]

It may be argued that decompression of the nerve in chronic cases would be futile. In humans, however, neurogenic muscle atrophy can be reversed in some cases if reinnervation occurs within 20 months.[4] Unfortunately no such time frames are available in horses. The limiting factor for recovery is the ability of the animal to restore the atrophied muscle. It has been recommended that exploratory decompression be performed when soft tissue healing has occurred and a "reasonable period of time" has elapsed for reinnervation of the muscle. Two to four months after the signs have appeared has been the recommended period to wait before attempting surgery.[8] One series, however, identified the earliest return to function and best end result in horses operated on *early*, after the acute swelling had decreased and muscle atrophy was first noticed.[7] Electromyography can be helpful in identification of early denervation.

Long-term results of decompression of the suprascapular nerve have been encouraging. In another series, 11 of 12 cases of sweeny improved following surgery, and although the muscle mass returned to normal in most horses, it was not uncommon for the dorsal one half of the supraspinatus muscle to remain atrophied.[7]

References

1. Stashak, T.S., (Ed.): Adams' Lameness in Horses, 5th ed. Philadelphia, Lea & Febiger, 1986.
2. Adams, O.R., et al.: A surgical approach to treatment of suprascapular nerve injury in the horse. J. Am. Vet. Med. Assoc. 187:1016, 1985.
3. Bora, F.W., and Unger, A.: The Inhibition of Scar after Tendon and Nerve Injury in Soft and Hard Tissue Repair. (T.K. Hunt et al. Eds.) Vol. 1, Surgical Science Series. New York, Praeger Scientific Publications, 1984, p. 586.
4. Leffert, R.D.: Surgery of the peripheral nerves and brachial plexus. In Current Techniques in Operative Neurosurgery. (H.H. Schmidek and W.H. Sweet Eds.) New York, Grune and Stratton, 1977.
5. Rooney, J.R.: Biomechanics of Lameness in Horses. Baltimore, Williams & Wilkins Co., 1969, p 114.
6. Schneider, R.K.: Personal communication, Phoenix, Arizona, 1985.
7. Schneider, J.E., et al.: Scapular notch resection for suprascapular nerve decompression in 12 horses. J. Am. Vet. Med. Assoc. 187:1019, 1985.
8. Stashak, T.S.: The nervous system: specific techniques. In Textbook of Large Animal Surgery. (P. Jennings Ed.) Philadelphia, W.B. Saunders, 1984, p. 1019.
9. Stashak, T.S.: Personal communication, 1985.

"Streetnail" Procedure

Infection of the navicular bursa (bursa podotrochlearis) is caused by penetration by any sharp object (e.g., nail) into the solar surface of the hoof at the middle third of the frog.[4] It also has been seen as an iatrogenic infection following injection of corticosteroids or other anti-inflammatory agents into the area of the navicular bursa.

Infection of the navicular bursa produces a very severe lameness resembling a fracture of one of the phalanges. The lameness will improve dramatically when the palmar/plantar nerves are blocked, but the horse will rarely approach complete soundness.

Radiographs are useful to rule out fractures. If a foreign body is present, it should be left in place until radiographs have been taken. They will give the clinician an indication of how close it has come to penetrating the bursa. If the tract made by the penetrating wound is still open, then injection of a suitable contrast agent up the track or insertion of a sterile metal probe also will help determine if the navicular bursa is involved. Infection of the bursa will cause radiographic changes in the navicular bone when the condition is long-standing. A diagnosis of infectious navicular bursitis is usually based on the presence of severe lameness associated with a puncture wound that has not responded to therapy. Horses with puncture wounds of the sole may respond to drainage of the wound within 24 to 48 hours. If improvement is not noticed in this time, and the wound is located in such a region of the sole that puncture of the bursa is possible, then septic navicular bursitis osteomyelitis and sepsis of the deep digital flexor tendon can occur.[4] Conservative methods of therapy are generally futile because of the location of the septic process, which will extend from the nevicular bursa into the deep digital flexor tendon and navicular bone. Surgery for infection of the navicular bursa has historically been called the penetrating "streetnail procedure" because of the cause of the infection. It consists of drainage of the bursa through a "window" cut in the frog, digital cushion, and deep flexor tendon.[1–4]

Anesthesia and Surgical Preparation

The foot is prepared by trimming the hoof with a pair of good quality nippers and a rasp. The foot is then placed in a medicated bandage and allowed to soak overnight, in preparation for surgery. The entire foot is again prepared for surgery in a routine manner following removal of this bandage. The procedure is best performed with the horse under general anesthesia with the affected limb uppermost. A tourniquet placed above the fetlock joint is essential to produce a relatively bloodless field and allow the surgeon to inspect the flexor tendon and navicular bone for damage.

Additional Instrumentation

A Stryker or similar oscillating saw or osteotome set and mallet and hoof-trimming equipment (knife, nippers, and rasp) are required.

A shoe with a removable steel plate will be necessary later in the convalescence.

Surgical Technique

A square hole is cut in the center third of the frog (Fig. 5-26A, B). In horses with a soft pliable frog a sharp scalpel will be adequate. Horses in dry parts of the country will have a very hard, tough frog and will require a Stryker or similar oscillating saw or osteotomes (Fig. 5-26C). The procedure should begin with a transverse incision through the frog at the junction of the caudal and middle third of the frog; external and perpendicular to the bearing surface of the frog. Another transverse incision is made as shown in Figure 5-26A and then connected with the first incision by two lateral incisions. The loosened portion of the frog and digital cushion are dissected free. The aperture should measure 7.5×2 cm and taper down to a smaller one as shown in Figure 5-26D. We have found that an external aperture smaller than this will result in a smaller internal aperture (in the deep flexor tendon), which will seal over and not provide adequate drainage. When the "core" of the frog and digital cushion have been removed, the condition of the deep flexor tendon will be evident. A small rectangular window is made in the deep flexor tendon, to complete the entry into the navicular bursa, by initially making two transverse incisions (Fig. 5-26E). A culture of the infected bursa should be taken at this time. Visibly obvious necrotic tendon should be removed at this point. This can result in a larger defect in the tendon. Care should be taken not to incise dorsal to the navicular bone thus injuring the distal sesamoid impar ligament, which will result in immediate entry into the distal interphalangeal (coffin) joint.

The flexor (distal) surface of the navicular bone will be visible, and its hyaline cartilage covering should be inspected by flexing and extending the distal interphalangeal joint. The defect in the frog and digital cushion should be vigorously flushed to remove tissue debris. It is then packed with gauze soaked with an antibacterial solution.

Postoperative Management

The convalescent period is long and will require almost daily attention for several weeks. Antibiotics are usually administered for one week postoperatively. Penicillin and an aminoglycoside antibiotic have been recommended.[4] Nonsteroidal antiinflammatory drugs will be required for at least a week to control pain because it is usually quite severe, at least initially. Tetanus prophylaxis must be provided.

The medicated gauze that has been placed in the defect is changed daily until a good healthy bed of granulation tissue has appeared. This will take 10 to 14 days. After this time, the dressing can be changed less frequently, depending on the amount of suppuration that is present initially. Nerve blocks may be required if the horse is very sensitive. Equally important during this time is to provide a good waterproof durable bandage around the hoof to prevent contamination of the surgical site. The horse should be kept in a clean dry stall, free of any moisture if possible.

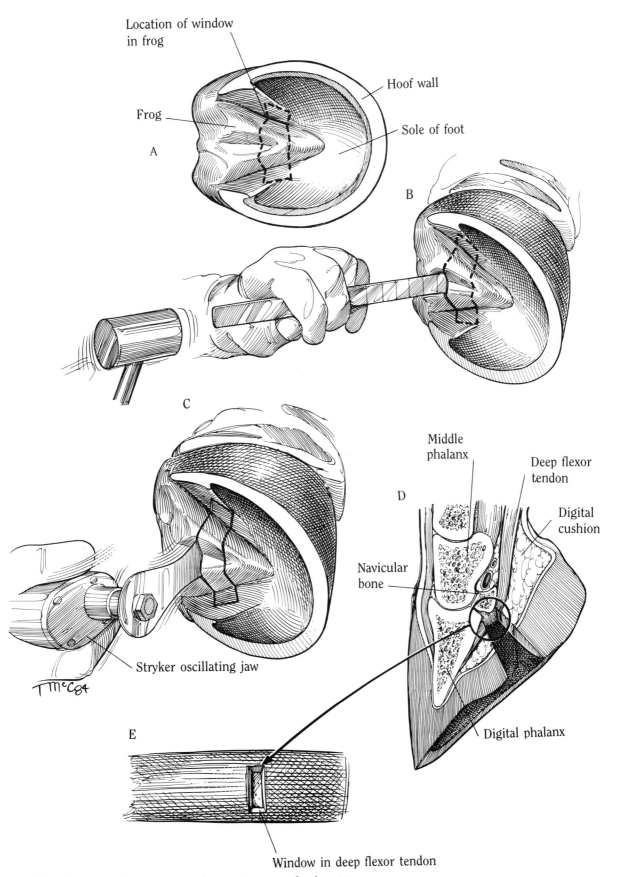

FIG. 5-26. "Streetnail" procedure for septic navicular bursitis.

When the defect has completely filled with granulation tissue and there is no evidence of fistula formation, a shoe with a removable steel plate can be applied. This will drastically reduce the amount of bandage material required to keep the foot clean and enable the horse to be turned out into a less restricted area. It is also useful in horses that do not tolerate the bandage or bandage changes well. Eventually, the regrown frog that has bridged the defect must be toughened sufficiently to allow the horse to be without the special shoe. Drying agents such as tincture of iodine are useful at this stage. Finally, a shoe with a leather pad can be applied and re-set much like a normal shoe, depending on the amount of sole growth.

Comments

The prognosis for future soundness for a penetrating wound of the navicular bursa should always be guarded to poor.[4] Frequently it is difficult to save the horse even for breeding purposes. Rotational laminitis in the opposite limb often leads to the demise of the horse. The key to success in the operation is *early* surgery as soon as penetration of the bursa is diagnosed or even suspected. The authors are aware of several cases that may have been saved if diagnosis had been made sooner. If the operation has been successful, the horse will gradually begin to put weight on the limb. It is important that nonsteroidal antiinflammatory drugs do not mask the signs of uncontrolled infection, further tissue necrosis, and overall patient deterioration. Although we recommend antibiotics, the key to success in this operation is ventral drainage of what is a "closed cavity" infection.

If the horse is still non-weight bearing some days after the operation, then continued necrosis of the deep flexor tendon and/or infectious arthritis of the coffin joint should be suspected. Development of an ascending cellulitis proximad indicates involvement of the tendon sheath and additional surgery (including drainage) should be considered. Advanced cases of tendon sheath involvement can result in rupture of the deep digital flexor tendon.[4]

References

1. Frank, E.R.: Veterinary Surgery, 7th ed. Minneapolis, Burgess Publishing Company, 1964, p. 222.
2. Guard, W.F.: Surgical Principles and Technics. Columbus, OH, W.F. Guard Publisher, 1953, p. 131.
3. Kersjes, A.W., Nemeth, F., and Rutgers, L.J.E.: Atlas of Large Animal Surgery. Baltimore, Williams & Wilkins, 1985, p. 90.
4. Richardson, G.L., O'Brien, T.R., Pascoe, J.R. et al.: Puncture wounds of the navicular bursa in 38 horses. A retrospective study. Vet. Surg. 15:156, 1986.

Surgery for Fibrotic Myopathy (After Bramlage)

Fibrotic myopathy in the horse refers to a gait abnormality that results from fibrosis of the semitendinosus muscle, with occasional involvement of the semimembranosus and biceps femoris muscles.[1,4] Fibrotic myopathy involving the gracilis muscle also has been reported,[2] and trauma with subsequent inflammation and fibrosis is considered the initiating factor.[1] External trauma can result in fibrotic myopathy, but the condition also may be work-related, particularly in Quarter Horses.[1,4] If bone forms in the affected tissues, the condition is termed ossifying myopathy.[1] Examination of case histories of 18 horses with fibrotic myopathy at our hospital revealed that 5 had developed the lameness secondary to intramuscular injections.[4] In this series all 5 had involvement of the left hindlimb, which may reflect that horses are handled from the left side and left-sided injections may have been given more commonly.[4] The condition may also be congenital.[3]

Earlier treatments described for these conditions include semitendinosus tenotomy and resection of the affected tissue, with surgical removal of restrictive adhesions.[1] This procedure was, in our practice, associated with a high incidence of complications. These complications included acute disruption of the skin incision, dehiscence of the wound during healing, prolonged hemorrhage from the wound, and necrosis under the quill sutures that were used to relieve tension across the skin incision.[4]

We have subsequently used a modified technique first described by Bramlage et al.[3] This technique entails a tenotomy of the tendinous insertion of the semitendinosus muscle. It is technically an easier procedure than partial myotenotomy and seems to be more effective in treatment of fibrotic myopathy of the semitendinosus muscle.[3]

Anesthesia and Surgical Preparation

The surgical procedure is performed with the patient under general anesthesia in lateral recumbency with the affected limb down. The area immediately caudodistal to the femorotibial joint is clipped and surgically prepared.

Surgical Technique

The semitendinosus tendon of insertion is palpated over the proximal medial tibia, caudal to the medial saphenous vein, and overlying the gastrocnemius muscle (Fig. 5-27A). An 8-cm vertical skin incision is made over the tendon, and the incision is carried through the subcutaneous and crural fascia until the tendon is exposed (Fig. 5-27B). A large forceps, such as curved Kelly or Crile forceps, is passed under the tendon to isolate it from the muscle, and the tendon is transected (Fig. 5-27C). Fascial layers are closed with interrupted synthetic absorbable sutures, and the skin is closed with interrupted nonabsorbable suture material. Tension sutures or support sutures are also recommended.

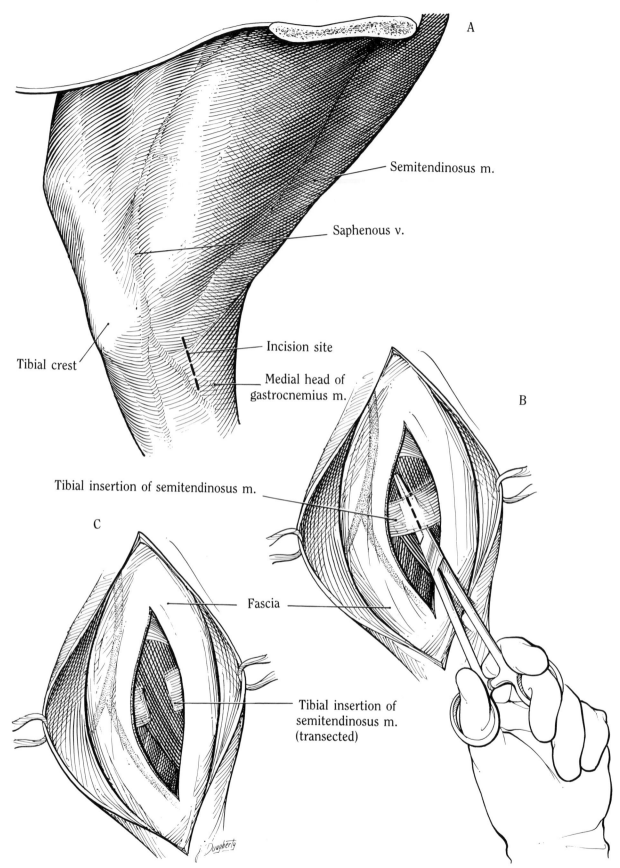

A — Semitendinosus m.

Saphenous v.

Tibial crest

Incision site

Medial head of gastrocnemius m.

B

Tibial insertion of semitendinosus m.

C

Fascia

Tibial insertion of semitendinosus m. (transected)

j. Daugherty

Fɪɢ. 5-27. Tenotomy of the tendinous insertion of the semitendinosus muscle for fibrotic myopathy.

Postoperative Management

The use of antibiotics is optional. No special treatment of the skin incision is required or recommended. The incision is too proximal to recommend pressure bandaging. Occasionally a seroma may form at the surgical site. If the seroma is large, it may require needle aspiration under aseptic conditions. Because of the high mobility of the skin in this area, partial dehiscence of the skin incision may occur, but uneventful healing by second intention usually follows. Phenylbutazone (2 to 3 g) is administered intravenously to reduce postoperative pain, although it would be ill-advised to recommend or encourage too much activity for the horse in the immediate postoperative period. Mild exercise can begin at two weeks with unrestricted exercise allowed after six weeks.[3] Skin sutures are removed 12 to 14 days after the operation.

Comments

Our initial experience with this technique was encouraging. Certainly the consequences of skin dehiscence of this smaller incision are not nearly as great as with the myotenotomy procedure previously described.[1,4] The surgical procedure is much less extensive, and there is less predisposition to re-formation of a scar that can result in recurrence of the gait abnormality.[3] However more cases must be accumulated to compare the effectiveness of this technique compared with earlier methods.

References

1. Adams, O.R.: Lameness in Horses, 3rd ed. Philadelphia: Lea & Febiger, 1974, pp. 320–322.
2. Bishop, R.: Fibrotic myopathy in the gracilis muscle of a horse. Vet. Med. Small Anim. Clin. 67:270, 1972.
3. Bramlage, L.R., Reed, S.M., and Embertson, R.M.: Semitendinosus tenotomy for treatment of congenital and acquired fibrotic myopathy in the horse. J. Am. Vet. Med. Assoc. 186:565, 1985.
4. Turner, A.S., and Trotter, G.W.: Fibrotic myopathy in the horse. J. Am. Vet. Med. Assoc. 184:335, 1984.

6

Surgery of the Upper Respiratory Tract

Prosthetic Laryngoplasty

The use of a prosthetic device for surgical correction of laryngeal hemiplegia was first described in 1970[10] and is now a time-honored technique, although various modifications are used by individual surgeons.[1,6,7,8,11,14,15,18] The principle of the technique is to place a suture or sutures between the muscular process of the arytenoid cartilage and the caudodorsal aspect of the cricoid cartilage to abduct the arytenoid cartilage and simulate the action of the paralyzed cricoarytenoideus dorsalis muscle. The technique is generally considered the best procedure to alleviate exercise intolerance and respiratory noise associated with laryngeal hemiplegia, particularly when endoscopic examination has revealed that the corniculate process of the arytenoid cartilage is displaced axially from the normal resting or intermediate position. The technique of laryngoplasty is always augmented with a ventriculectomy. If a ventriculectomy has previously been performed, the ventricle is reopened to promote the development of an arytenoid-thyroid cartilage adhesion with the arytenoid cartilage in the abducted position.

Success rates with the technique of laryngoplasty have been quoted at 80 to 90%,[7,10,14] but some authors consider the success rate to be considerably less than that.[2,3,4] It has been stated that the majority of cases have a marked improvement in respiratory capacity and that the majority of these will not produce noise during exercise,[7] but this assessment is controversial.[16] Even when the arytenoid cartilage is abducted less than desired, the success rate exceeds that of ventriculectomy alone.

Anesthesia and Surgical Preparation

A prosthetic laryngoplasty is performed under general anesthesia. The horse is placed in lateral recumbency with the affected (usually left) side up. The head and neck must be fully extended, and a pad is placed under the laryngeal region to improve the surgical presentation (Fig. 6-1A). After completion of the laryngoplasty, the horse is moved into dorsal recumbency for the laryngeal ventriculectomy.

Prior to surgery, phenylbutazone is administered to minimize laryngeal edema. Procaine penicillin is also commenced preoperatively and tetanus toxoid is administered. The neck is clipped prior to surgery, and the immediate surgical site is shaved either just before or just after induction of anesthesia.

Surgical Technique

A 10- to 12-cm skin incision is made parallel and ventral to the linguofacial vein extending rostrad from the sternomandibularis muscle (Fig. 6-1A). Electrocautery or ligation is used to control hemorrhage. The incision is continued through the fascia to establish a plane of dissection below the linguofacial vein and dorsal to the omohyoideus muscle. This plane of dissection can be continued, using finger dissection to expose the lateral aspect of the larynx with the overlying thyropharyngeus and cricopharyngeus muscles so that the cleavage plane between these two muscles can be identified (Fig. 6-1B). Malleable retractors are used dorsally to facilitate surgical exposure. Care is taken to avoid the thyrolaryngeal vascular pedicle. The fascial septum between the thyropharyngeus and cricopharyngeus muscles is then divided, using Metzenbaum scissors, to expose the muscular process of the arytenoid cartilage in the more dorsal part of the incision (Fig. 6-1C). A plane of dissection is then established in a caudal direction under the cricopharyngeus muscle. Scissors or an elevator are used to fashion a tunnel to the caudal aspect of the cricoid cartilage. Fascia over the dorsal caudal portion of the cricoid cartilage is then removed to expose the most axial portion of the cricoid cartilage. Necessary portions of the larynx are now exposed and ready for placement of the prosthetic suture.

A number of suture materials have been and can be used for the prosthesis, but the material should be nonabsorbable, and some attention to tissue reactivity is appropriate to minimize the risk of postoperative infection. The elastic material Lycra, which was initially described,[10] has been replaced by nonelastic materials by most surgeons. One of us (CWM) prefers two separately tied strands of no. 2 Mersilene, and the other (AST) prefers no. 5 Polydek (Deknatel).

Different suture configurations have been used. In many instances a single suture is placed but there is some evidence supporting the advantage to two sutures.[16] In some instances the two sutures are passed through a single hole in the muscular process, but in others they are placed through two separate holes. A technique using two sutures with the material placed through one hole in the muscular

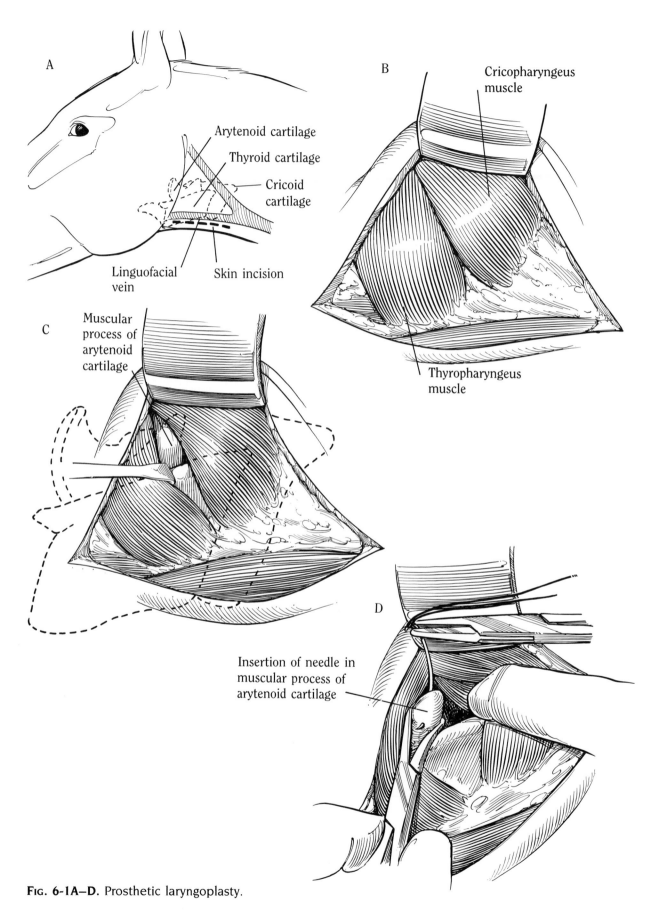

A

Arytenoid cartilage
Thyroid cartilage
Cricoid cartilage

Linguofacial vein   Skin incision

B

Cricopharyngeus muscle

Thyropharyngeus muscle

C

Muscular process of arytenoid cartilage

D

Insertion of needle in muscular process of arytenoid cartilage

FIG. 6-1A–D. Prosthetic laryngoplasty.

process first and two separate holes in the cricoid cartilage second will be described. Other surgeons place the suture in the cricoid cartilage first; these are merely differences in technique.

The first step in placement of the suture is to grasp the arytenoid cartilage below the tip of the muscular process using towel clamps and pull it up to facilitate insertion of a ½ circle needle containing the suture (Fig. 6-1D). The needle is then passed in a medial to lateral direction through the muscular process slightly rostral of center (in an attempt to maximize the part of arytenoid cartilage caudal to the suture and through which the suture has to migrate before loss of tension). A double suture strand is placed in this fashion: The suture is divided at the end of placement so that two separate strands are obtained. One end of each suture is now passed caudad under the cricopharyngeus muscle (Fig. 6-1E).

The landmark for placement of the suture in the cricoid cartilage is a notch immediately adjacent to the dorsal midline of the larynx, and this can be palpated with a finger. Placement of the suture (or one of the sutures if a double technique is used) through this area is important to mechanically achieve maximum abduction of the arytenoid cartilage. It has been shown that better abduction can be obtained with less tension if the prosthesis is anchored in the cricoid cartilage close to its dorsal spine.[16] If the prosthesis is placed too laterally, it begins to produce adduction of the vocal cord as well as inadequate abduction of the corniculate portion of the arytenoid cartilage. This is apparently related to the complex range of movement of the cricoarytenoid joint. Placement of this suture in the cricoid cartilage can be facilitated by grasping the caudolateral aspect of the larynx with a towel forceps and elevating and rotating this part laterad. Exposure of this axial portion of the cricoid cartilage may also be facilitated by extubation of the larynx at this time. The same round-bodied, ½ circle needle is threaded, and the tip is placed behind the cricoid cartilage in the region of this axial notch and carefully advanced submucosally along the inner surface of the cricoid cartilage to avoid penetration of the laryngeal mucosa (Fig. 6-1F). The cricoid cartilage is penetrated approximately 1 to 1.5 cm rostral to the caudal border. The carotid artery and the esophagus are reasonably close to the dorsal aspect of the larynx but are easily avoided if malleable retractors and the towel clamp are used. If the needle penetrates a smaller thyrolaryngeal vessel during this process, bleeding is controlled with sponges and pressure. The second suture strand is placed 8 to 10 mm lateral to the first.

The prosthetic sutures are tied using hand ties and moderate tension. Figure 6-1G illustrates the position with one suture, and Figure 6-1H the situation with two. (An alternative is to make two separate passages with the needle and suture through the muscular process of the arytenoid cartilage.) More tension is generally required to abduct the arytenoid cartilage in older patients. Neither of us uses intraoperative monitoring of abduction with an endoscope.

The incision between the thyropharyngeus and cricopharyngeus

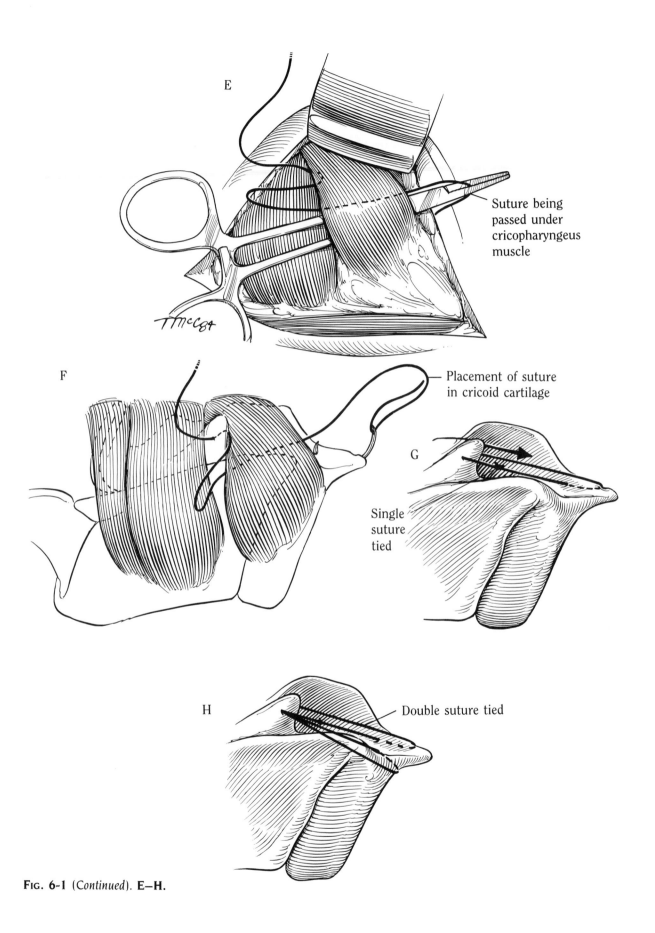

E

Suture being
passed under
cricopharyngeus
muscle

F

Placement of suture
in cricoid cartilage

G

Single
suture
tied

H

Double suture tied

FIG. 6-1 (Continued). **E–H.**

muscles is closed with a simple continuous pattern using 2/0 synthetic absorbable suture material (Fig. 6-1I). The fascia adjacent to the linguofacial vein and omohyoid muscle is reapposed using a simple continuous pattern of 0 synthetic absorbable material (Fig. 6-1J). The subcutaneous tissue is reapposed, and the skin is closed with nonabsorbable suture material using a simple interrupted pattern (Fig. 6-1J).

An alternative surgical approach to the larynx dorsal to the maxillary vein has been described.[8,10] It does give excellent access to the muscular process of the arytenoid cartilage but is a more difficult approach to the cricoid cartilage and is not recommended.

Following completion of the laryngeal prosthesis, the horse is positioned in dorsal recumbency while a laryngotomy and laryngeal ventriculectomy are performed (described in our previous text[17]). During the laryngotomy a brief check should be made to ensure that the laryngeal mucosa has not been penetrated with a prosthetic suture. If a previous ventriculectomy has been performed, the healed opening of the saccule is incised and as much mucosa removed as possible. At the completion of the ventriculectomy the laryngotomy incision is not sutured.

Postoperative Management

Procaine penicillin is continued for five days postoperatively. The laryngeal wound is cleaned twice daily, and care is taken not to contaminate the primary incision line over the laryngeal prosthesis. The animal is confined to a stall for the two to three weeks it takes for the wound to heal. After this time the horse is hand-walked. Training may be resumed eight weeks after surgery. A tracheostomy is not performed unless there is a critical or specific indication for it immediately postoperatively.

Potential Complications and Comments

Potential complications of laryngoplasty include wound dehiscence, infection of the synthetic implant, development of a chronic cough, and expulsion of food material from the nose. Wound infection and dehiscence are minimized with good technique and appropriate selection of suture material. Any dehiscence and infection would lead typically to the formation of a chronic sinus tract associated with the suture material. Dead space is left between the larynx and the fascia associated with the linguofacial vein and omohyoid muscle, but the use of a drain prophylactically is not considered appropriate. A chronic cough is generally attributed to the lateral fixation of the arytenoid cartilage and inability of the larynx to protect the trachea from the aspiration of ingesta.[5,9,10,13] Pharyngeal dysfunction associated with surgical trauma could be a factor in some instances.[5] Excessive arytenoid abduction is believed to allow retention of ingesta in the lateral food channel and passage of ingesta into the larynx during swallowing. Coughing was noticed in 26 of 68 (38%) horses in one series.[4] If nasal return of food or water occurs, it is likely due to pharyngeal dysfunction.[5]

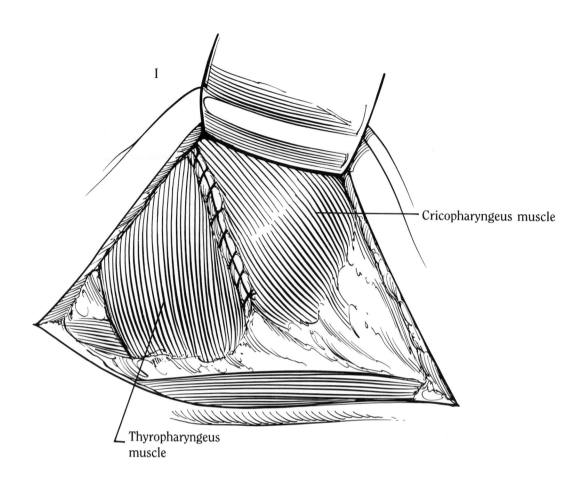

Cricopharyngeus muscle

Thyropharyngeus
muscle

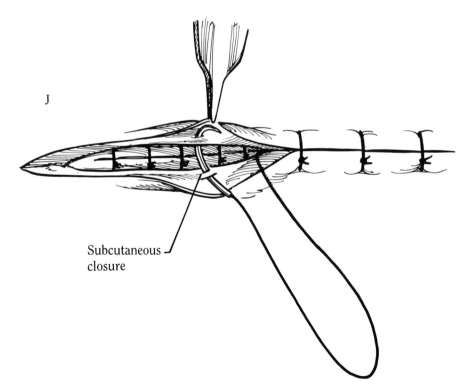

Subcutaneous
closure

FIG. 6-1 (Continued). **I, J.**

It is recognized that the suture will migrate through the laryngeal cartilage, and long-term success is dependent on some degree of permanent adhesion/fibrosis to maintain abduction after the prosthesis fails to provide tension between the arytenoid and cricoid cartilages. The placement of the suture in the muscular process of the arytenoid cartilage as far rostral as possible is one attempt to maximize the time for the suture to migrate through the cartilage. There is also a report of using a piece of Teflon between the cricoid suture and the cricoid cartilage and a buttress suture to provide forward tension to the arytenoid suture in order to minimize the migration.[4] Whether a second suture, lateral to the first, is of value is debatable.

When a laryngeal prosthesis has failed, repeating the operation is an alternative that can be successful.[13] More commonly, a partial arytenoidectomy is performed. Partial arytenoidectomy has been used by the first author as a primary treatment in some cases of laryngeal hemiplegia. Partial arytenoidectomy using a sophisticated laser technique has also been used by one surgeon as an initial surgical treatment for laryngeal hemiplegia.[12]

References

1. Baker, E.J.: Laryngeal hemiplegia in the horse. Compend. Cont. Educ. 5:S61, 1983.
2. Barber, S.M., Fretz, P.B., Bailey, J.V., and McKenzie, N.T.: Analysis of surgical treatments with selected upper respiratory tract conditions in horses. Vet. Med. 79:678, 1984.
3. Cook, W.R.: Idiopathic laryngeal paralysis in the horse; a clinical and pathological study with particular reference to diagnosis, aetiology and treatment. Ph.D. Thesis, University of Cambridge, 1976.
4. Goulden, B.E., and Anderson, L.G.: Equine laryngeal hemiplegia. Part III. Treatment by laryngoplasty. N.Z. Vet. J. 30:1, 1982.
5. Greet, T.R.C., Baker, G.J., and Lee, R.: The effect of laryngoplasty on pharyngeal function in the horse. Eq. Vet. J. 11:153, 1979.
6. Haynes, P.F.: Surgical complications in upper respiratory surgery. In Proceedings of AAEP, 1978, p. 223.
7. Haynes, P.F.: Surgery of the equine respiratory tract. In Practice of Large Animal Surgery. (P.B. Jennings, Ed.), Philadelphia, W.B. Saunders, 1984, pp. 388–487.
8. Johnson, J.H.: Laryngoplasty for advanced laryngeal hemiplegia. VM/SAC 65:347, 1970.
9. Johnson, J.H.: Complications in equine laryngeal surgery. Arch. Am. Coll. Vet. Surg. 4:9, 1975.
10. Marks, D., MacKay-Smith, M.P., Cushing, L.S., et al.: Use of a prosthetic device for surgical correction of laryngeal hemiplegia in horses. J. Am. Vet. Med. Assoc. 157:157, 1970.
11. Merriam, J.P.: Laryngoplasty—An evaluation of three abductor muscle prostheses. Proceedings of the 19th Meeting of the American Association of Equine Practitioners, 1974, pp. 123–131.
12. Montgomery, T.C.: Personal communication, 1984.
13. Raker, C.W.: Complications related to the insertion of the suture to retract the arytenoid cartilage to correct laryngeal hemiplegia in the horse. Arch. Am. Coll. Vet. Surg. 4:64, 1975.
14. Raker, C.W.: Laryngeal hemiplegia. In Equine Medicine and Surgery, 3rd ed. Santa Barbara, CA, American Veterinary Publications, Inc., 1982, p. 758.
15. Speirs, V.C.: Abductor muscle prostheses in the treatment of laryngeal hemiplegia in the horse. Aust. Vet. J. 48:251, 1972.
16. Speirs, V.C., Bourke, J.M., and Anderson, G.A.: Assessment of the efficacy of an abductor muscle prosthesis for treatment of laryngeal hemiplegia in horses. Aust. Vet. J. 60:294, 1983.
17. Turner, A.S., and McIlwraith, C.W.: Techniques in Large Animal Surgery. Philadelphia, Lea & Febiger, 1982.
18. Wheat, J.D.: Surgery of the larynx. Am. Coll. Vet. Surg. Forum, 1980.

Partial Arytenoidectomy

Partial arytenoidectomy is indicated to increase the effective airflow through the larynx in cases of chondritis or chondroma of the arytenoid cartilage(s) or ossification of the laryngeal cartilages.[1-6,8,9] It is also indicated in cases of laryngeal hemiplegia that have not responded to the conventional treatments of laryngoplasty and ventriculectomy. It is also indicated, in some surgeons' opinions, in lieu of laryngoplasty to avoid (1) the postoperative side effects such as aspiration of ingesta and coughing or (2) the short-lived effectiveness of laryngoplasty in athletic horses that has been the experience of some surgeons.[3] Currently, the most common indication is chondritis of the arytenoid cartilage. The object of partial arytenoidectomy is to remove the diseased portion of the arytenoid cartilage to improve the aerodynamics of the larynx. It has been stated that it is desirable to leave some of the corniculate process intact (if not obviously abnormal) to add stability and facilitate effective closure of the laryngeal orifice during swallowing.[4] However, the real need to retain any portion of the corniculate cartilage is still uncertain. We feel that if epiglottic function is normal, it is doubtful that the rima glottidis or caudal commissure of the larynx needs to be completely sealed upon adduction.

In the method described here the corniculate process is completely removed and the technique is intended to provide maximum diameter of the airway. The muscular process and articular facet (articulation with the cricoid cartilage) of the arytenoid cartilage are left intact.

The use of ventriculectomy with focal excision of intraluminal lesions has been described as a moderately successful and transiently effective means of treating mild cases of arytenoid chondritis.[1] Although rest from exercise may be sufficient to cause regression of the lesion, resumption of athletic stress most certainly will cause further irritation and consequently recurrence, and any conservative management is generally temporary. When there is any degree of luminal compromise and exercise ability is necessary, the arytenoidectomy technique is recommended. Partial arytenoidectomy is used both as an attempt to return a racing animal to athletic performance and also as a salvage procedure in other cases where the extent of the condition compromises the patient's ability to breathe, even at rest. Bilateral arytenoidectomy can be performed as a single procedure in cases of bilateral chondritis. An alternative is to perform a unilateral arytenoidectomy on the most severely affected side, as this can be effective in returning some horses to racing.

Anesthesia and Surgical Preparation

Partial arytenoidectomy is performed through a laryngotomy incision with the horse positioned in dorsal recumbency. Inhalation anesthesia is administered by an endotracheal tube placed through a midcervical tracheostomy incision (Fig. 6-2A). When there is obstruction of the rima glottidis, preoperative placement of a tracheostomy tube

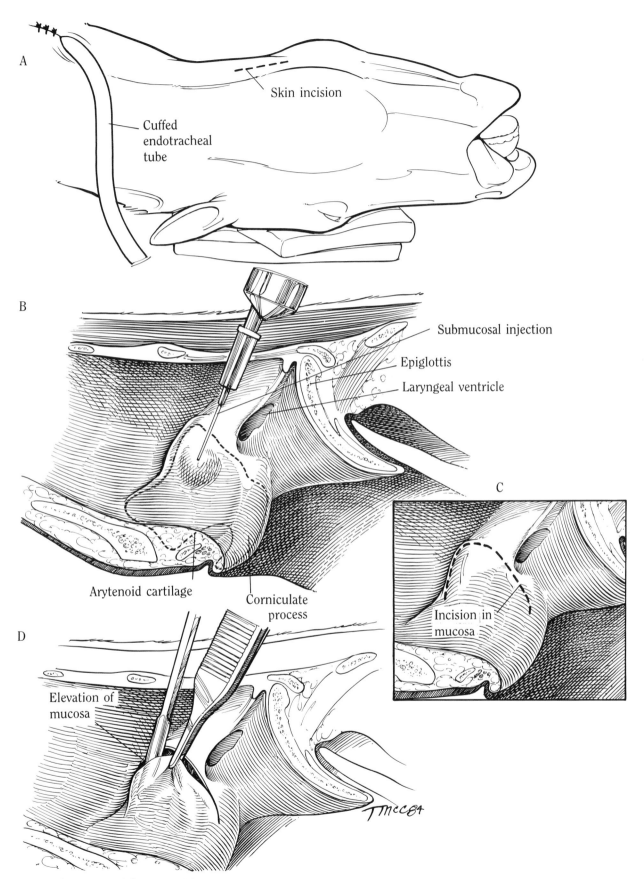

Fig. **6-2A–D.** Partial arytenoidectomy.

may be necessary. In patients without respiratory compromise at rest, the tracheostomy is performed immediately following induction of anesthesia. Prior to surgery, patients are administered phenylbutazone, perioperative antibiotics such as procaine penicillin, and tetanus toxoid. The area of the neck is clipped. Final preparation of the surgical site is performed after induction of anesthesia.

Surgical Technique

Directly following induction of anesthesia the midcervical region is surgically prepared quickly, a tracheostomy is performed between the tracheal rings,[7] and a cuffed endotracheal tube is inserted (Fig. 6-2A). The laryngotomy site is then aseptically prepared for the operation.

A ventral laryngotomy is performed.[7] Extension of the laryngotomy by splitting the thyroid cartilage and the cricoid cartilage is not considered necessary.[1] The use of two Weitlaner retractors can assist in providing maximum exposure. A submucosal injection of 1:10,000 epinephrine to help control oozing and assist in elevation of the mucous membrane during the operation may be made at this time (Fig. 6-2B). However, it has minimal effectiveness when there is extensive chondritis and adhesion of the laryngeal mucosal membrane to the arytenoid cartilage and is not used by us. The lines of incision in the mucosa depend on the nature of the lesion. If healthy, intact muscosa is present, an incision may be made through the mucosa along the ventral free border of the arytenoid cartilage and continued along the caudal border of the cartilage to below the articular facet (Fig. 6-2C). When there is active sepsis and involvement of significant mucosa over the cranial portion of the body of the arytenoid cartilage (the common situation in our experience) an H-type incision is made and the central portion of mucosa is removed (Fig. 6-2E). Undermined mucosa from over the corniculate portion is later retracted caudad to fill the defect. This technique is now favored by the first author for all cases and is illustrated in Figs. 6-2E–J.

The mucous membrane over the luminal side of the arytenoid cartilage is then dissected away with a nasal or periosteal elevator (Figs. 6-2D, F). The dissection is continued forward over the corniculate portion. All efforts are made to keep the mucosa intact, but it is easily disrupted in regions of pathologic change. In minor cases, a suture is used to obliterate the hole; in more involved cases, the mucosal sliding technique is necessary. When the mucosa has been freed from the luminal side of the involved arytenoid cartilage, the lateral surface of the cartilage is dissected free of the soft tissues (vestibularis, vocalis and cricoarytenoideus lateralis muscles and lateral ventricle) using scissors (Fig. 6-2G). Dissection around the corniculate portion is completed. The arytenoid cartilage is then grasped with towel forceps and retracted in a rostral direction to enable separation of the cartilage immediately below the level of the muscular process and articular facet. This separation usually requires heavy scissors. Retraction is continued in a rostral direction while the remaining soft tissue attachments along the dorsal surface of the arytenoid cartilage are divided with scissors to complete removal of the

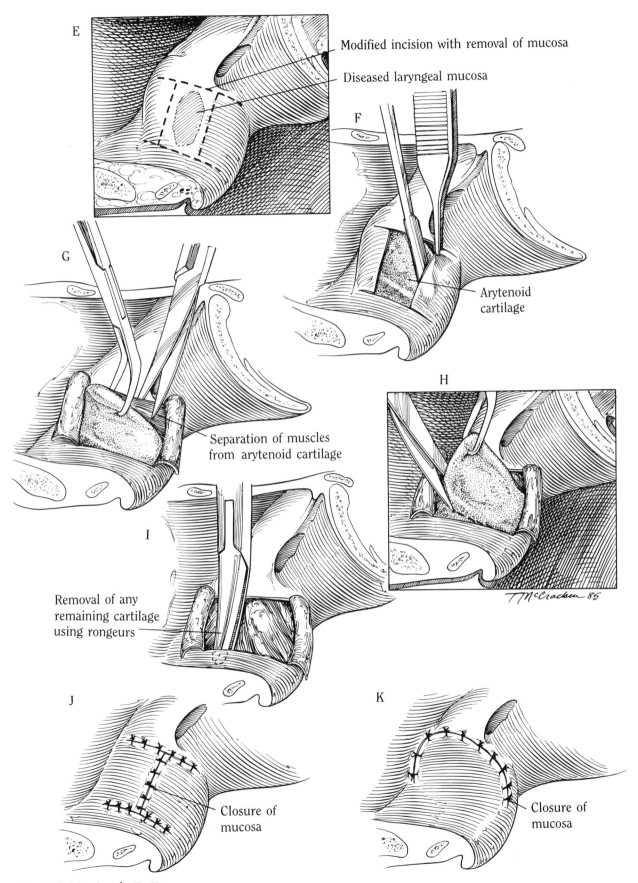

E

Modified incision with removal of mucosa

Diseased laryngeal mucosa

F

Arytenoid cartilage

G

Separation of muscles from arytenoid cartilage

H

I

Removal of any remaining cartilage using rongeurs

T. McCracken 85

J

Closure of mucosa

K

Closure of mucosa

FIG. 6-2 (Continued). **E–K.**

arytenoid cartilage (Fig. 6-2H). The latter maneuvers may involve removal of the arytenoid cartilage in more than one portion. Any remaining cartilage in the dorsal portion of the larynx can be removed with a set of rongeurs (Fig. 6-2I). Following removal of the arytenoid cartilage, the lateral ventricle on that side is also removed. An alternative is to remove it at the beginning of the procedure. The mucosal incision is then closed in a simple interrupted pattern using 3/0 polyglactin 910 (Vicryl) with a small half-inch swaged on taper point circle needle. Figures 6-2J and 6-2K illustrate the two alternative techniques of closure used depending on the initial mucosal incisions made. The ventral laryngotomy incision is allowed to heal by second intention.

Postoperative Management

A tracheotomy tube is secured in place during recovery. This tube is left in place for three to five days depending on the patency of the laryngeal airway. Moderate swelling of the intraluminal surgical site can be anticipated to reach a maximal extent at 48 to 72 hours postoperatively.[2] Phenylbutazone and a suitable antibiotic such as procaine penicillin are continued for five days postoperatively. Feeding is resumed 12 hours postoperatively. Sequential endoscopic examinations are performed to assess the airway. Some dehiscence of the suture line may occur, particularly when there has been marked compromise of the mucosa. These sites will heal, however, generally without complication. The surgical site should appear excellent endoscopically at 45 to 60 days.

Comments

The rationale that has been proposed for leaving the corniculate cartilage intact (subtotal arytenoidectomy) is to protect the laryngeal lumen from aspiration of ingesta.[4] It is considered that this cartilage will be held laterally with fibrosis. However, as presented above, removal of the corniculate cartilage has also produced good results in our experience and allows maximal use of the mucosa for closure when the "H" incision is used. It is also important to note that one should not be overly concerned about the immediate postoperative appearance of the surgical site, since this will be improved considerably on subsequent examinations.

Subtotal arytenoidectomy has also been performed using CO_2 laser combined with an operating microscope and microsurgical instruments.[3] This technique emphasizes hemostasis, reduced surgical trauma, and primary closure of the entire surgical wound. The primary tissue benefits achieved are more rapid healing and improved tissue function due to decreased scarring. We think the technique is a progressive step to be emulated, but it requires specialized equipment as well as specialized training.

References

1. Haynes, P.F.: Surgery of the equine respiratory tract. In Practice of Large Animal Surgery. (P.B. Jennings, Ed.) W.B. Saunders, Philadelphia, 1984, p. 388.

2. Haynes, P.F., Snyder, T.G., McClure, J.R., and McClure, J.J.: Chronic chondritis of the equine arytenoid cartilage. J. Am. Vet. Med. Assoc. 177:1135, 1980.
3. Montgomery, T.C.: Personal Communication, 1985.
4. Raker, C.W.: The arytenoid cartilages. In Equine Medicine and Surgery, 3rd ed. (R.A. Mansmann, E.S. McAllister, and P.W. Pratt, Eds.) Santa Barbara, CA, American Veterinary Publications, Inc., 1982, p. 766.
5. Shapiro, J., White, N.A., Schlafer, D.H., and Rowland, G.N.: Hypertrophic ossification of the laryngeal cartilages of a horse. J. Eq. Med. Surg. 3:320, 1979.
6. Trotter, G.W., Aanes, W.A., and Snyder, S.P.: Laryngeal chondroma in a horse. J. Am. Vet. Med. Assoc. 178:829, 1981.
7. Turner, A.S., and McIlwraith, C.W.: Techniques in Large Animal Surgery. Philadelphia, Lea & Febiger, 1982.
8. Wheat, J.D.: Surgery of the larynx. Am. Coll. Vet. Surg. Surgical Forum, Chicago, 1980.
9. White, N.A., and Blackwell, R.B.: Partial arytenoidectomy in the horse. Vet. Surg. 9:5, 1980.

Surgical Relief of Epiglottic Entrapment

Epiglottic entrapment is the envelopment of the apex and lateral margins of the epiglottis by the arytenoepiglottic folds.[4] The condition has also been referred to as hyperplasia of the ventral epiglottic mucosa.[2] The arytenoepiglottic folds extend from the lateral aspect of the arytenoid cartilage to the ventrolateral aspect of the epiglottis. It has been noted recently that this fold of respiratory mucosa is continuous with the glossoepiglottic fold in the subepiglottic area and that the latter also contributes to the entrapping tissue.[4] Surgical removal (or at least, surgical sectioning) of this abnormally placed tissue is indicated when the condition is compromising respiratory capacity. It is to be noted that horses can race successfully with an entrapped epiglottis and that epiglottic entrapment has been found as an *incidental endoscopic finding* in horses with neither decreased exercise tolerance nor abnormal respiratory noise.[9]

Recently, unhooking or splitting of the entrapped tissue using a long curved hooked instrument per nasum under direct endoscopic visualization has become popular at race tracks. The resection technique described here is now generally performed when the former methods have been unsuccessful.

Preoperative radiographs of the pharyngeal region with specific measurements of the epiglottis are recommended prior to selecting a case for surgery. Short thyroepiglottic lengths have been found in animals with epiglottic entrapment, as well as with dorsal displacement of the soft palate.[7] The prognosis is decreased in such cases.[4,5] The length of the epiglottic cartilage can be predicted from a lateral radiograph by measurement from the body of the thyroid cartilage to the tip of the epiglottis (thyroepiglottic length). For effective radiographic demonstration of the epiglottis, both the introduction of air into the oral cavity as a negative contrast medium[7] and the use of a pharyngogram with positive contrast material[4] have been described. Thyroepiglottic length in healthy Thoroughbreds is 8.76 ± 0.44 cm.[7] In a series of 9 Thoroughbreds with epiglottic entrapment the thyroepiglottic length was 6.59 ± 0.33 cm.[7] It is important that a shortened epiglottis be recognized prior to surgery so that the client is aware that the prognosis is less favorable than when the epiglottis is apparently normal.[1,4]

Both the oral cavity and a ventral pharyngotomy have been used as approaches for operations on epiglottic entrapment.[1,10] The arytenoepiglottic folds have been either trimmed or simply incised when the oral approach is used, but the technique is less reliable than removal of the entrapped tissue via laryngotomy. The ventral pharyngotomy approach involves more extensive surgery (technique illustrated separately) and is not considered to have any advantages over the laryngotomy technique.[8,10] Resection of the arytenoepiglottic folds by ventral laryngotomy is the preferred technique and the one described here. It is considered to be the most effective, and good visualization is achieved.

Anesthesia and Surgical Preparation

The horse is placed under general anesthesia in dorsal recumbency. Intravenous anesthesia has been used as a sole anesthetic agent,[4] but inhalation anesthesia with the tube withdrawn at the time of surgical removal of the entrapping tissue is used more commonly. If a prolonged or difficult surgical procedure is anticipated, prior placement of the endotracheal tube through a midcervical tracheostomy (described with arytenoidectomy) is an alternative.

Phenylbutazone, preoperative antibiotics such as procaine penicillin, and tetanus toxoid are administered preoperatively. The ventral pharyngeal/laryngeal area is clipped prior to the operation.

Surgical Technique

A ventral laryngotomy is performed.[11] The epiglottis and entrapping arytenoepiglottic folds lie rostral and deep to the laryngotomy incision (Fig. 6-3A). An index finger is inserted down and hooked around the lateral edge of the epiglottis to help bring it up toward the laryngotomy incision. At this time a pair of sponge forceps or Allis tissue forceps are inserted and manipulated with the other hand to grasp the entrapping tissue near the apex of the epiglottis. Traction is then used to evert the apex of the epiglottis (it will come with the entrapping fold because of its attachment to the ventral surface of the epiglottis) into the laryngotomy opening (Fig. 6-3B, C). The arytenoepiglottic folds are then removed with scissors (Fig. 6-3C, D). Only the central portion of the fold is excised rather than a complete excision from the margins. Figure 6-3B illustrates an axial "notching" incision commencing on one side and extending across to the opposite side. Some authors feel that resection of the entire fold can potentiate epiglottic dysfunction and the development of dorsal displacement of the soft palate.[2,6] Care is also taken that the incision line is at least 5 to 10 mm away from the junction of the arytenoepiglottic fold with the epiglottis to ensure that the epiglottic mucosa or cartilage is not traumatized. Such damage could potentially lead to granuloma formation. As the entrapping folds are removed, the epiglottis will return to its normal position. The laryngotomy is left to heal by second intention.

Postoperative Management

The laryngotomy wound is cleaned once or twice daily until it has healed (two to three weeks). When it is healed, hand-walking can be performed, but no training is initiated for at least four to six weeks. Endoscopic examination prior to this is recommended.

Comments

In an early report for surgical treatment of this condition, 8 out of 9 horses operated on returned satisfactorily to training, racing, or pleasure work.[1] Since that time a number of complications to the operation have been recognized including dorsal displacement of the soft

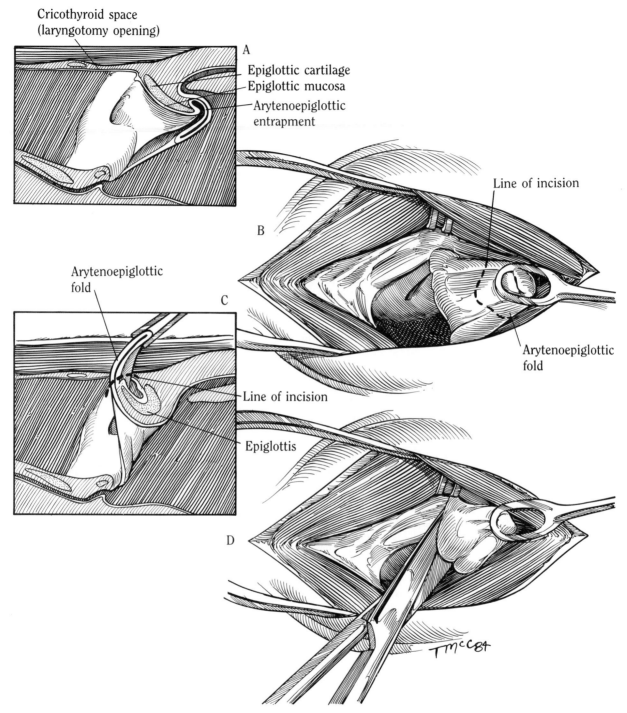

Cricothyroid space
(laryngotomy opening)

Epiglottic cartilage
Epiglottic mucosa
Arytenoepiglottic
entrapment

Line of incision

Arytenoepiglottic
fold

Arytenoepiglottic
fold

Line of incision

Epiglottis

Fig. 6-3. Surgical relief of epiglottic entrapment.

palate, re-entrapment of the epiglottis, and granuloma formation on the epiglottis.[3]

The most common postoperative complication associated with surgical removal of epiglottic entrapment is the development of dorsal displacement of the soft palate postoperatively.[4,5] The relationship of dorsal displacement of the soft palate to epiglottic entrapment and epiglottic shortening has been documented, and it is considered that dorsal displacement of the soft palate will occur with higher frequency in epiglottic entrapment cases when the epiglottis is hypoplastic or shortened.[5,7] The occurrence of dorsal displacement of the soft palate postoperatively may be associated simply with the inadequate ability of a smaller epiglottis to retain the soft palate in its correct position. It has been suggested that a shortened epiglottis may allow the soft palate to separate from the larynx easily, whereas an entrapped hypoplastic epiglottis presents a larger contact area to retain the soft palate in position.[8] It has also been suggested that there could be impairment of epiglottic function as a result of its distorted position during its entrapment.[1,4] More recently, it has been suggested that excessive formation of subepiglottic scar tissue associated with excessive removal of arytenoepiglottic fold tissue may prevent proper reflection of the epiglottis and promote dorsal displacement of the soft palate.

Postoperative dorsal displacement of the soft palate (DDSP) may resolve spontaneously in 10 to 14 days,[4] or it may persist. If the condition does persist, surgical intervention to correct the dorsal displacement of the soft palate should be considered but is frequently unrewarding. Because of the frequency of DDSP as a sequel to the epiglottic entrapment operation, trimming of the soft palate at the same time as the epiglottic entrapment is corrected has been recommended.[7] It is the clinical impression of one experienced surgeon that this improves the success rate.[8] It is now suggested that removal of less tissue at the time of the entrapment operation is more the key in preventing the problem (assuming a normal epiglottic length).[6] The use of the more recently described technique of myectomy of the sternohyoid and omohyoid muscles may be preferable (this technique is described separately in this text). If DDSP is recognized preoperatively, it would be appropriate to perform the myectomy concurrently with the operation on the entrapped epiglottis. One author reports that in an uncomplicated entrapment (normal epiglottic size and no evidence of DDSP) the success rate may approach 75%.[4] In patients with concurrent DDSP or in those predisposed to DDSP because of a short epiglottis (7 cm or less), the success rate may not exceed 50%.[4]

Re-entrapment may also occur as a postoperative complication. Although it may be suggested that an adequate amount of tissue had not been resected, the situation has occurred in animals following consistent technique.[3] Granuloma formation characterized by tissue proliferation in the area of the epiglottis (probably from excessive tissue resection) has also been seen as a complication. Resection of any such masses generally carries a poor prognosis.

The suggestion that excessive tissue resection can promote epiglottic dysfunction and DDSP has been mentioned previously. Evidence has been provided that sectioning of the entrapment without excessive tissue removal may improve results.[6] The results of a new technique of electrosurgical sectioning of 5 entrapments via endoscopy have been encouraging.[6] It has been suggested that unsuccessful results with a cutting hook may be explained by the entrapment not being completely incised but rather being pulled off so that it later re-entraps. It would seem at this stage that removal of less rather than more tissue (no matter what the method) is appropriate.

References

1. Boles, C.L., Raker, C.W., and Wheat, J.D.: Epiglottic entrapment by arytenoepiglottic folds in the horse. J. Am. Vet. Med. Assoc. 172:338, 1978.
2. Cook, W.R.: Some observations on form and function of the equine upper airway in health and disease. Larynx. Proceedings 27th Annual Convention of the American Association of Equine Practitioners, 1981, pp. 393–451, 1982.
3. Haynes, P.F.: Surgical failures in upper respiratory surgery. Proceedings of the 24th Annual Convention American Association Equine Practitioners, 1978, p. 223, 1979.
4. Haynes, P.F.: Surgery of equine respiratory tract. In The Practice of Large Animal Surgery. (P.B. Jennings, Ed.) Philadelphia, W.B. Saunders, 1984.
5. Haynes, P.F.: Dorsal displacement of the soft palate and epiglottic entrapment: Diagnosis, management and interrelationship. Comp. Cont. Educ. 5:S379, 1983.
6. Jann, H.W., and Cook, W.R.: Transendoscopic electrosurgery for epiglottal entrapment in the horse. J. Am. Vet. Med. Assoc. 187:484–492, 1985.
7. Linford, R.L., O'Brien, T.R., Wheat, J.D., and Meagher, D.M.: Radiographic assessment of epiglottic length and pharyngeal and laryngeal diameters in the Thoroughbred. Am. J. Vet. Res. 44:1660, 1983.
8. Raker, C.W.: The epiglottis. In Equine Medicine and Surgery, 3rd ed. (R.A. Mansmann and E.S. McAllister) Santa Barbara, CA, American Veterinary Publications, 1982.
9. Raphel, C.F.: Endoscopic findings in the upper respiratory tract of 479 horses. J. Am. Vet. Med. Assoc. 181:470, 1982.
10. Speirs, V.C.: Entrapment of the epiglottis in horses. J. Eq. Med. Surg. 1:267, 1977.
11. Turner, A.S., and McIlwraith, C.W.: Techniques in Large Animal Surgery. Philadelphia, Lea & Febiger, 1982.

Myectomy of the Sternohyoid, Sternothyroid, and Omohyoid Muscles

Myectomy is a simple procedure that hardly fulfills the criterion for an "advanced technique" but is described here because it is not presented in our previous textbook of basic techniques. The rationale behind this procedure is based on the concept of *laryngopalatal subluxation* in the pathogenesis of the majority of the cases of dorsal displacement of the soft palate.[1,5] It has been suggested that excessive contraction of the sternothyrohoid and omohyoid muscles during forced inspiration might lead to an overretraction of the larynx resulting in laryngopalatal subluxation.[1] The hypothesis also correlates with the observed movements of the larynx during forced inspiration induced by nasal occlusion.[5] The sternothyroid and sternohyoid muscles originate on the cartilage of the manubrium and extend along the ventral aspect of the neck to insert upon the thyroid cartilage of the larynx and the basihyoid bone. The omohyoid muscle originates from subscapular fascia and inserts on the basihyoid bone. The abnormally vigorous contraction of these muscles may be a reaction in a horse that is suffering from other respiratory disease or may be the result of overaction or spasm of the muscle in a normal horse caused by nervous excitement when a willing horse is suddenly asked to give its best.[1]

It has been suggested that myectomy of the omohyoid and sternothyrohyoid muscles close to their insertion may prevent laryngeal retraction that results in dorsal displacement of the soft palate.[5] In a preliminary trial on 21 horses it was shown that 17 of them (71%) were benefited by the operation.[2] The actual value of the myectomy is somewhat controversial, but we consider that it offers a relatively benign initial treatment for dorsal displacement of the soft palate. The operation can be performed while the horse is standing, and the horse can be continued in training. This procedure has some advantages over the staphylectomy, which has its own potential complications and requires a longer period of convalescence.

Anesthesia and Surgical Preparation

A myectomy can be performed with the horse in the standing position with its head elevated to place some tension on the ventral cervical muscles and facilitate their identification. If the operation is being done in conjunction with another procedure, such as relief of epiglottic entrapment, it will be performed under general anesthesia. The proximal half of the neck is clipped. We use a surgical site just caudal to the larynx in the cranial portion of the neck in order that the axial portion of the omohyoid muscle can be removed as well as the sternothyroid and sternohyoid muscles. If the surgery is performed while the horse is standing, the patient is sedated. Local anesthesia is administered in the form of a "U-block."

Surgical Technique

A 12- to 15-cm midline incision is made from the caudal border of the larynx distad (Fig. 6-4A). This incision is continued through the subcutaneous tissue to expose the paired sternohyoid muscles. Dissection is continued between the muscle bellies on the midline using scissors until the trachea is reached, and then finger dissection is used in a lateral direction to undermine this musculature as well as the axial portion of the omohyoid muscle that borders on the sternohyoid muscle (Fig. 6-4B). Once the sternohyoid and central portion of the omohyoid muscles are undermined, they are incised at the proximal and distal portions of the incision so that a 10-cm portion is removed in the stretched position (Fig. 6-4C). The transecting incisions are made with a blade and continue into the omohyoid muscle until close to the jugular groove. They are not extended beyond this because of the risk of damaging vital structures. This procedure is repeated on the opposite side to leave the thin, straplike sternothyroid muscles lying against the trachea on either side (Fig. 6-4D). A similar segment is also transected from these. A quarter-inch (1 cm) Penrose drain is then placed across the incision as illustrated in Figure 6-4E, and the subcutaneous fascia is closed, using a simple continuous suture of 2/0 polyglactin 910 (Vicryl). The skin is closed with simple interrupted sutures of nonabsorbable material (2/0 nylon), and a stent bandage of rolled gauze (e.g., Kling) is sutured over the incision.

Postoperative Management

The Penrose drain is removed at five days, and the stent bandage is removed at the same time. Sutures are removed 12 to 14 days following surgery. Training can be resumed at this stage.

Comments

A number of surgeons using this technique have limited their muscle resection to the sternohyoid and sternothyroid muscles.[3] This technique has less potential for hemorrhage and seroma formation. The additional resection of the axial portion of the omohyoid muscle is an attempt to nullify any potential retraction action of this muscle. While it is recognized that the more lateral portions of the muscle are necessarily left intact, the muscle fibers run obliquely, and it is thought that some effect of the muscle is negated by transection of the axial portion. These opinions are, however, subjective.

Opinions vary on the success rate of this procedure, but it does appear to have an overall success approaching that of partial resection of the soft palate.[3] Raker has reported on horses failing to respond to staphylectomy that have responded favorably to myectomy.[7] The advantages of the procedure are that it can be performed in the standing patient, and the results of the procedure can be evaluated upon return to work within 2 weeks following the myectomy. It is to be recognized that DDSP is the most nebulous of the upper respiratory tract lesions and the treatment is correspondingly so.

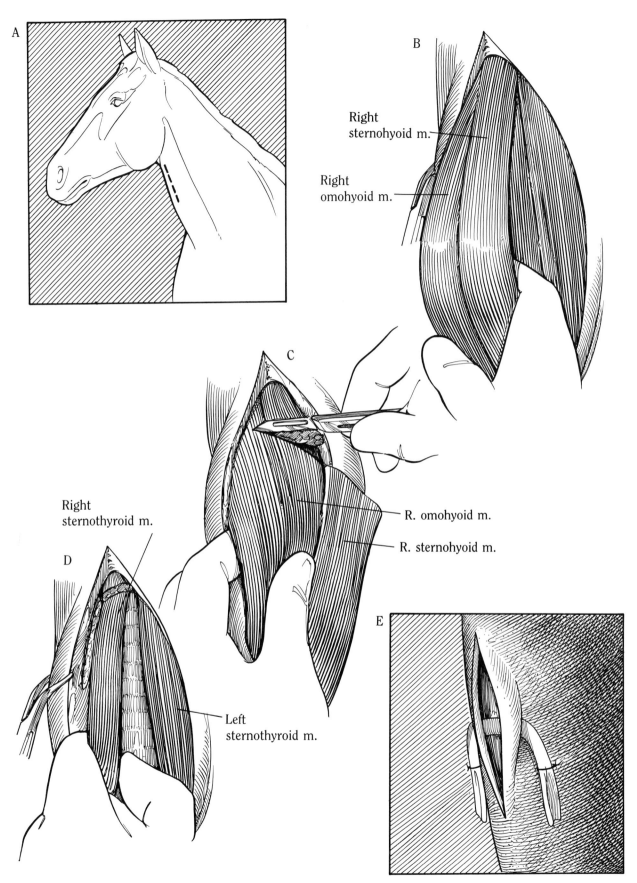

A

B

Right
sternohyoid m.

Right
omohyoid m.

C

R. omohyoid m.

R. sternohyoid m.

D

Right
sternothyroid m.

Left
sternothyroid m.

E

FIG. 6-4. Sternohyoid, sternothyroid, and omohyoid myectomy.

It is also to be noted that dorsal displacement of the soft palate may be associated with significantly shortened thyroepiglottic lengths [6.43 ± 0.4 cm compared to the normal of 8.76 ± 0.44 cm in 24 healthy Thoroughbreds[6]]. Displacement of the soft palate associated with epiglottic shortening does not carry a good prognosis, and the value of the myectomy in these cases is questioned.[4] In these cases it has been suggested that partial resection of the soft palate is the initial procedure of choice in that it may reduce the bulk of tissue that obstructs the airway.[4]

References

1. Cook, W.R.: Some observations on form and function of the equine upper airway in health and disease: I The Pharynx. *In* Proceedings 27th Annual Convention of the American Association of Equine Practitioners in 1981. 1982, p. 5.
2. Cook, W.R., and Chandler, N.: Unpublished material, 1977.
3. Haynes, P.F.: Surgery of the equine respiratory tract. *In* The Practice of Large Animal Surgery. (P.B. Jennings, Ed.) Philadelphia, W.B. Saunders, 1984.
4. Haynes, P.F.: Persistent dorsal displacement of the soft palate associated with epiglottic shortening in two horses. J. Am. Vet. Med. Assoc. 179:677, 1981.
5. Heffron, C.J., and Baker, G.J.: Observations on the mechanism of functional obstruction of the nasopharyngeal airway in the horse. Eq. Vet. J. 11:142, 1979.
6. Linford, R.L., O'Brien, T.R., Wheat, J.D., and Meagher, D.M.: Radiographic assessment of the epiglottic length and pharyngeal and laryngeal diameters in the Thoroughbred. Am. J. Vet. Res. 44:1660, 1983.
7. Raker, C.W.: The nasopharynx. *In* Equine Medicine and Surgery, Vol. 3. (R.A. Mansmann and E.S. McAllister, Eds.) Santa Barbara, CA, American Veterinary Publications, 1982, p. 747.

Ventral Pharyngotomy and Excision of a Subepiglottic Cyst

Ventral pharyngotomy has been reported to provide surgical access to the oropharynx and for surgical manipulation of epiglottic entrapment and cleft of the soft palate.[1,5] It has been suggested as a possible alternative to approach a subepiglottic cyst when the conventional laryngotomy approach involves twisting as well as retraction on the epiglottis.[2,7] Although the pharyngotomy approach has disadvantages of being a deep incision with limited visibility, it does provide direct access to the subepiglottic surface.

Anesthesia and Surgical Preparation

Ventral pharyngotomy is performed under general anesthesia with the patient in dorsal recumbency. The ventral aspect of the pharynx, the caudal mandibular area, and the cranial cervical area are clipped and prepared. Phenylbutazone, perioperative antibiotics, and tetanus toxoid are administered preoperatively.

Surgical Technique

A ventral midline incision is made rostral to the body of the thyroid cartilage (immediately rostral to the site for ventral laryngotomy) (Fig. 6-5A). The incision is continued between the sternohyoid muscles to expose the deeper omohyoid muscles. These are also separated axially, and the incision is continued through the thyrohyoid ligament (Fig. 6-5B). The hyoepiglottic muscle is divided on the midline deep within the incision. This division reveals the glossoepiglottic fold, and an incision through this fold enables entry into the oropharynx (Fig. 6-5C). Figure 6-5D illustrates the surgical entry in cross section. The rostral extent of the incision is limited by the basihyoid bone, and division of this to obtain additional exposure for cleft palate repair has been reported by one author.[1] Weitlaner retractors facilitate exposure during the surgical approach.

If a subepiglottic cyst is the indication for the pharyngotomy, the surface mucosa is grasped with a pair of Allis tissue forceps and the mucosa divided. Submucosal dissection is then performed to enucleate the cyst. Rupture of the cyst is avoided if at all possible. Because of poor surgical exposure, the subepiglottic surface is not closed. Following removal of the cyst, excessive mucosa may be trimmed, and the wound can be left to heal by granulation.

The pharyngotomy incision is left to heal by second intention.

Comment

It is to be noted that where satisfactory exposure for cleft palate repair in 3 horses was reported using a pharyngotomy approach, the hyoid bone was also sectioned and the most caudal section of the root of the tongue was split. For exposure of clefts involving the rostral half of the soft palate, extensive pharyngotomy is coupled with man-

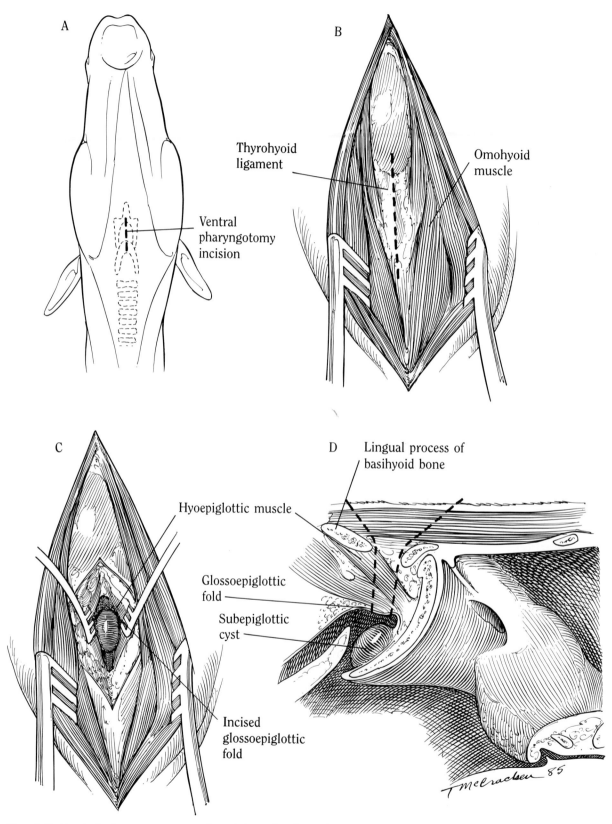

FIG. 6-5. Ventral pharyngotomy and excision of subepiglottic cyst.

dibular symphysiotomy.[4] In most reports of surgical treatment of pharyngeal cysts, laryngotomy has been the approach used.[3,6]

References

1. Cook, W.R.: Some observations on diseases of the ear, nose and throat in the horse, and endoscopy using a flexible fiberoptic endoscope. Vet. Rec. 94:533, 1974.
2. Haynes, P.F.: Surgery of the equine respiratory tract. In The Practice of Large Animal Surgery. (P.B. Jennings, Ed.) Philadelphia, W.B. Saunders, 1984, pp. 388–487.
3. Koch, E.B., and Tate, L.P.: Pharyngeal cysts in horses. J. Am. Vet. Med. Assoc. 173:858, 1978.
4. Nelson, A.W., Curley, B.M., Kainer, R.A.: Mandibular symphysiotomy to provide adequate exposure for intraoral surgery in the horse. J. Am. Vet. Med. Assoc. 159:1025, 1971.
5. Spiers, V.C.: Entrapment of the epiglottis in horses. J. Eq. Med. Surg. 1:267, 1977.
6. Stick, J.A., and Boles, C.: Subepiglottic cyst in three foals. J. Am. Vet. Med. Assoc. 177:62, 1977.
7. Raker, C.W.: The nasopharynx. In Equine Medicine and Surgery, 3rd ed. (R.A. Mansmann, E.S. McAllister, and P.W. Pratt, Eds.) Santa Barbara, CA, American Veterinary Publications, 1982, p. 747.

Extradiverticular Ligation of the Internal Carotid Artery for Guttural Pouch Mycosis

Guttural pouch mycosis is a fungal infection within the guttural pouch that may erode into a major artery such as the internal carotid artery. This erosion can result in a fatal epistaxis.[1] Other clinical signs seen in association with guttural pouch mycosis can be attributed to involvement of various nerves that run adjacent to the pouches. These signs include pharyngeal paralysis, dysphagia, laryngeal hemiplegia, dorsal displacement of the soft palate, Horner's syndrome, and facial paralysis.[1] Guttural pouch mycosis may also manifest as nasal catarrh, abnormal head posture, mild colic, and subparotid abscessation.[1] The signs of the infection are variable and will depend on which nerve or blood vessel is affected. Endoscopic examination of the interior of the guttural pouch will usually demonstrate the lesions on the roof of the diverticulum. The lesions may vary in extent, color, and texture. Some have a black or white furry appearance; others consist of a flat brown diphtheritic plaque, slightly elevated above the mucosa of the guttural pouch. An *Aspergillus sp.* is the most frequent fungus involved.[4] In lesions that have recently hemorrhaged the pouch may be entirely filled with blood, making endoscopic visualization of the lesion virtually impossible. The relevant anatomy is illustrated in Figure 6-6A.

The condition may be unilateral or bilateral. The interiors of both pouches always must be examined, therefore, to formulate an accurate prognosis.

The underlying cause behind initiation of the fungal growth is unclear. It is felt that an underlying defect such as an aneurysm in the wall of the internal carotid artery just before it enters the base of the skull may create favorable conditions for initiation of certain species of fungus that normally reside within the pouch.[2] The external carotid artery may also be involved, but this site is far less frequent than the internal carotid artery.

If the horse has had a history of an acute profuse epistaxis, conservative therapy (flushes, antifungal agents [topical and systemic], hypotensive agents) are usually futile. To delay surgical treatment only increases the likelihood of a fatal hemorrhagic episode. We therefore recommend operating as soon as practical.

Surgical treatment for guttural pouch mycosis by arterial ligation has been reported.[1-7] It was originally proposed that ligation of the artery on both sides of the lesion was necessary, because ligation on the cardiac side of the area of fungal growth did not take into account the retrograde blood flow from the circle of Willis. Continued hemorrhage could lead to exsanguination and death. Because of the anatomic difficulty associated with ligating the internal carotid artery on both sides of the lesion, Cook proposed using an extradiverticular (without opening the pouch) approach.[2] It is believed that in most cases ligation of the artery on the cardiac side of the lesion causes enough drop in the blood pressure at the site of fungal erosion that hemorrhage is averted and that a thrombus, extending to the cranial

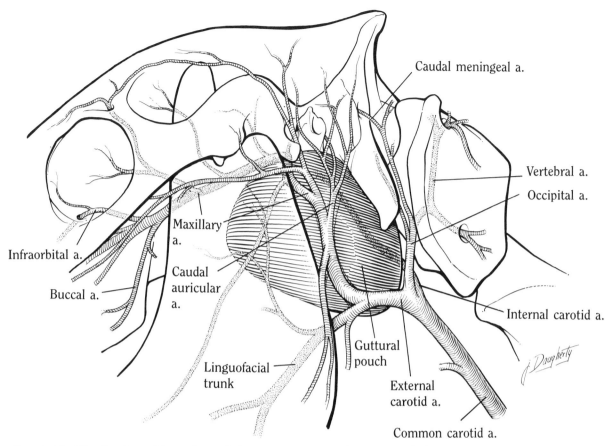

FIG. 6-6A. Distribution of branches of the common carotid artery, including relevant ones in the vicinity of the guttural pouch.

side of the lesion, prevents retrograde bleeding from the circle of Willis[1] (Fig. 6-6A).

Another technique of managing hemorrhage from the internal carotid artery is to use a balloon-tipped catheter.[3] The catheter is introduced distal to a ligature on the carotid artery close to its origin. The tip is advanced beyond the site of infection; then the balloon is inflated so that the infected segment of artery is isolated from the cerebral vascular system. This technique is probably the ideal method of treatment but comparative success figures are not available. It is recommended that the reader consult the literature if this technique is to be used.[3]

Anesthesia and Surgical Preparation

With the large volumes of blood that can be lost by the horse with guttural pouch mycosis, patients frequently are severely anemic. Packed cell volumes (PCV) between 10 and 20 are not uncommon.[1] Blood transfusion in these cases should be considered prior to general anesthesia. This will mean cross matching and location of a suitable donor as soon as possible. If the PCV is borderline (20 to 30), then we recommend collecting and storing the blood appropriately until the time of the operation. It should be available immediately if problems arise during the procedure. The ligation procedure is performed under general anesthesia with the patient in lateral recumbency and the affected side uppermost. Ideally, to ascertain the exact location of the lesion and source of the hemorrhage, a *carotid arteriogram* is performed first. This is especially critical if the lesion is not in the usual position on the internal carotid artery. When there is active bleeding and immediate ligation is necessary to prevent exsanguination, this step should be eliminated because time is critical. If the lesion has hemorrhaged but is no longer continuing to do so (temporary stabilization), the angiogram should be performed with the horse under general anesthesia immediately prior to surgical ligation.

Additional Instrumentation

CAROTID ANGIOGRAM. This requires a polypropylene catheter (14 guage), a soluble contrast agent such as iothalamate meglumine* or diatrizoate meglumine,† and sterile ⅛-inch umbilical tape.

ARTERIAL LIGATION. Malleble retractors and nonabsorbable suture material (e.g., no. 2 nylon) are needed.

Surgical Technique

CAROTID ANGIOGRAM. An 8 to 10 cm skin incision is made parallel to and dorsal to the jugular furrow in the middle of the neck on the affected side (Fig. 6-6B). Careful blunt dissection is used to isolate the common carotid artery, and two pieces of sterile umbilical tape are passed under the artery at each end of the isolated segment. Care is taken to avoid excessive traumatization of the recurrent laryngeal nerve or the vagosympathetic trunk that is near the carotid artery.

A section of artery is exteriorized by placing gentle traction on the umbilical tape ligatures, simultaneously occluding flow in the artery. A small longitudinal incision (just enough to admit the 14-gauge polyethylene catheter) is made into the lumen of the artery using a no. 15 scalpel blade. The sterile 14-gauge polyethylene catheter (primed with Ringer's solution, extracellular fluid, or physiologic sterile saline solution) is threaded up the carotid artery in preparation for injection of the contrast agent (Fig. 6-6C). The appropriate size of loaded x-ray cassette is positioned, and the x-ray machine is aligned. Ten to 15 ml of the contrast agent are injected *rapidly* in a bolus, and immediately *after* all the solution is injected, the film is taken.

Following completion of the angiogram, the incision in the common carotid artery is closed with a simple continuous suture of 5/0 polypropylene or nylon. The tension on the umbilical tape ligatures should be released to check for any leakage at the incision site. If leakage is significant, one or more simple interrupted sutures should be added to correct the problem. Closure consists of a synthetic ab-

---

*Conray. Diagnostic Products Division, Mallinckrodt, St. Louis, MO 63134.
†Angiovist 370. Berlex, Wayne, NJ 07470.

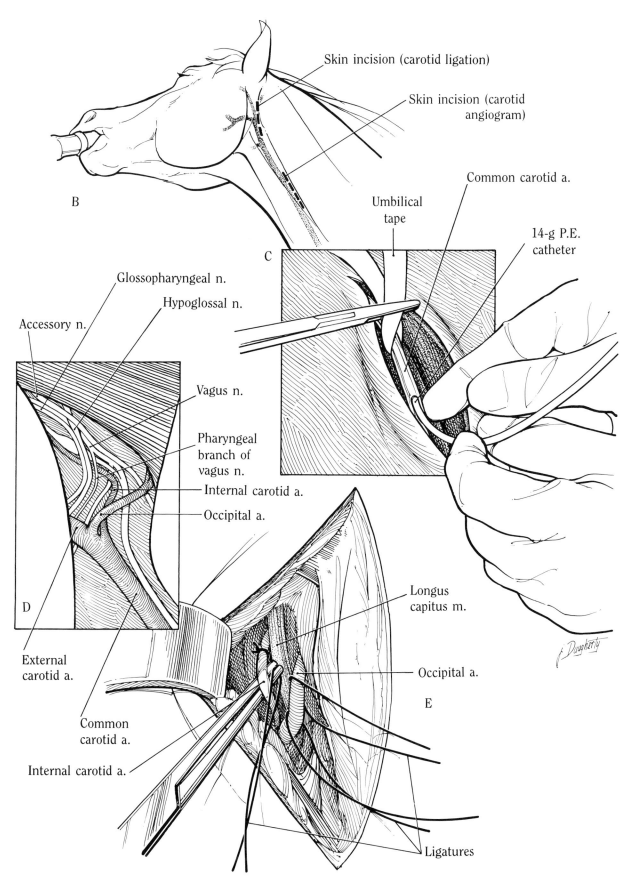

Labels in figure:

Skin incision (carotid ligation)

Skin incision (carotid angiogram)

Common carotid a.

Umbilical tape

14-g P.E. catheter

B

C

Glossopharyngeal n.

Hypoglossal n.

Accessory n.

Vagus n.

Pharyngeal branch of vagus n.

Internal carotid a.

Occipital a.

External carotid a.

Common carotid a.

Internal carotid a.

D

Longus capitus m.

Occipital a.

E

Ligatures

Fig. 6-6 (*Continued*). **B–E.** Carotid angiogram and extradiverticular ligation of the internal carotid artery.

231

sorbable suture in the subcutaneous tissue and a nonabsorbable suture in the skin.

ARTERIAL LIGATION. The surgical approach to the internal carotid artery at its origin from the carotid is similar to the hyovertebrotomy approach to the guttural pouch, except that the incision is slightly more ventral and caudal.[7]

An 8 to 10-cm incision is made parallel and just cranial to the wing of the atlas (Fig. 6-6B). The skin incision exposes the parotid salivary gland and the overlying parotidoauricular muscle. The ventral part of the parotidoauricular muscle is incised, and a dissection plane for the parotid gland is established by incising the fascia on its caudal border. The parotid gland is reflected craniad. The caudal auricular nerve crosses obliquely in the dorsal aspect of the surgical field and is reflected caudad if necessary. Reflection of the parotid gland reveals the occipitohyoid and digastric muscles craniodorsally and the rectus capitis cranialis muscle caudodorsally. The mandibular salivary gland is identified ventrally. Blunt dissection through aerolar tissue exposes the dorsolateral wall of the guttural pouch and the pharyngeal branch of the vagus nerve. In most cases the ventral dissection will reveal the origin of both the internal carotid and the occipital arteries (Fig. 6-6D).

Because of the anatomic variation in this area it may be impossible to distinguish the internal carotid from the occipital artery. The occipital artery is usually more superficially located in the surgical site and tends to be larger. However, to ensure against inadvertent ligation of the wrong artery, we are currently recommending ligation of *both* the occipital and internal carotid arteries unless angiographic monitoring is used during the operation. Identification of the arteries as one dissects through the aerolar tissue can be facilitated by palpation of a pulse in the vessel with the index finger. The artery(ies) is individually identified and the surrounding fascia freed from the vessel walls. Each vessel is double ligated at a convenient location above its origin from the common carotid artery (Fig. 6-6E). We use a nonabsorbable monofilament synthetic suture such as no. 2 nylon. Silk would also be satisfactory. Absorbable suture materials have also been used successfully.[3]

Because the ligation procedure does not enter the lumen of the guttural pouch, the wound can be regarded as a sterile one, and primary intention healing can be anticipated. Closure of the hyovertebrotomy incision utilizes a synthetic absorbable suture in the fascia associated with the parotid gland, and the skin is closed with a monofilament nonabsorbable suture material or stainless steel staples. Rapid clean healing of the surgical site is one advantage of this extradiverticular approach over those that ligate the artery by exposing the interior or the guttural pouch.

Postoperative Management

Tetanus prophylaxis should be provided, but we do not consider postoperative antibiotics to be necessary unless the surgeon has suspected a break in aseptic technique during either the angiogram or the ligation procedure.

In our experience the fungal lesion within the guttural pouch usually resolves soon after the internal carotid artery has been ligated with no additional treatment. Fiberoptic examination of the lesions on the roof of the pouch as soon as one week after the affected artery has been ligated frequently reveals a greatly diminished growth of the fungus with evidence of scarring and fibrosis.

The horse should be confined to a box stall for two to three weeks following the operation. Stress should be minimized. The skin sutures or stainless steel staples can be removed two weeks after surgery. Exercise should not be resumed until fiberoptic examination of the interior of the pouch has demonstrated complete absence of fungal growth.

Comments

We are aware of cases of guttural pouch mycosis that exsanguinated because of inadvertent ligation of either the wrong artery or of a nerve instead of an artery. The most common error seems to be failure to differentiate the internal carotid artery from the occipital artery.

One advantage of the extradiverticular approach to the internal carotid artery is that it is a relatively simple and quick procedure provided the surgeon is familiar with the local anatomy. Also, it can be done in the face of a fatal hemorrhagic episode.

Arterial ligation should be considered in *all* cases of guttural pouch hemorrhage because a fatal epistaxis can occur at any time, without any predisposing causes such as strenuous exercise. In other words, we recommend ligation as soon as the diagnosis is made, since a horse with guttural pouch mycosis typically will have one or two hemorrhages before a fatal episode occurs.[5]

It is recognized that ligation of the artery on only one side of the lesion does not eliminate completely the potential for retrograde hemorrhage from the circle of Willis. Cases of unsuccessful ligation of the internal carotid artery at its bifurcation from the common carotid artery have been reported, although the surgeon admitted that, in one case, the pulse in the internal carotid was greatly diminished.[4]

The question arises about the potential interference to circulation of the brain when a case of bilateral guttural pouch mycosis is presented for surgical treatment. In cases with bilateral involvement our colleagues and we have ligated both internal carotid arteries without neurologic sequelae. We therefore recommend ligating both vessels at the one operation rather than risking exsanguination and death due to continued erosion of the artery by the fungus.

Epistaxis associated with lesions in the external carotid artery has been seen. Such cases emphasize the need for an angiogram to ensure ligation of the appropriate vessel.

References

1. Cook, W.R.: Observations on the aetiology of epistaxis and cranial nerve paralysis in the horse. Vet. Rec. 78:396, 1966.

2. Cook, W.R.: American College of Veterinary Surgeons Annual Forum, Chicago, 1978.
3. Freeman, D.E., and Donawick, W.J.: Occlusion of internal carotid artery in the horse by means of a ballon-tipped catheter: clinical use of a method to prevent epistaxis caused by guttural pouch mycosis. J. Am. Vet. Med. Assoc. 176:236, 1980.
4. Haynes, P.F.: Surgery of the equine respiratory tract. *In* Textbook of Large Animal Surgery (P. Jennings, Ed.) Philadelphia, W.B. Saunders, 1984, p. 463.
5. McIlwraith, C.W.: Surgical treatment of epistaxis associated with guttural pouch mycosis. VM/SAC 73:67, 1978.
6. Owen, R. ap R.: Epistaxis prevented by ligation of the internal carotid artery in the guttural pouch. Eq. Vet. J. 61:143, 1974.
7. Owen, R. ap R.: Ligation of the internal carotid artery to prevent epistaxis due to guttural pouch mycosis. Vet. Rec. 104:100, 1979.
8. Turner, A.S., and McIlwraith, C.W.: Techniques in Large Animal Surgery. Philadelphia, Lea & Febiger, 1982, p. 194.

Surgical Management of Guttural Pouch Tympany (Tympanites)

Tympany (tympanites) of the guttural pouch usually results from a failure of the pharyngeal orifice of the eustachian tube to allow escape of air; the defective orifice acts much like a one-way valve, with air entering the pouch but unable to leave it.[1-6] The condition is seen in foals and young horses. It is considered that there is a congenital defect of the pharyngeal opening. The exact cause has been attributed to excessive mucous membrane attached to the medial lamina of the auditory tube cartilage or an abnormally large and redundant plica salpingopharyngea.[2] The condition has been seen with a higher incidence in fillies.[1] It is usually unilateral, but bilateral cases have been observed.[5]

The animal usually has a nonpainful tympanic swelling of the parotid region. It may be difficult to determine which in fact is the distended side because distention will appear on both sides, especially if it is severe, and may lead the surgeon into thinking it is a bilateral problem.[1] Percussion of the tympanic swelling will enable one to determine that the swelling is gas and not fluid.

The foal is usually bright and alert with a normal temperature, pulse, and respiration. Upon exertion there may be signs of upper airway obstruction if the distention is great. Nursing foals may have dysphagia in severe cases, resulting in an accompanying aspiration pneumonia (with fever and moist rales). Milk may appear from the nostrils and a fluid line may be evident on lateral radiographs.[1] A dorsoventral radiograph may help determine which side is involved.

Examination of the pharynx with a fiberoptic endoscope will reveal a bulging of the pharyngeal walls. Catheterization of the affected pouch during endoscopic examination will result in immediate reduction in the size of the parotid swelling. The pouch will gradually reinflate when the catheter is removed. If swelling in the parotid area is still evident following deflation of one side, then a bilateral condition should be considered.[5]

Conservative treatment of guttural pouch tympany is unsuccessful and surgical management provides the most satisfactory treatment. Two methods of surgical treatment have been utilized. One involves enlargement of the pharyngeal orifice,[3,4,6] and the other involves creation of a fistula between the left and right pouches. The latter is the preferred method and appears to be more successful.[1,2,4,5] It is described here. It allows the pharyngeal orifice on the healthy side to provide atmospheric pressure to both guttural pouches.[4] Bilateral cases are managed with a combination of both surgical techniques.[1]

Anesthesia and Surgical Preparation

The technique is performed under general anesthesia with the animal in lateral recumbency with the affected guttural pouch uppermost.

Preoperative antibiotics should be administered if aspiration pneumonia is suspected. The surgical approach (through Viborg's triangle as illustrated in Figure 6-7A) is clipped and prepared for surgery in a routine manner.

Additional Instrumentation

The procedure requires a flexible fiberoptic endoscope or rigid endoscope of suitable diameter that can enter the normal guttural pouch. Malleable retractors will facilitate visualization of the interior of the guttural pouch.

Surgical Technique

The guttural pouch is approached through Viborg's triangle, which is the area defined by the tendon of the sternomandibular muscle, the linguofacial (external maxillary) vein, and the caudal border of the vertical ramus of the mandible. A 4 to 6 cm skin incision is made, (the size of the skin incision will depend on the size of the patient), just dorsal to and parallel with the linguofacial vein from the border of the mandible caudad (Fig. 6-7A, B). The subcutaneous tissue is separated, and the base of the parotid gland is reflected dorsad. Care should be taken to avoid trauma to the parotid gland, linguofacial vein, and the branches of the vagus nerve ventral to the floor of the guttural pouch. In the distended tympanic state, the location of the wall of the guttural pouch is greatly facilitated because entry into a normal uninflated pouch is quite difficult. The guttural pouch membrane is grasped and incised with scissors (Fig. 6-7C).

Identification of the septum and interior of the guttural pouch is greatly facilitated by the use of an endoscope, preferably a flexible fiberoptic endoscope. A rigid endoscope (cystoscope) or a Chambers mare catheter can also be used. The endoscope or catheter is inserted into the nostril of the "normal" side (lowermost) and passed into the normal guttural pouch.

When the affected guttural pouch is entered, the pouch will collapse immediately. With the illumination of the endoscope, its tip will be identified shining through the thin median septum between the pouches. The median septum is grasped with a pair of Allis tissue forceps and a generously sized fistula (2 cm × 2 cm) is created by resecting a portion of the septum with Metzenbaum scissors (Fig. 6-7D).

If the condition is bilateral a long (9-inch) pair of Allis tissue forceps or sponge forceps is passed rostrad through the auditory tube to its pharyngeal orifice. The cartilaginous flap is palpated with the index finger and then grasped with the forceps. A piece of tissue (2.5 cm × 1.5 cm) is resected. Failure to remove enough tissue and subsequent inflammation and swelling of the new orifice will result in a recurrence of the condition and possibly empyema. This surgical procedure is performed in addition to fenestration of the septum. Primary closure of the guttural pouch can be considered if the infection within the pouch has not become purulent. If it has, the pouch should be left

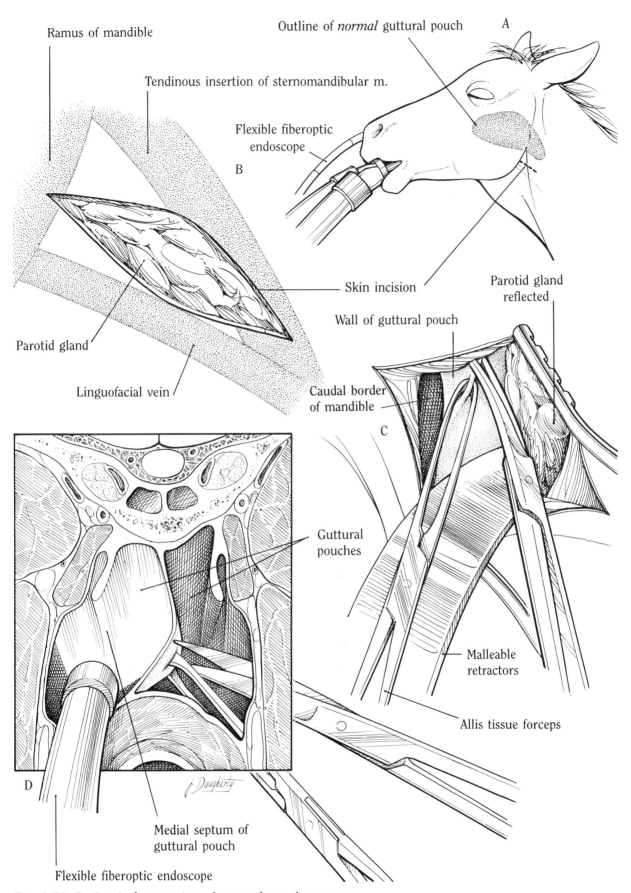

Ramus of mandible

Tendinous insertion of sternomandibular m.

Outline of *normal* guttural pouch

A

Flexible fiberoptic endoscope

B

Skin incision

Parotid gland

Linguofacial vein

Parotid gland reflected

Wall of guttural pouch

Caudal border of mandible

C

Guttural pouches

Malleable retractors

Allis tissue forceps

D

j Daugherty

Medial septum of guttural pouch

Flexible fiberoptic endoscope

Fɪɢ. 6-7A–D. Surgical correction of guttural pouch tympany.

open for drainage, and the wound allowed to heal by second intention.

Postoperative Management

The incision site through Viborg's triangle should be cleaned daily and then flushed with a *dilute* antiseptic solution for three to four days. Strong irritating solutions should never be flushed into the guttural pouch because of the risk of damage to the major nerves and blood vessels that are in close proximity to the guttural pouch. Tetanus prophylaxis should be provided.

In a case uncomplicated by aspiration pneumonia or guttural pouch empyema, antibiotics are optional. Broad-spectrum antibiotics would be required if these conditions did exist.

Comments

In the absence of pneumonia or guttural pouch empyema, the prognosis for a unilateral case of tympanites is excellent. The surgical procedure is relatively quick and easy to perform, and an immediate improvement will be noticed if sufficient fenestration between the pouches has been created. If immediate improvement in the foal's condition is not evident, then bilateral involvement should be suspected.[1]

References

1. Freeman, D.F.: Diagnosis and Treatment of Diseases of the Guttural Pouch (Part I). Compend. Con. Educ. Pract. Vet. 2:503, 1980.
2. Haynes, P.F.: Surgery of the equine respiratory tract. *In* Textbook of Large Animal Surgery, Vol. I. (P. Jennings, Ed.). Philadelphia, W.B. Saunders, p. 462.
3. Mason, T.A.: Tympany of the eustachian tube diverticulosis (guttural pouch) in a foal. Eq. Vet. J. 4:153, 1972.
4. Milne, D.W., and Fessler, J.F.: Tympanites of the guttural pouch in a foal. J. Am. Vet. Med. Assoc. 161:61, 1972.
5. Raker, C.W.: Diseases of the guttural pouch. Mod. Vet. Pract. 57:549, 1976.
6. Wheat, J.D.: Tympanites of the guttural pouch of the horse. J. Am. Vet. Med. Assoc. 140:453, 1962.

Nasal Septum Resection

Resection of the nasal septum is indicated if its thickening or deviation is causing upper airway obstruction. The causes of thickening of the nasal septum in the horse are chronic inflammation secondary to trauma, infection, congenital cystic degeneration, or, rarely, neoplasia.[1] In athletic horses during strenuous exercise, high airflow through the nares is essential; otherwise, exercise intolerance is likely to occur. Fiberoptic examination and radiographic evaluation of the skull are important adjuncts to the physical examination when such a case is encountered. This should enable the surgeon to evaluate the extent and site of the septal deformity.[1,3]

Anesthesia and Surgical Preparation

Because the surgical procedure is accompanied by considerable hemorrhage, preoperative physical evaluation should include a complete blood count and a hemogram. A crossmatch for blood transfusion is indicated in *every case*. For marginally anemic horses blood should be taken from the appropriate donor and be readily available in the surgery.[2] Blood may also be obtained from the patient and stored for autotransfusion.[2] Anemic horses should receive a blood transfusion or, alternatively, the cause of the anemia should be diagnosed, treated, and corrected before the surgery is performed. The procedure is an elective one, and practice on a cadaver head is recommended. This will enable the surgeon to proceed as rapidly as possible to minimize blood loss. There is no other surgery that exemplifies the adage "time is of the essence" more than nasal septum removal in the horse. In addition, all horses, regardless of anesthetic risk, should receive judicious fluid replacement in the form of balanced polyionic solutions throughout the operation to minimize hypotension.

Nasal septum resection is performed under general anesthesia with the patient in left or right lateral recumbency. The area between the medial canthi of the eyes and rostral ends of the facial crests is clipped in preparation for the trephination of the nasal cavity. The midcervical area should be clipped in preparation for a tracheostomy. Both areas are given an initial scrub prior to a final scrub when the horse is recumbent under general anesthesia.

Additional Instrumentation

This procedure requires a guarded chisel. These chisels may not be readily available from commercial instrument manufacturers but are readily made by any metal worker/blacksmith. An osteotome or bone gouge also has been recommended.[2] Also needed are a 1-inch trephine, Ochsner or Doyen forceps, sterile cotton gauze that has

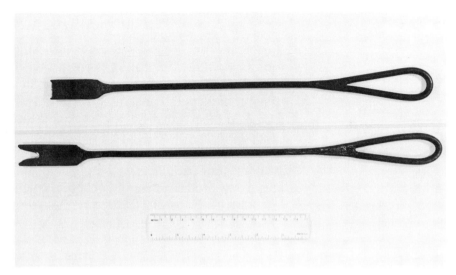

Two different types of guarded chisels that are suitable for nasal septum removal.

been soaked in a 1:10,000 solution of epinephrine, a tracheostomy tube, and vulsellum forceps.

Surgical Technique

An 8- to 10-cm skin incision is made exactly on the midline of the face commencing immediately rostral to the frontal sinuses (where the nasal bones begin to diverge slightly caudal to the level of the rostral aspect of the facial crest;[2]) (Fig. 6-8A). The skin edges are retracted with towel clamps, and the periosteum is quartered and reflected. A 25-mm (1 inch) circular trephine hole is made directly on the midline of the face, and the bone is removed and discarded. The nasal septum will now be visible. Ochsner or Doyen forceps are then inserted through the trephine hole, perforating mucous membrane with each blade on either side of the septum, until the floor of the nasal passage is felt. The forceps should be directed perpendicularly and then closed on the nasal septum (Fig. 6-8B).

Moving to the external nares, the surgeon palpates the nasal septum through the uppermost nostril to determine how much of the rostral portion of the septum is unthickened and can be preserved. The surgeon then incises through the rostral aspect of the septum from dorsal to ventral, just caudal to the alar cartilages. This incision should be convex, with the convex surface facing rostrally. This will maintain the support to the alar cartilages. (Fig. 6-8C, D).

At this point, surgery must proceed rapidly, as hemorrhage will be profuse. With the guarded chisel, the dorsal and ventral attachments of the septum are severed by forcing the chisel along the nasal septum until it meets the forceps. This may take a few attempts, as the chisel may slip off the septum or the septum may be sufficiently thickened as to require several firm thrusts of the instrument to completely sever all dorsal and ventral attachments (Fig. 6-8E). The cau-

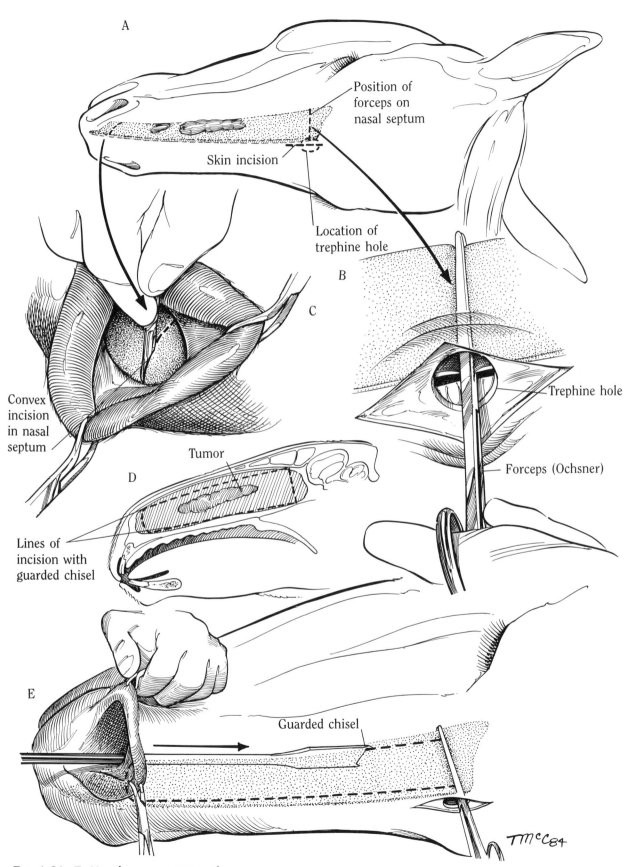

A

Position of
forceps on
nasal septum

Skin incision

Location of
trephine hole

B

C

Trephine hole

Convex
incision
in nasal
septum

Forceps (Ochsner)

Tumor

D

Lines of
incision with
guarded chisel

E

Guarded chisel

TMᶜC84

Fig. 6-8A–E. Nasal septum removal.

dal attachment is severed rostral to the Ochsner or Doyen forceps with a chisel or osteotome. The septum is then grasped firmly with vulsellum forceps and extracted from the nasal cavity. If the septum is still firmly anchored in the nasal cavity, further attempts should be made to sever it dorsally and ventrally with the guarded chisel. Attachments at the caudal end of the septum can be severed with scissors introduced into the trephine hole.

Gauze soaked in 1:10,000 epinephrine solution is then packed into the nasal cavity from the trephine hole and through the external nares. The packing should be inserted as tightly as possible to achieve a tamponade effect to reduce the hemorrhage. The gauze can be anchored at the nostrils by horizontal mattress sutures using no. 2 nylon, but it should not require anchoring at the trephine hole. The nostrils can also be closed with these sutures to prevent the packing from falling out.

Prior to extubation of the horse, a tracheostomy is performed, and a suitable tracheostomy tube is inserted and *anchored securely* in place. It should be recognized that if the tracheostomy tube is dislodged the horse may be asphyxiated because the nasal cavity will be completely occluded.

Postoperative Management

Tetanus immunization is administered. Antibiotics are administered for four to five days postoperatively.

The packing should be removed 48 to 72 hours after surgery, using appropriate restraint of the horse. Flushing the nasal cavity may be indicated. This will aid removal of dried blood and tissue debris. Any large tissue fragments or clots can be removed gently with sponge forceps. Flushing can be achieved using water at ambient temperature or physiologic saline solution in a bulb syringe.[3]

The trephine hole is cleaned once or twice daily with gauze sponges and allowed to heal by second intention. The tracheostomy site is managed similarly. Horses that have been scheduled for athletic endeavors should be examined with a fiberoptic endoscope to monitor the healing process. The horse will require approximately two months' rest before returning to work.[3]

Comments

Although the surgery is technically relatively easy to perform, complications are common. In the largest series of cases published to date, complications included persistence of noise and respiratory difficulty, excessive granulation tissue and adhesions at the caudal incised edge, and inability to remove the entire resected septum.[3] In an attempt to minimize these it has been recommended that the caudal edge of the septum be amputated by making a *more oblique cut* ensuring removal of more septum. The oblique cut edge is just rostral to the ethmoid and sphenopalatine sinus and dorsal to the soft palate. Excessive granulation tissue in this region is less likely to cause narrowing or adhesions to the conchae, which would result in airflow turbulence, because the nasal passage is much wider at this point.[3] If the original cause of thickening of the nasal septum was a neoplastic process, then recurrence of the tumor is always a possibility.

The complication arising from the removal of too much cartilage rostrally is a flattening of the bridge of the nose near the nasal diverticula. This is more likely to occur if the surgery is performed in foals under six months of age. We have seen inadequate development of the entire nasal bones and premaxilla in a foal that required nasal septum removal at two months of age.

References

1. Haynes, P.F.: The respiratory system. In The Practice of Large Animal Surgery. (P. Jennings, Ed.) Philadelphia, W.B. Saunders, 1984, p. 400.
2. Nelson, A.E., Herring, D.S., and Robertson, J.D.: Contribution of the nasal septum to the radiographic anatomy of the equine nasal cavity. J. Am. Vet. Med. Assoc. 186:590, 1985.
3. Tulleners, E.P., and Raker, C.W.: Nasal septum resection in the horse. Vet. Surg. 12:41, 1983.

Bone Flap Technique for Sinus Exploration

A thorough exploration of the paranasal sinuses of the horse is occasionally required and is best performed with the use of a bone flap.[1,3,4] Compared to the traditional trephine technique, this technique allows a larger volume of the sinus to be examined. The end result is more satisfactory cosmetically than multiple trephine holes where the actual circular pieces of bone and skin have been discarded.[3,4]

The bone flap technique is most useful for cases of chronic primary sinusitis in which the mucosa of the sinus has become very thickened and the infection has resisted long-term antibiotics and lavage. The exposure will allow curettage of considerable amounts of the thickened sinus membrane that would otherwise be inaccessible through a trephine hole. The bone flap technique is also useful when exposure to the roots of several check teeth is required for repulsion. A trephine hole is still the preferred method to gain access to the tooth roots if one or two teeth are to be repelled.

Although the prognosis is generally poor, access to tumors (e.g., squamous cell carcinoma, adenocarcinoma) of the sinuses is feasible by this method.[3] Usually metastases have occurred to regional lymph nodes by the time the diagnosis has been made.[3] Biopsy of different areas of the lesion is possible to evaluate its extent. The sinus flap technique is the approach of choice for ablation and curettage of congenital cystic lesions of the paranasal sinuses.[1,3,4]

Anesthesia and Surgical Preparation

The surgery is performed with the horse under general anesthesia with the affected side uppermost. The ability to tilt the horse to allow drainage of blood and exudate to come out the external nares rather than back down the trachea is useful, but not essential. The surgical site over the affected sinus is clipped and prepared for surgery in a routine manner.

Additional Instrumentation

The bone flap technique requires a hand drill and a 3.2-mm drill bit, an osteotome or chisel, a small mallet, stainless steel wire, and curettes. Other instruments such as dental punches may be required, depending on the reason for the sinus exploration.

Surgical Technique

Maxillary Sinus

A curved skin incision is made to create a flap as shown in Figure 6-9A. The incision is made over the rostral, ventral and caudal borders of the maxillary sinus. The skin and subcutaneous tissue are reflected dorsad, revealing the levator labii maxillaris and levator nasolabialis muscles. These muscles are reflected dorsad (usually) or ventrad, depending on the exact location and extend off the boundaries of the flap.

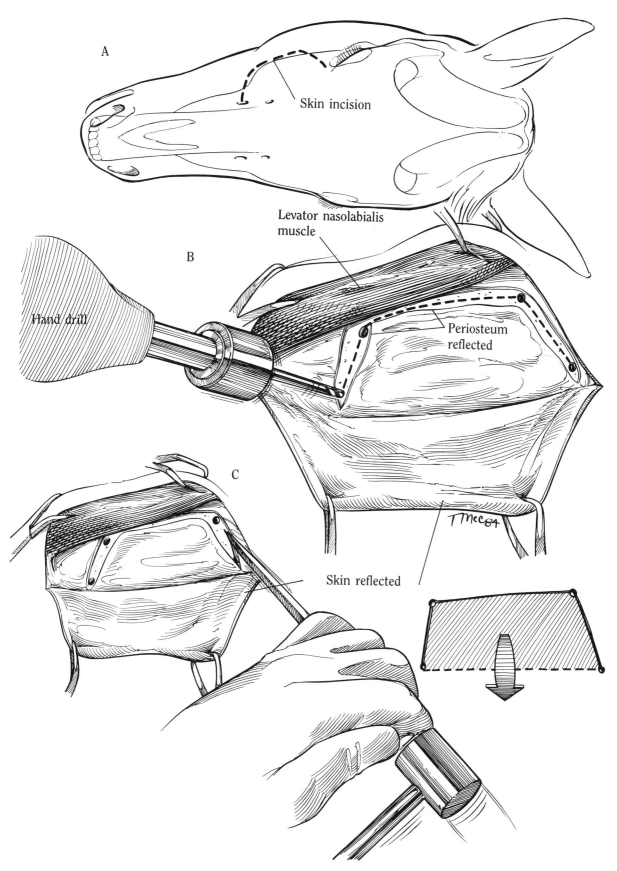

FIG. 6-9A–C. Bone flap technique for sinus exploration.

245

The periosteum is incised on the same three sides as the skin incision and reflected back 5 to 6 mm. The bone is then cut along the same margins. A variety of instruments have been recommended to cut the bone. An oscillating (e.g., Stryker) saw or burr attached to a surgical air drill has been suggested, but both these instruments leave a bony defect when it comes time to reattach the bone flap. A simpler way is to drill four holes and connect them on three sides with an incision made by a chisel or osteotome (Fig. 6-9B). The incision by the chisel is made on an oblique angle to the bone surface such that the external surface of the flap is slightly larger than the inner surface of the flap (Fig. 6-9C). This produces a better dovetail pattern and a more secure closure. During this procedure care should be taken not to damage the osseous nasolacrimal duct, which is located dorsally in the maxillary sinus. The bone flap created is then carefully elevated along the dorsal margin, using the intact periosteum as a hinge (Fig. 6-9D). If the bone has become pathologically thickened, then this maneuver may be difficult.

When the flap has been reflected back, surgery within the sinus can then be carried out. For example, teeth can be repelled, thickened hypertrophic sinus mucosa can be removed, or a biopsy of a suspicious lesion can be done. Bacterial cultures can be taken at this time. If an embryologic sinus cyst is present, it is important to ablate the cyst and establish drainage of the cyst or maxillary sinus into the nasal cavity. The cyst wall is broken down, and the lining should be trimmed out with scissors or curetted out. Drainage into the nasal cavity is then established as described below.

Following the appropriate surgery, the bony flap is repositioned and gently pressed back into position. If the incision in the bone has been beveled and there has been no loss of bone, closure of the periosteum with simple interrupted sutures will be all that is required. A synthetic absorbable suture material can be used for the periosteum. If the bone flap is unstable, it must be wired in place by predrilling holes in the corners of the flap and adjacent parent bone. The wires should not be tightened so vigorously as to cut through the bone. The subcutaneous tissues and skin are closed using a suture material and pattern of the surgeon's choice.

Frontal Sinus

The bone flap technique can be used to expose the frontal sinus or caudal part of the dorsal conchae (turbinate bone). The size of the flap can be tailored to the size of the lesion and the amount of exposure required.

Drainage of Sinuses

Essential to surgery for septic conditions of the sinus is adequate postoperative drainage.[2] In long-standing cases of sinusitis it will be necessary to reestablish drainage or reopen the nasomaxillary orifice.

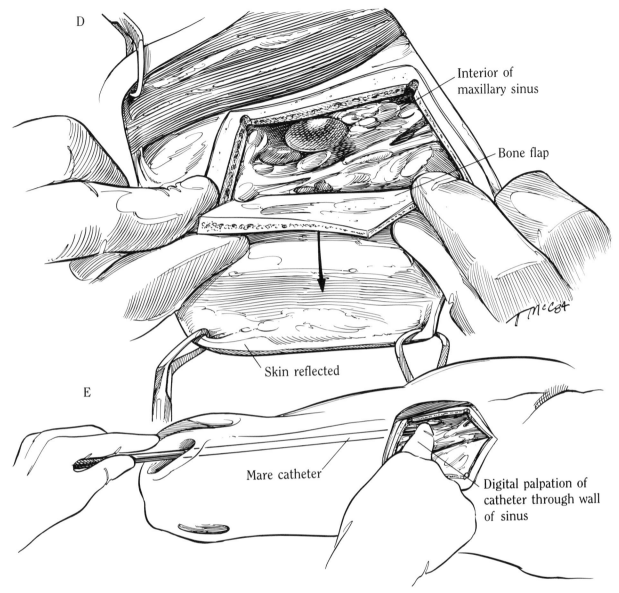

D

Interior of
maxillary sinus

Bone flap

Skin reflected

E

Mare catheter

Digital palpation of
catheter through wall
of sinus

FIG. 6-9 (*Continued*). **D–E.**

This can be achieved by placing a finger into the sinus and palpating the floor of the rostral compartment of the maxillary sinus, medial and rostral to the tooth roots. A catheter is then passed up the nasal cavity on the same side and forced through the conchae and wall of the sinus as determined by the position of the surgeon's finger (Fig. 6-9E). The opening should be enlarged by spreading scissors to ensure that it will not swell shut and prevent drainage into the nasal cavity.

Drainage can be established in a similar way for the frontal sinus. It should always be done as the last step in the surgical procedure because of the potential hemorrhage.

When drainage must be created in the floor of the maxillary or frontal sinuses using this method, it is wise to thread a piece of gauze (seton) through the new (or reopened) orifice exiting out the external nares. This will help to maintain patency.[2] The seton can be anchored to a roll of gauze on the side of the face, exiting a small hole made in the bone flap. This will be left in place for three to four days and then removed completely. If extensive flushing is required, a polyethylene catheter can be passed through a small hole made in one of the edges of the bone flap and anchored to the face with nonabsorbable retention sutures. It can also be placed through a separate hole into the sinus using a Steinmann pin or drill.

The wound should be covered with nonadherent dressing and several gauzes. Then the entire face should be bandaged with an elastic adhesive bandage, being careful to avoid the eyes.

Postoperative Management

Antibiotics and tetanus prophylaxis are provided postoperatively. Phenylbutazone may be indicated in certain cases. Most sinus infections benefit mainly from drainage, and antibiotics should be regarded as adjunctive therapy. If tooth removal is anticipated, however, a perioperative course of antibiotics is advisable because of the possibility of bacterial endocarditis.

The sinus should be irrigated twice daily until the discharge has become noticeably less purulent. Very dilute povidone-iodine (Betadine) solution is satisfactory, although the mechanical rinsing and drainage is probably more important than the content of the flush. Flushing should continue for at least 10 days. The gauze set is removed after four or five days.

Comments

The size of the flap can be varied to fit the extent of the lesion. If teeth are to be repelled, then the flap can be small, but if the surgery is needed for access to resect a tumor or ablate a congenital maxillary sinus cyst or remove chronically thickened sinus mucosa, a larger flap may be required. The flap must be secured fairly snugly; otherwise, it will loosen and remain unstable, not regain its blood supply, and possibly sequester. The end result will be a large defect that will lack underlying bony support. Sequestration of the bone flap will be evident if the skin margins fail to heal.

Any sinus surgery is accompanied by hemorrhage. If curettage of the sinus membrane is required, hemorrhage will be copious. At this point in the surgery it is helpful to tilt the table to allow the blood to run from the sinus out the nostril (via the nasomaxillary orifice).

The healing of the bone flap and associated skin is usually excellent despite the purulent infection within the underlying sinus, presumably because of the extensive blood supply to the head.

References

1. Cannon, J.H., Grant, B.D., and Sande, R.D.: Diagnosis and surgical treatment of cystlike lesions of the equine paranasal sinuses. J.A.V.M.A. 169:610, 1976.
2. Guard, W.F.: Surgical Principles and Technics. Columbus, WF Guard, 1953, p. 84.

3. Haynes, P.F.: Surgery of the respiratory tract. In The Practice of Large Animal Surgery. (P. Jennings, Ed.) Philadelphia, W.B. Saunders, 1984, p. 400.
4. McAllister, E.S.: Paranasal sinus flap. In Equine Medicine and Surgery, 3rd ed., Vol. 2. (R.A. Mansmann and E.S. McAllister, Eds.) Santa Barbara, CA, American Veterinary Publications 1982, p. 729.
5. Wheat, J.D.: Sinus Drainage and Tooth Repulsion in the Horse. Proceedings of 19th Annual Convention American Association of Equine Practitioners, 1983. 1984, p. 171.

Surgical Repair of Depression Fractures of the Skull

Fractures of the facial bones and cranial vault are seen occasionally in horses. Fractures of the cranial vault are usually fatal because of the associated neurologic problems.[3] Fractures of the facial bones in horses are amenable to various reconstructive techniques.[1,2,4–6]

Fractures of the facial bones in horses should be repaired because facial deformity, bone sequestration, and sinusitis may occur. Cosmetic results are important in show animals. Reconstruction should be preferably an elective procedure when the animal has been physiologically stabilized.[6] The exception would be a fracture of the orbital rim causing excessive tension on the optic nerve because the eye is being proptosed. In such circumstances, emergency reconstruction of the orbital rim and return of the eye to its socket are required to minimize the chance of permanent blindness. The other indication for immediate surgery is a fracture of the cranium with a deterioration in vital signs, progressive papillary dilation, and depressed conciousness, or an open fracture extending into the cranial vault.[3]

Anesthesia and Surgical Preparation

Epistaxis frequently occurs when the nasal mucosa has been torn; hence blood loss may make the animal an anesthetic risk. In such cases the horse should be stabilized prior to surgery. Correction of any fluid or electrolyte imbalance before anesthesia is important. Blood transfusions are generally not necessary in most skull fractures, but those with extensive trauma should at least be crossmatched with a suitable available donor.

Most depression fractures of the facial bones are open because the mucous membrane of the sinus or nasal cavity is frequently lacerated. It is advisable to begin antibiotic therapy, especially if surgery is to be delayed while the horse is being physiologically stabilized. We have used procaine penicillin G. We have no evidence that antibiotics are an essential part of management. Because of the rich blood supply to the head, it is our opinion that surgical management (debridement, fracture reduction, irrigation, and wound closure) is the key to success in such fractures.

If there has been severe impairment of the function of the nasal cavity due to displacement of bone and soft tissues, tracheostomy may be indicated. The tracheostomy site should be clipped and prepared for surgery in a routine manner. Following induction of anesthesia, the horse can then be intubated through the tracheostomy. Alternatively, intubation can be performed in the normal manner through the mouth, and a suitable tracheostomy tube inserted through a tracheostomy when the horse is standing following the recovery from anesthesia.

The procedure is always performed with the horse under general anesthesia and in lateral recumbency. The location of the depression fracture will dictate whether the horse will be positioned in right or left lateral recumbency (Fig. 6-10A).

Additional Instrumentation

This procedure requires periosteal elevators, 18- or 20-gauge stainless steel wire, wire twisters, a hand drill, and small drill bits.

Surgical Technique

Because of the variability in the configuration of depression fractures, it is impossible to describe a standard technique but rather discuss general principles.

Large curvilinear skin incisions or generous S-shaped incisions extending well beyond the margins of the involved bones should be used to expose the fracture site[6] (Fig. 6-10A). Reduction of the fracture with the aid of a periosteal elevator should be done patiently, being careful not to detach bone fragments from their blood supply (Fig. 6-10B). We have found that during reduction of the fracture it is advantageous to elevate as many points of contact under the fragment as possible to minimize the chances of the fragment splitting into smaller pieces. Once reduction has been achieved, if the fragments are unstable, they can be maintained in position with 18- to 20-gauge stainless steel wire (Fig. 6-10C, D). Holes should be drilled in the loose fragments, with the appropriately sized drill bit, approximately 0.5 cm from the fracture edge. The fragment(s) should be supported during the drilling process. Corresponding holes in the surrounding stable bone also should be drilled. Pieces of wire should now be inserted and preplaced. Reduction of the fracture can now be commenced. When reduction of the fracture is satisfactory, the wire sutures are secured by twisting. The wire twists should be bent over and be smooth to the touch, thereby avoiding pressure necrosis on the overlying skin flap. Care must be taken not to twist the wire too tightly or it will cut through the fragile bone. Small pieces of bone devoid of periosteum that cannot be rigidly stabilized should be discarded because of potential formation of sequestra. Defects may exist when the repair is completed, but the final appearance is usually satisfactory if the surrounding bones are flush with the normal contours of the face.

If a very large defect exists because bone fragments have become loose and devoid of periosteum or are missing, the surgeon may consider filling the defect with synthetic mesh.* This technique has been used also for filling a defect remaining after removal of an everted sinus in a horse.[7] To secure the mesh, holes are drilled around the edge of the defect, and the mesh is sutured in place, using interrupted horizontal mattress sutures of a suitable braided synthetic suture material such as Mersilene. The sutures are placed through the mesh and the holes. The edges of the mesh can be sutured to the subcutaneous tissue with a synthetic absorbable suture material.[7]

*Marlex Mesh, Davol Inc., Providence, RI.

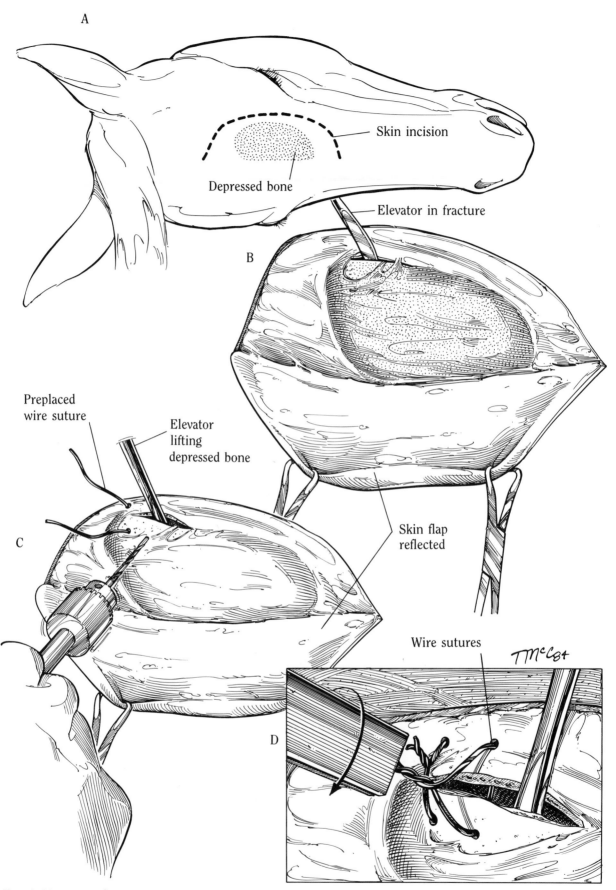

A

Skin incision

Depressed bone

Elevator in fracture

B

Preplaced
wire suture

Elevator
lifting
depressed bone

C

Skin flap
reflected

Wire sutures

D

TMcC84

Fig. 6-10. Surgical repair of depression fracture of the skull.

Following reduction of the fracture or implantation of the mesh, the skin is sutured. The use of a synthetic intradermal suture improves the cosmetic appearance. However, this pattern can be used only when tension of the incision has been relieved by a strong subcutaneous suture layer and the wound edges are almost in apposition prior to beginning this suture.[6]

Fractures of the orbital rim also can be reconstructed by the principles described above.

Postoperative Management

Head bandages are recommended during the early postoperative period. A nonadherent dressing is applied and held in position with a cotton gauze bandage that is applied to the head in a figure-8 pattern. This is then covered with elastic adhesive bandage. The bandage should allow normal mastication, maintain firm even pressure along the surgical site, and keep dust and feed material from entering the wound. The bandage will also help to minimize chances of subcutaneous emphysema that is caused by air escaping from the nasal cavity. The bandage should be monitored carefully to ensure that it does not slip and cause mechanical irritation to the eyes. The bandage should be removed in four to five days.

Antibiotics should be continued until the bandage is removed and the surgeon has had an opportunity to assess the healing of the incision(s). If sinusitis and nasal discharge develop, antibiotic therapy may be indicated for longer periods. If a nasal discharge persists for longer than two or three weeks, radiographs may be indicated to rule out the possibility of formation of sequestra or the presence of a foreign body.

References

1. Turner, A.S.: Surgical management of depression fractures of the equine skull. Vet. Surg. 8:29, 1979.
2. Levine, S.B.: Depression fractures of the nasal and frontal bones of the horse. J. Eq. Med. Surg. 3:186, 1979.
3. Stashak, T.S.: The nervous system: Specific techniques. In Textbook of Large Animal Surgery. (P. Jennings, Ed.) Philadelphia, W.B. Saunders, 1984, p. 1005.
4. Koch, D.B., Leitch, M., and Beech, J.: Orbital surgery in two horses. Vet. Surg. 9:61, 1980.
5. Little, C.B., Hilbert, B.J., and McGill, C.A.: A retrospective study of head fractures in 21 horses. Aust. Vet. J. 62:89, 1985.
6. Turner, A.S.: Large animal orthopedic surgery. In Textbook of Large Animal Surgery. (P. Jennings, Ed.) Philadelphia, W.B. Saunders, 1984, p. 897.
7. Martin, G.S., and McIlwraith, C.W.: Repair of a frontal sinus eversion in a horse. Vet. Surg. 10:149, 1981.

Modified Forssell's Operation for Cribbing

Crib biting in the horse is a vice characterized by the placement of the upper incisors on a solid object, arching of the neck, depressing the tongue, elevating the larynx, and pulling backward. If the horse swallows air, the vice is called wind sucking. There is usually an audible grunt. The sequelae to these habits are poor performance, weight loss, erosion of incisor teeth, and flatulent colic. Above all, it is a vice that is objectionable and irritating to most owners. Why horses commence cribbing or wind sucking is unknown. It is a vice that is learned or acquired, and the most common cause cited is boredom or frustration. In our experience, one of the most common reasons for presentation of a horse that crib bites is owner annoyance rather than weight loss, colic, and property destruction (the more traditional side effects of the vice).[4]

Surgical methods of treatment have included the Forssell's procedure, which involves removal of portions of the sternomandibular, omohyoid, sternohyoid and sternothyroid muscles. This technique has since been modified and is described here. Creation of a therapeutic buccal fistula (buccostomy) has also been described. The disadvantages of this procedure include spontaneous closure of the buccostomy or daily care of the tube used to prevent such closure. The surgical technique involving sectioning of the ventral branch of the accessory nerve (cranial nerve XI) has been used. This nerve innervates the sternomandibular muscle, the largest and most powerful muscle involved in cribbing. The nerve is transected bilaterally. The disappointing results with this method obtained by various surgeons in the U.S. and overseas[1] prompted us to adopt the modification of Forssell's procedure, whereby excision of a portion of the sternothyrohyoid and omohyoid muscles is combined with bilateral removal of a 10- to 12-cm section of the accessory nerves.[4]

Anesthesia and Surgical Preparation

The modified Forssell's technique is performed with the horse under general anesthesia and in dorsal recumbency, with the head positioned at about a 30-degree angle to the horizontal. The ventral neck and throat region is clipped, shaved, and scrubbed for aseptic surgery in a routine manner.

Additional Instrumentation

This procedure requires malleable retractors (1-inch width), a 1-inch Penrose drain, and a hand towel (the latter will be used as a stent bandage to minimize incisional swelling).

Surgical Technique

A skin incision approximately 30 cm long is made on the ventral aspect of the neck, and the skin edges are reflected laterad (Fig. 6-11A). This exposes the ventral surfaces of the paired bellies of the omohyoid and sternothyrohyoid muscles (Fig. 6-11B), as well as the

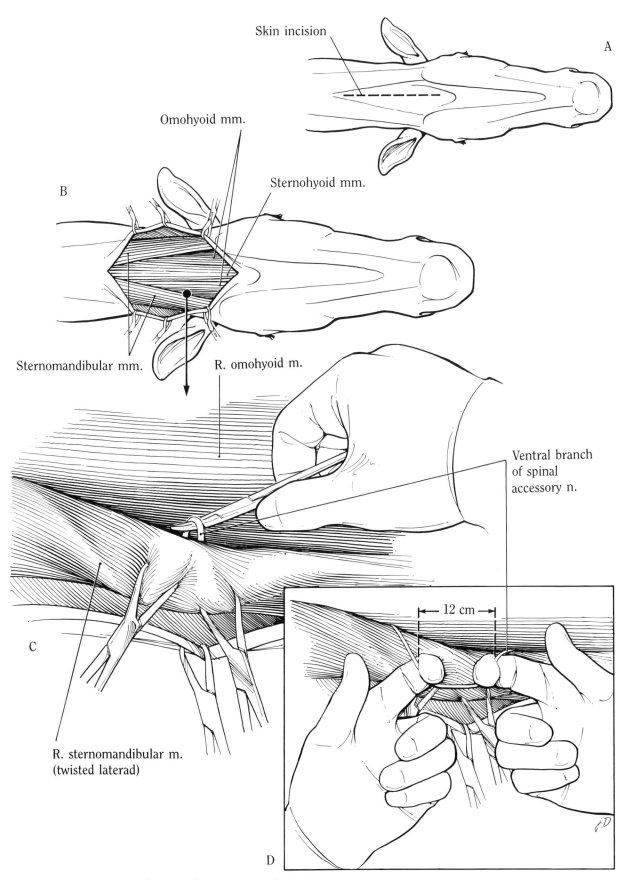

Skin incision

Omohyoid mm.

Sternohyoid mm.

A

B

Sternomandibular mm.

R. omohyoid m.

Ventral branch
of spinal
accessory n.

C

R. sternomandibular m.
(twisted laterad)

12 cm

D

FIG. 6-11A–D. Modified Forssell's operation for cribbing.

cranial ends of the sternomandibular muscles. Hemostasis is controlled by electrocoagulation or torsion and ligation.

A plane of dissection is established on the medial side of the sternomandibular muscle, about 5 cm caudal to the musculotendinous junction (Fig. 6-11B, C). The ventral branch of the accessory nerve is located on the dorsomedial aspect of this muscle by carefully rolling the muscle belly laterad. To aid in locating the nerve one can dissect down to the aponeurosis of the sternomandibular muscle and identify a constant muscular branch from the common carotid artery, which crosses between the sternomandibular and omohyoid muscles. Just beneath this vessel, the ventral branch of the accessory nerve emerges from within the neck and extends laterad.[4] Sudden contracture of the muscle indicates that the nerve has been located.

Curved hemostats are placed under the nerve (Fig. 6-11C). The nerve is then elevated until both fingers can be inserted under the nerve. By forcefully elevating and separating the fingers, a sizable portion of the nerve can be exteriorized and removed (at least 12 cm) (Fig. 6-11D). This maneuver is then performed on the opposite side. Maintaining hemostasis up to this point minimizes staining of the areolar tissue and fascial planes, thus simplifying location and identification of the nerve.

Following bilateral neurectomy, the myectomy is performed. A 30-cm section of the combined bellies of the omohyoid and sternothyrohyoid muscles is removed. These muscle bellies are isolated in the cranial end of the incision, immediately ventral to the larynx. The muscles are freed from the larynx and fascial attachments to the linguofacial vein and thyroid gland. A pair of straight scissors, Ochsner or similar forceps is passed under the muscle bellies prior to transection to ensure inclusion of all parts of the muscle bellies (Fig. 6-11E). The muscle bellies are then grasped and "peeled" caudad, and areolar connective tissue attaching them to the trachea is sharply dissected away. The bellies of the sternothyroid muscles and the ventral aspect of the trachea are then visible. The omohyoid muscles are now sectioned obliquely and the sternohyoid muscles are sectioned at the caudal extremity of the incision (Fig. 6-11F). The sternothyroid muscles on the ventral surface of the trachea (Fig. 6-11F) are then removed, using scissors or a scalpel.

Closure consists of a simple continuous suture in the subcutaneous tissue with synthetic absorbable material, along with insertion of a 1-inch diameter Penrose drain. The Penrose drain can emerge from the incision itself (Fig. 6-11G), but a better surgical principle is to place the ends through generous stab incisions at either end of the incision. Skin closure is performed with nonabsorbable suture material in an interrupted pattern of the surgeon's choice. We routinely use skin staples* to reduce the operative time associated with closure of this long incision and find them satisfactory. To help eliminate dead space, a stent bandage (hand towel) is sutured over the incision, using

---

* Proximate. Ethicon, Inc., Sommerville, NJ.

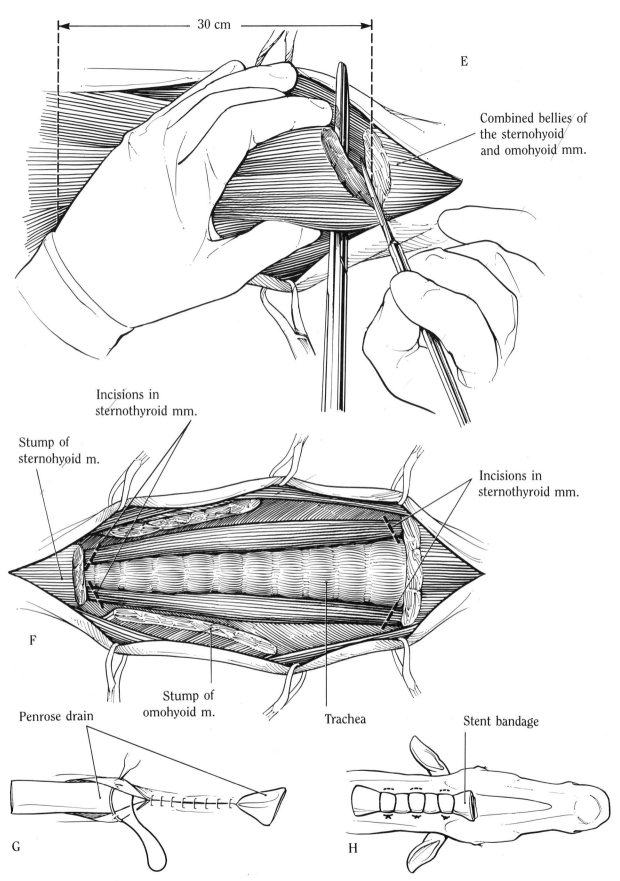

E

Combined bellies of
the sternohyoid
and omohyoid mm.

Incisions in
sternothyroid mm.

Stump of
sternohyoid m.

Incisions in
sternothyroid mm.

F

Penrose drain

Stump of
omohyoid m.

Trachea

Stent bandage

G

H

FIG. 6-11 (*Continued*). **C–F.**

nonabsorbable suture material in a horizontal or vertical mattress pattern (Fig. 6-11H).[4]

Postoperative Management

After surgery, the horse is confined to a box stall or turned into a small corral. The stent bandage is removed three to four days after surgery. The Penrose drain is maintained for three to seven days. An antibiotic (procaine penicillin G) is administered until 24 hours after the drain is removed. Tetanus prophylaxis is provided. The drain sites are cleaned daily, and skin sutures or staples are removed approximately two weeks after surgery.

Comments

In a retrospective study of 35 horses, 20 (57%) were not cribbing one year following surgery.[4] Marked improvement was noted in another 11 (there was noticeable reduction in the frequency of crib biting). Some horses in this latter group would apply the incisor teeth to an object but did not arch the neck and go through the motions of cribbing. Four of 35 horses returned to cribbing in the same manner as before surgery. One of these would arch the neck but not make the characteristic "grunt." This horse gained considerable weight after surgery. Several cribbing brood mares had lost considerable weight and had failed to ovulate. After surgery they either stopped cribbing or continued to crib at a much reduced frequency and gained weight. They began to have regular estrous cycles and some were bred successfully. In 34 cases, the final cosmetic result was regarded as excellent as judged by the owner. One owner reported that the "scar" from surgery was still visible.[4]

The modified myectomy and neurectomy technique appears to be superior to neurectomy alone. The poor results achieved with neurectomy alone are believed attributable to the variable innervation of the sternomandibular muscle, which receives additional ventral cervical branches beyond the site of section of the ventral branch of the accessory nerve.[3]

This method differs slightly from a modification of this technique wherein myectomy is performed prior to neurectomy.[2] We believe the ventral branch of the spinal accessory nerve is identified more readily before the surgical field has become obscured by the blood from the transected stumps of the muscle bellies. Similarly, we believe meticulous control of hemorrhage is important until the nerves are located. The outstanding advantage with this method is that good cosmetic results and quicker wound healing can be achieved when compared with the original more radical Forssell's technique.[4] Virtually all of the owners questioned were pleased with the cosmetic appearance of the surgical site.[4] The Forssell procedure produces a thin neck and a step-like defect where the sternomandibular muscle bellies are transected distally.

References

1. Firth, E.C.: Bilateral ventral accessory neurectomy in windsucking horses. Vet. Rec. 106:30, 1980.
2. Greet, T.R.C.: Windsucking treated by myectomy and neurectomy. Eq. Vet. J. 14:299, 1982.
3. Huskamp, B., Henschel, E., and Arenhoevel, H.: Technik and Ergebnisse einer modernen Kopperoperation. Prak. Tierarz. 64:110, 1983.
4. Turner, A.S., White, N.A., and Ismay, J.: Modified Forssell's operation for cribbing in the horse. J. Am. Vet. Med. Assoc. 184:309, 1984.

7

Surgery of the Gastrointestinal Tract

Caudal Molar Extraction

Removal of teeth is indicated in cases of infundibular necrosis, fractures, abscesses, periodontal disease, and chronic ossifying periostitis. Infection of the teeth may occur secondary to fractures of the skull (mandible and maxilla) that involve the roots of the teeth. When the disease involves the mandibular teeth, swelling and chronic drainage from the ventral border of the mandible is usually present. Involvement of the caudal molar (sixth cheek tooth) of the mandible is unusual because of the extreme caudal location of this tooth. Removal is performed in a slightly different manner than that for the more rostral teeth.

Anesthesia and Surgical Preparation

Repulsion of the caudal molar of the mandible should be performed with the horse under general anesthesia and with the affected tooth uppermost. A mouth speculum is placed on the horse and opened sufficiently to allow admission of the surgeon's hand. The hair is clipped over the entire masseter muscle on that side, and a routine surgical preparation is performed (described in our previous textbook[3]).

Additional Instrumentation

Caudal molar extraction requires a mouth speculum, mallet or hammer, chisels or osteotomes, curved dental punches, and umbilical tape.

Surgical Technique

The location of the sixth lower cheek tooth necessitates trephination over the lateral surface of the mandible. A line is drawn from the center of the table surface of the tooth to the point of greatest curvature of the ramus of the mandible (Fig. 7-1A). An incision is made on this line through the skin and masseter muscle in the direction of its fibers. The incision should be liberal enough to allow the muscle to be separated from the bone. The skin and muscle incision is terminated at least 4 cm from the border of the mandible to avoid severing the branches of the facial nerve and maxillary artery that spread out over the surface of the masseter muscle from above, ventrad and rostrad. The root of the sixth cheek tooth can be identified by its bulging appearance. To gain access to the tooth root, an opening is made with a chisel. The opening is further elongated to give better direction for the punch and lessen the chances of fracturing the medial bony plate of the mandible (Fig. 7-1B). With careful guidance of the chisel it is possible and preferable to provide access to the root of this tooth without ever using a trephine. When sufficient lateral body plate of the mandible has been removed, the surgeon introduces one hand into the mouth, locates the diseased tooth, and determines the tooth's path in the jaw. The punch is then placed onto the root of the tooth, and an assistant begins to tap the punch with a mallet. The first few blows with the mallet should be sufficient to seat the punch into the root of the tooth (Fig. 7-1C). To allow the punch access to the diseased teeth, the opening may have to be enlarged by removing a little more of the lateral cortex of the mandible with the chisel.

Once the punch is seated, the assistant delivers steady blows to the punch. The mallet blows will produce a characteristic ringing sound when the punch is seated properly, and the surgeon will feel the vibrations of these blows transmitted through the tooth to his hand. If the punch slips off the tooth, it needs to be repositioned. After some time, the surgeon will feel the gradual loosening of the tooth with the hand that is in the horse's mouth. Subsequent blows with the mallet should be less forceful as the tooth is being driven from the alveolus. Removal of the crown of the tooth with molar cutters may be required in young horses before it can be delivered from the mouth.

Following tooth repulsion, any fragments should be removed from the alveolus with forceps. The alveolus may require curettage if diseased bone surrounds the tooth. To prevent the socket from being packed with food material, it should be filled with a suitable material, such as dental wax, dental acrylic, gutta-percha, or gauze rolls, until the socket is almost filled with granulation tissue. If gauze rolls are used, a roll that will fit snugly into the hole is made and tied around the center with umbilical tape, leaving two long ends. The ends are passed through the socket and trephine hole, the gauze is wedged firmly into the cavity, and the umbilical tape is brought to the exterior. The umbilical tape is then secured to the skin by tying it to another gauze roll. The ends should be kept long, so that the gauze roll in the alveolus can be replaced without having to thread the new piece of umbilical tape back through the trephine hole.

Hoof acrylic (methylmethacrylate) is used by some surgeons to pack the alveolus. It is prepared by mixing the powder with the liquid

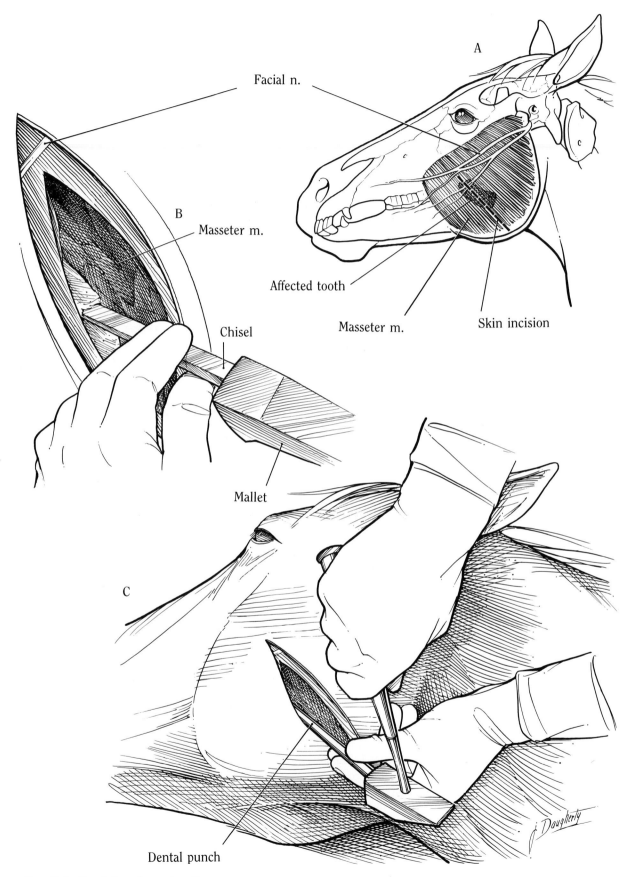

A

Facial n.

B

Masseter m.

Chisel

Mallet

Affected tooth

Masseter m.

Skin incision

C

Dental punch

FIG. 7-1. Caudal molar extraction.

catalyst and working it into a dough-like consistency. It is then packed into the socket from the oral side and extended about 1 cm below the gingival margins.

After the socket has been attended to, the dorsal two thirds of the masseter muscle is opposed with synthetic absorbable sutures. The proximal two thirds of the skin incision is closed with synthetic monofilament nonabsorbable sutures, leaving the ventral aspect open to ensure drainage. To completely close the incision in the masseter muscle would be inviting problems because the potential contamination from the oral cavity could result in abscessation and/or cellulitis if the incision were not free to drain.

Postoperative Management

The horse should be placed on antibiotics preoperatively and for about one week postoperatively. If a gauze pack has been placed in the alveolar socket, it should be changed every other day for two weeks. While the gauze is out of the socket, it should be flushed with warm antiseptic solution. The new gauze should be tied to the umbilical tape, wedged back into the socket, and secured to the skin by tying it to another gauze roll. This maneuver is best done with the mouth speculum in place and sedation with a drug such as xylazine. It necessitates placing the hand into the mouth to remove the old gauze roll and to reposition the new gauze roll. This does present a management problem, and the procedure is not without risk to the surgeon if the horse resents manipulation in this area. For these reasons, packing the socket with an acrylic at the time of surgery is preferred as a more practical solution. The socket eventually fills with granulation tissue. The biggest problem we have found with this technique is difficulty in anchoring the acrylic firmly in the socket. If it loosens and falls out, the horse must be reanesthetized, the socket flushed and all feed material removed, and the acrylic reinserted.

References

1. Guard, W.F.: Surgical Principles and Techniques. Columbus, Ohio, W.F. Guard, 1953.
2. Frank, E.R.: Veterinary Surgery, 7th ed. Minneapolis, Burgess Publishing Company, 1964.
3. Turner, A.S. and McIlwraith, C.W.: Techniques in Large Animal Surgery, Philadelphia, Lea & Febiger, 1982.

Esophagotomy for Removal of an Esophageal Foreign Body

Treatment of esophageal obstruction can involve medical, manipulative, and surgical methods; a fixed protocol is not appropriate. Many cases of obstruction with feed materials will resolve themselves spontaneously or with simple medical support. Gentle manipulation with a stomach tube combined with lavage can be useful in clearing feed obstructions. However, the long-term presence of an impaction can cause pressure necrosis of the esophageal mucosa and subsequent stricture formation; overzealous manipulations with a stomach tube can have similar effects and even cause perforation of the esophagus. Foreign bodies that do not respond to conservative management should be definitively identified by radiographic and/or endoscopic examination.[2] Inert, firm, rough-surfaced, or sharp foreign bodies require surgical intervention to avoid extensive esophageal damage.

Longitudinal esophagotomy with primary closure of the incision results in minimal complications when performed in a region of normal esophagus.[4] The surgeon should always remember that a well-performed esophagotomy is less traumatic than prolonged pressure and bruising to the esophageal wall. The reader is reminded that the esophagus has properties quite distinct from the remainder of the gastrointestinal tract and these are important surgically. The esophagus is not covered by serosa (this tissue layer promotes a rapid seal due to exudation of fibrin following intestinal surgery). The musculature of the esophagus is weak and holds sutures poorly, but the mucosa is relatively strong (in the remainder of the gastrointestinal tract the mucosa is weak and the submucosa is the strongest layer). Nonabsorbable suture material is used to close the mucosa rather than catgut which is absorbed too quickly to be of value. Some surgeons now use polypropylene for all layers.[5] Blood vessels to the esophagus are short and easily damaged, requiring care and imposing limitations in mobilizing the esophagus.

Anesthesia and Surgical Preparation

The esophagotomy is performed under general anesthesia with the horse placed in dorsal recumbency. Prior to induction of the anesthesia, the horse's neck is clipped for a ventral midline approach. A nasogastric tube is also placed as far as the foreign body to facilitate identification of the esophagus during the surgical approach. Following anesthetization, the midline of the neck is shaved, and a routine surgical preparation is performed.

Surgical Technique

An 8- to 10-cm skin incision is made on the ventral midline over the area of the obstruction. This will provide sufficient exposure to make a 5-cm incision in the esophagus. The paired sternohyoid muscles are divided on the midline to expose the trachea. The fascia on the left side of the trachea is then bluntly dissected to locate the esophagus (Fig. 7-2A). The ventral wall of the esophagus is exposed with careful dissection of adventitial tissue, and the left carotid sheath containing the carotid artery and vagus nerve is identified and retracted laterad (Fig. 7-2A). A longitudinal incision is made through the esophagus with a scalpel (Fig. 7-2B). The surgeon attempts to incise a normal esophageal wall, but this will depend on the site, mobility, and extent of the obstruction.

Following removal of the foreign body (Fig. 7-2C) the mucosa of the esophagus is examined. If it appears normal, it is closed with 3/0 polypropylene or nylon suture material in a simple continuous pattern with the knots tied within the lumen (Fig. 7-2D). The esophageal musculature is closed with 2/0 nonabsorbable monofilament material or synthetic absorbable material in a simple interrupted pattern (Fig. 7-2E). A one-quarter inch fenestrated suction drain (Redi-Vacette perforated tubing, one-quarter inch (6.4 mm) OD, Orthopedic Equipment, Bourbon, Indiana) is placed beside the esophagus and exited through the skin caudal to the skin incision (Fig. 7-2F). It is maintained for 48 hours to remove serum and blood from the surgical site. Retention of the drain beyond this period is contraindicated unless there is salivary leakage. The muscle and fascia of the neck incision are closed with synthetic absorbable material or synthetic nonabsorbable material in a simple interrupted pattern. The skin is closed with simple interrupted sutures of nonabsorbable material (Fig. 7-2F).

If removal of the foreign body is necessary through an obviously diseased segment of the esophagus, the esophagotomy incision is not closed. An esophagotomy tube may be placed directly through the esophagotomy incision.

Postoperative Management

When an esophagotomy with a primary closure has been performed through healthy mucosa, extraoral alimentation is not used postoperatively. Food is withheld for 48 hours, and then small quantities of pelleted feed in a slurry are given. Normal feeding is resumed in 8 to 10 days. As discussed previously, the drain is removed in 48 hours unless saliva is leaking from the drain. Detection of salivary leakage heralds the occurrence of dehiscence. If this does occur, the approach incision is opened to avoid spread of infection down into the thorax (a major potential complication). In the early period of convalescence, parenteral electrolyte solutions may be used to maintain hydration if necessary.

If the esophagotomy is performed through a compromised esophagus, extraoral alimentation is given through either an esophagostomy tube placed through a separate aboral incision or an esophagostomy tube placed directly into the initial esophagotomy incision. Cervical esophagostomy has been documented as a safe and convenient means of tube feeding in the horse[1,3] and is preferred over the use of a nasogastric tube or pharyngostomy tube. A complete pelleted diet (7 g/kg in 5 L water t.i.d.) is satisfactory for extraoral alimentation.[3] Ten

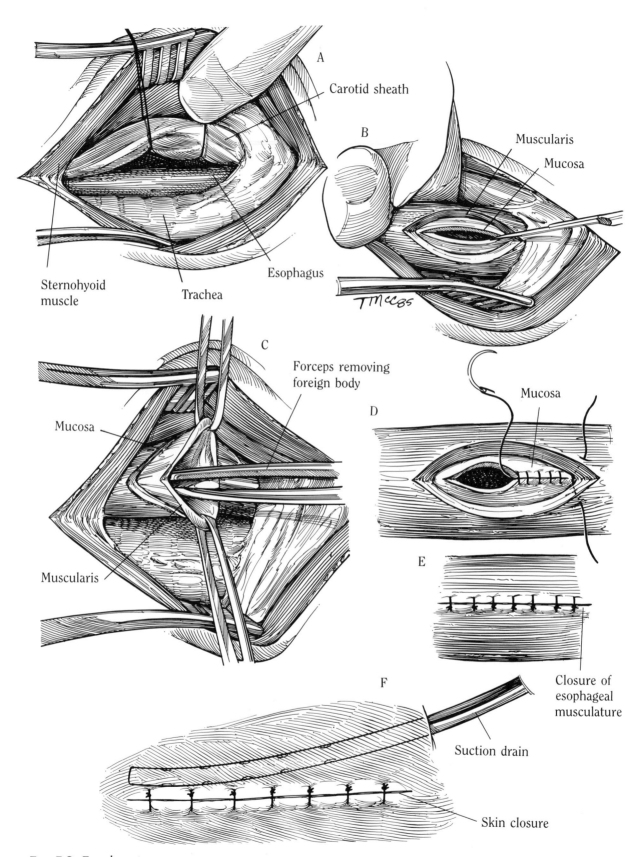

A
Carotid sheath

B
Muscularis
Mucosa

Sternohyoid muscle

Trachea

Esophagus

C
Forceps removing foreign body

Mucosa

D
Mucosa

Muscularis

E
Closure of esophageal musculature

F
Suction drain

Skin closure

Fig. 7-2. Esophagotomy.

days of extraoral alimentation is sufficient in most esophageal surgery cases. The tubes are removed, and the stoma is left to heal by second intention.

Comments

The use of a primarily sutured esophagotomy through healthy mucosa has definite advantages. It heals significantly faster than nonsutured esophagotomies, and the latter group also tends to develop traction diverticula.[4]

References

1. Freeman, D.E., and Naylor, J.M.: Cervical esophagostomy to permit extraoral feeding of the horse. J. Am. Vet. Med. Assoc. 172:314, 1978.
2. Stick, J.A.: Surgery of the esophagus. Vet. Clin. North. Am. Large Anim. Pract. 4:33, 1982.
3. Stick, J.A., Derksen, F.J., and Scott, E.A.: Equine cervical esophagostomy: Complications associated with duration and location of feeding tubes. Am. J. Vet. Res. 42:727, 1981.
4. Stick, J.A., Krehbiel, J.D., Kunze, D.J., et al.: Esophageal healing in the pony: Comparison of sutured vs. non-sutured esophagotomy. Am. J. Vet. Res. 42:1506, 1981.
5. Stick, J.A.: Personal communication, 1985.

Surgical Correction of Displacements and Abnormalities of the Small Intestine

In keeping with the concept of this text as a surgical atlas, the presentations of this and the next section will be limited to a brief description of specific abnormalities and manipulations to correct them. The inexperienced surgeon needs to augment this material with more detailed discussions of the pathogenesis, pathophysiology, diagnosis, and medical management of these conditions available elsewhere in textbooks[8,10,11] and journal publications.

When a specific procedure such as enterotomy or jejunocecal anastomosis is given as a treatment method (or part of the treatment), the reader is referred to the sections where these techniques are specifically presented. When the surgical diagnosis and manipulative treatments for a condition are straightforward and diagrams are considered unnecessary, only a brief summary of the presentation and treatment will be given.*

Simple Obstruction of the Small Intestine
Impaction of the Small Intestine

Primary impactions of the small intestine are of two types: impaction of the ileum with feed material[4,8] and generalized impaction of the small intestine with *Parascaris equorum*.[11,18]

Cases of ileal impaction with feed material present with clinical signs of simple obstruction of the small intestine. At laparotomy, ingesta are found impacted from the ileocecal orifice orad for 30 to 90 cm.[4] The small intestine cranial to the impaction will be distended with gas and fluid. Treatment in most cases involves massage of the feed material into the cecum with or without prior injection of saline solution into the mass to soften the ingesta. In occasional severe cases, enterotomy may be necessary to remove the impacted feed material. In severe cases ileocecal bypass (side-to-side anastomosis) or resection and jejunocecal anastomosis (if bowel compromise is present) may be necessary. Conservative management in early cases may be feasible.[8] Some degree of postoperative ileus can be anticipated following surgical correction.

Ascarid impaction usually occurs shortly after anthelmintic treatment. The small intestine may be partially or completely obstructed with these worms, and rupture of the intestine can occur in severe cases. Surgical relief of the obstruction through enterotomy is indicated for complete obstruction or any obstruction that has not responded to administration of mineral oil. In some cases laparotomy reveals that the intestine has already ruptured. In addition to the normal physiologic changes associated with small intestinal obstruc-

---

* In this textbook the authors have chosen to use cranial and caudad to describe position in the gastrointestinal tract in preference to proximal and distal (common usage but inaccurate) and oral and aboral (implies directional movement).

tion and fluid sequestration, it has been suggested that dead ascarids cause a toxic or allergic effect that may exacerbate any systemic deterioration.[18]

Pedunculated Lipoma

Pedunculated lipomas of the small intestinal mesentery may cause simple obstruction when the long pedicle of the lipoma encircles the small intestine. They more commonly cause a strangulating obstruction and are a problem of older horses. Laparotomy is needed to confirm the diagnosis of a pedunculated lipoma, whether it is simple or strangulated. Distention of the small intestine cranial to the obstruction will be present, and usually there will be evidence of a chronic duration. Because of this, normal motility may not return to the bowel cranial to the obstruction following removal of the lipoma, and in these cases resection and anastomosis of such nonfunctional intestine may be necessary if it is feasible.[11]

Adhesions

Adhesions may cause simple obstruction of the small intestine. They are most commonly seen following peritonitis or abdominal surgery. Simple obstructions associated with adhesions are commonly partial, and there may be a history of recurrent colic. The treatment of the adhesions usually involves either separation or cutting of the adhesions so that a patent lumen and normal bowel configuration are reestablished. In other instances, intestinal resection and anastomosis (in some cases a side-to-side anastomosis leaving the strictured bowel in situ is the most appropriate method) are performed. The severed or separated surfaces must be oversewn to minimize further formation of adhesions. The prognosis is always guarded because of the potential for reformation of adhesions.

Abdominal Abscesses

Abdominal abscesses may produce compression or stricture of a portion of the small intestine. The majority of abdominal abscesses involve the mesentery, and systemic spread from respiratory infection is considered the most common cause of the abscessation.[21] *Streptococcus equi*, *Streptococcus zooepidemicus*, and *Corynebacterium pseudotuberculosis* are the most common isolates. The condition is commonly a medical one, and long-term administration of penicillin has been used successfully in the treatment of internal abdominal abscesses.[21] Surgical treatment is indicated in some instances if a surgical colic is deemed to be present and if abscesses can be drained intraoperatively or marsupialized without peritoneal contamination. Intestinal resection and anastomosis with abscess removal may be appropriate in selected cases of localized obstruction associated with abscessation.[30]

Muscular Hypertrophy of the Ileum

Muscular hypertrophy of the distal ileum (at the ileocecal valve) may cause intestinal obstruction. The condition has been associated with stenosis of the ileum secondary to a mucosal lesion, strongyle larvae migration, neurogenic stenosis with prolonged closure of the ileocecal valve, and ileocecal intussusception.[6] The condition is classified as primary idiopathic hypertrophy when predisposing lesions are not found at necropsy.[9] The clinical signs will vary depending on whether the obstruction is incomplete or complete. Diagnosis is confirmed at laparotomy. Ileal myotomy has been used as a treatment,[6] but jejunocecal anastomosis is used more frequently.

Neoplasia

With the exception of pedunculated lipomas, neoplasms of the intestines are rare. Lymphosarcoma can involve the small intestine and small intestinal mesentery, and squamous cell carcinoma may metastasize throughout the abdomen involving the small intestine and small intestinal mesentery. These situations are not considered surgical cases, but surgery may be the means by which diagnosis is achieved.

Duodenitis-Cranial Jejunitis Syndrome

The duodenitis-cranial jejunitis syndrome is now well recognized in Europe and the United States.[2,7] There are clinical signs of a simple cranial obstruction of the small intestine with gastric reflux of fluid. There is a functional ileus of the proximal small intestine with a secondary overloading of the stomach.[7] The irony of this condition is that while the clinical signs suggest a lesion requiring surgical intervention is present, the stresses of general anesthesia and surgical manipulation have been found to produce a higher death rate than when conservative therapy is utilized.[2] The condition can be suggested on rectal examination by palpating a distended transverse duodenum. It may be difficult to differentiate the condition from other causes of small intestinal obstruction, and diagnosis can be achieved only at surgery in some cases. Conservative management is generally considered the treatment of choice and includes systemic antibiotics, flunixin meglumine (Banamine) for relief of pain and to combat the effects of endotoxin, and supportive fluid therapy. Some horses have required up to 10 days of critical care before gastric reflux ceased and normal eating can be allowed.[2] Clostridiosis or salmonellosis have been suggested etiologic factors, but as yet no definitive cause is known.

A technique of duodenocecostomy has been used in Europe to facilitate drainage of accumulating fluid into the cecum in several cases and has been reported as a successful procedure.[7] If performed, it involves a right flank approach between the 17th and 18th ribs with removal of the 18th rib. A side-to-side anastomosis of the duodenum to the base of the cecum is performed, using two layers of sutures in the serosa and muscularis and a cutting suture in the mucosa. The originator of the technique suggests that early closure of the stoma is facilitated by not involving mucosa in the suture line.[7]

Duodenal Stenosis

Duodenal stenosis is an uncommon condition that has been reported in foals four months and younger.[12,23] In all cases the strictures have been reported in the region of the *ansa sigmoidea* (lesser curvature of the duodenum) and two of three cases involved the normal stricture between the two dilated portions of the sigmoid (ampulla duodeni and ampulla hepatopancreatica). Both congenital and traumatic etiologies have been proposed. The clinical signs are similar to pyloric stenosis and include recurrent dysphagia, regurgitation, salivation, mild intermittent colic with metabolic alkalosis, depression, anorexia, and unthriftiness. Surgical correction of a case has utilized a longitudinal enterotomy over the stenotic area with closure in a transverse fashion.[12] Surgical exposure of the site is difficult but is possible in the foal. The enterotomy technique is inadequate for a longer stenotic segment, and in these cases duodenal myotomy or gastroduodenostomy (side-to-side anastomosis) should be considered. For a stricture in the distal part of the duodenum, a duodenojejunostomy or gastrojejunostomy (side-to-side anastomosis) should be considered (these techniques are as described for a side-to-side jejunocecal anastomosis on p. 311).

Strangulating Obstruction of the Small Intestine
Intussusception

An intussusception is the invagination of a segment of intestine (intussusceptum) and its mesentery into the adjacent distal segment of bowel (intussuscipiens) (Fig. 7-3A). The small intestine is the most common site of occurrence for this condition, which also can involve the jejunum, ileum, or terminal ileum (ileocecal intussusception). The condition occurs more frequently in young horses,[19,27] but not exclusively. The initial clinical signs are usually characterized by signs of complete obstruction of the small intestine. The superimposed signs of bowel strangulation develop at later stages. The condition is easily recognized at laparotomy with systematic exploration of the small intestine starting at the ileocecal valve. Reduction of the intussusception may be possible but can be precluded by excessive swelling of the intussuscipiens or serosal adhesions. While intussusceptions have been treated by reduction alone, the authors recommend that resection of all intussusceptions should be a general consideration even when the intussuscipiens is apparently viable. Progressive mucosal degeneration can still develop.[16] The surgeon must remember that the ileal artery, which runs along the mesenteric border of the ileum,

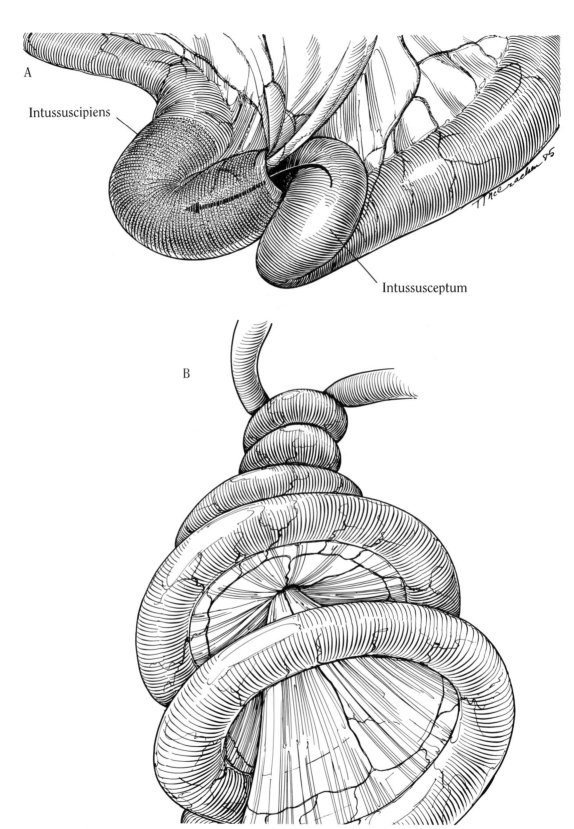

A

Intussuscipiens

Intussusceptum

B

FIG. 7-3. Strangulating obstruction of the small intestine. **A.** Intussusception of small intestine. **B.** Volvulus of small intestine.

is the sole source of blood supply for the ileum if the intussusception involves this area. Peritonitis (from necrosis of the bowel segment), stenosis, or adhesions are all potential developments if the intussuscepted portion is not resected. For intussusceptions involving the jejunum, resection and end-to-end anastomosis may be appropriate. If the ileum is involved in the intussusception, a jejunocecal anastomosis is performed.

Chronic small intestinal intussusception has also been reported in the foal. In the case of one reported in the ileum, a side-to-side anastomosis of ileum to cecum without resection was performed. If viable bowel is present, this procedure offers advantages in terms of eliminating any risk of contamination with an open resection and anastomosis.[24]

As with all the strangulating obstructions described in this section, ancillary therapy to combat the affects of ischemia and endotoxemia is important.

Volvulus

Small intestinal volvulus is produced by a 180-degree or greater rotation of a segment of jejunum and/or ileum about the long axis of the mesentery. Rotations of up to 180 degrees may occur physiologically without producing disturbances. Volvulus may occur as a primary displacement or may be secondary to a preexisting lesion such as incarceration of the small intestine in the mesentery, epiploic foramen, gastrosplenic ligament, mesodiverticular band, Meckel's diverticulum, or adhesions. The ileum is commonly involved. Incarceration involving the caudal segments of the small bowel (terminal jejunum and ileum) has been assigned a specific name "volvulus nodosus" by European workers.[8] The clinical signs associated with this condition are acute and severe.

Treatment of the volvulus involves surgical reduction and intestinal evacuation. At laparotomy, discolored, thickened and distended loops of bowel are usually found at the incision, and the direction of the volvulus is usually ascertained by palpating the mesentery at the base of the twist (Fig. 7-3B). In severe volvulus involving the entire small intestinal tract the mesentery is twisted in a cordlike spiral up to the mesenteric root. The more times the intestine is rotated, the higher up in the mesentery the constriction occurs. Any primary lesion must also be recognized and addressed. Tearing of the mesentery with incarceration may also occur secondarily to the volvulus. Which malposition to correct first depends on the individual case. Correction of the volvulus is performed by rotating all affected loops in the appropriate direction. Following reduction, nonviable bowel is resected if feasible. Sectioning of intestine with temporary closure may be necessary to correct the displacement. Following reduction, nonviable bowel is resected and an end-to-end anastomosis or jejunocecal anastomosis performed as appropriate. Resection of greater than 50% of the small intestine is not indicated, and the patient should be euthanized.[26]

The prognosis in cases of volvulus is commonly poor because of the rapid deterioration of the patient and excessive intestinal involvement in many instances.

Internal Hernias

An internal hernia is a displacement of organs through a normal or pathologic opening within the abdominal cavity.[13] Internal herniation of the small intestine usually results in incarceration. Herniation may occur through a normal opening (epiploic foramen) or a pathologic opening (acquired or congenital mesenteric defects, tears in the greater or lesser omentum or gastrosplenic ligament, or defects in the broad ligament or foramina formed by fibrous bands or adhesions). Herniation through the ductus deferens also has been described.[8] The clinical signs are generally typical of strangulating obstruction of the small intestine. In some instances, however, strangulation has not yet occurred at the time of laparotomy and the intestine is still viable.

EPIPLOIC FORAMEN INCARCERATION

The epiploic foramen that separates the omental bursa from the major peritoneal cavity is bounded dorsally by the caudal lobe of the liver and the caudal vena cava and ventrally by the right lobe of the pancreas, gastropancreatic fold, and portal vein. The foramen is limited cranially by the hepatoduodenal ligament and caudally by the junction of the pancreas and mesoduodenum.[20] Herniation of small intestines through the epiploic foramen can occur in a right-to-left direction from the peritoneal cavity through the foramen into the omental bursa (also called herniation from the lateral side)[8] or in a left-to-right direction where the omental bursa is involved in the herniation and is torn (also called herniation from the medial side). Herniation from right to left is the most commonly recognized form in the United States (12 of 15 cases in one report),[29] but in a European report, incarceration from medial to lateral was reported as more common.[8] These hernias are illustrated in Figure 7-3C and D. The incarcerated portion of bowel is distended. A special, rare form of epiploic foramen incarceration whereby a portion of the small intestinal wall protrudes through the epiploic foramen from the lateral side has been described from Europe and has been called a Littre's hernia.[8]

Surgical treatment of incarceration of small intestine in the epiploic foramen is made difficult because the condition is not always associated with signs typical of intestinal incarceration.[29] The degree of pain may be highly variable, but analysis of peritoneal fluid can be useful. Failure to diagnose the condition early and intervene surgically has caused a low success rate.[29]

The condition is confirmed at laparotomy during systematic exploration of the small intestine. Although the condition may be recognized by palpating the region of the epiploic foramen, the condition is more consistently characterized by locating the ileocecal fold and following the ileum craniad until the incarceration is encountered. The

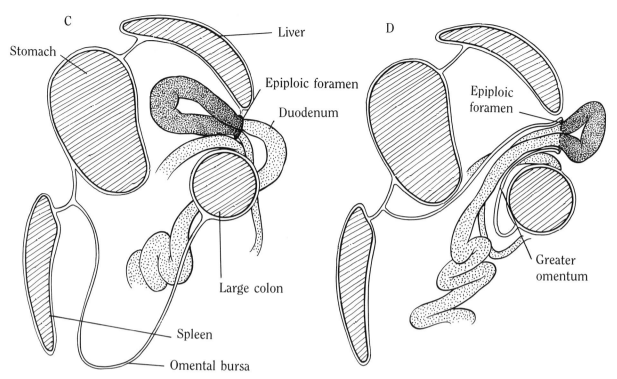

FIG. 7-3 (*Continued*). **C.** Right to left hernia of small intestine through epiploic foramen. **D.** Left to right hernia through epiploic foramen.

incarceration may involve midjejunum or distal jejunum and/or ileum. A large portion of the small intestine may be incarcerated. If the incarceration is from right to left, reduction is made from the right side of the abdominal cavity, and the intestine is pulled out of the omental bursa through the epiploic foramen. Reduction in this fashion is usually possible, but the strangulated intestine can become edematous to the point that reduction may not be feasible. Cautious manipulation and traction should be performed because of the vascular structures associated with the epiploic foramen. Prior decompression or even sectioning of the intestine and evacuation may be required in an exceptional case. A left-to-right incarceration needs to be retracted back into the omental bursa side. Resection and anastomosis of devitalized bowel is usually required, and end-to-end anastomosis of jejunum or jejunocecal anastomosis is performed as appropriate. Closure of the epiploic foramen is not practical. The prognosis depends on the promptness of surgical intervention and the amount of compromised bowel.

MESENTERIC INCARCERATION

Incarceration through an acquired rent in the mesentery usually occurs through the ileal mesentery. It has been assumed that these tears occur at the same time as the incarceration. However, spontaneous tears of the mesentery associated with physiologic invaginations of the small intestine due to hyperperistalsis may occur. In these cases, the mesentery of the intussusceptum becomes stretched and possibly torn.[8] The herniated piece of intestine can become incarcerated and strangulated by the hernial ring (Fig. 7-3E). Volvulus may occur secondary to this condition (Fig. 7-3F). The clinical signs are typical of strangulation obstruction of the small intestine. They will generally be more severe if there is an associated volvulus.

The condition is recognized at laparotomy. If volvulus of the herniated segment of bowel is found, it should be corrected first. Reduction of the mesenteric hernia may require prior evacuation of the herniated portion of the intestine as well as enlargement of the hernial ring. The strangulated jejunum or ileum is resected, and an end-to-end or jejunocecal anastomosis is performed as appropriate. Effective

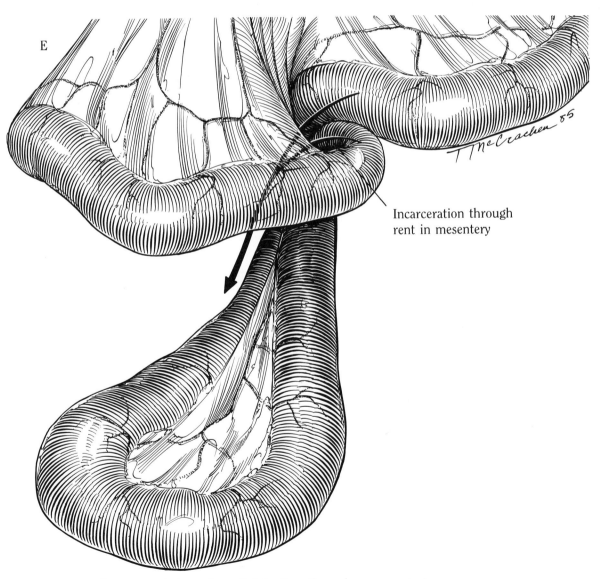

E

Incarceration through rent in mesentery

FIG. 7-3 (*Continued*). **E.** Herniation of small intestine through a mesenteric rent.

F

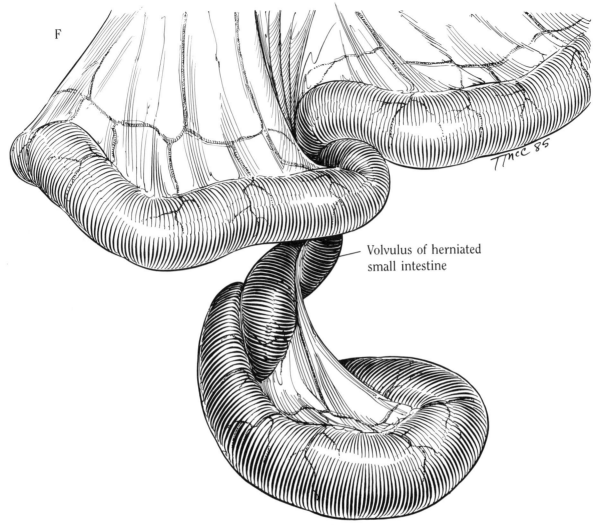

Volvulus of herniated small intestine

FIG. 7-3 (*Continued*). **F.** Volvulus of small intestine secondary to mesenteric herniation.

closure of the mesenteric rent can be difficult, and care must be taken to avoid damaging any mesenteric vessels.

MESENTERIC INCARCERATION IN ASSOCIATION WITH AN ANOMALOUS MESODIVERTICULAR BAND

A mesodiverticular band is formed by persistence of a distal segment of a vitelline artery and its associated embryonic mesentery (Fig. 7-3G). The band extends from one side of the small intestinal mesentery to the antimesenteric surface of the intestine (usually jejunum), and a triangular hiatus is thus formed between the mesodiverticular band, jejunal mesentery, and jejunum (Fig. 7-3G). Entrapment of intestine in this hiatus can result in herniation of the intestine through the jejunal mesentery.[5] Secondary volvulus of the incarcerated portion may also occur. Treatment of this condition consists of

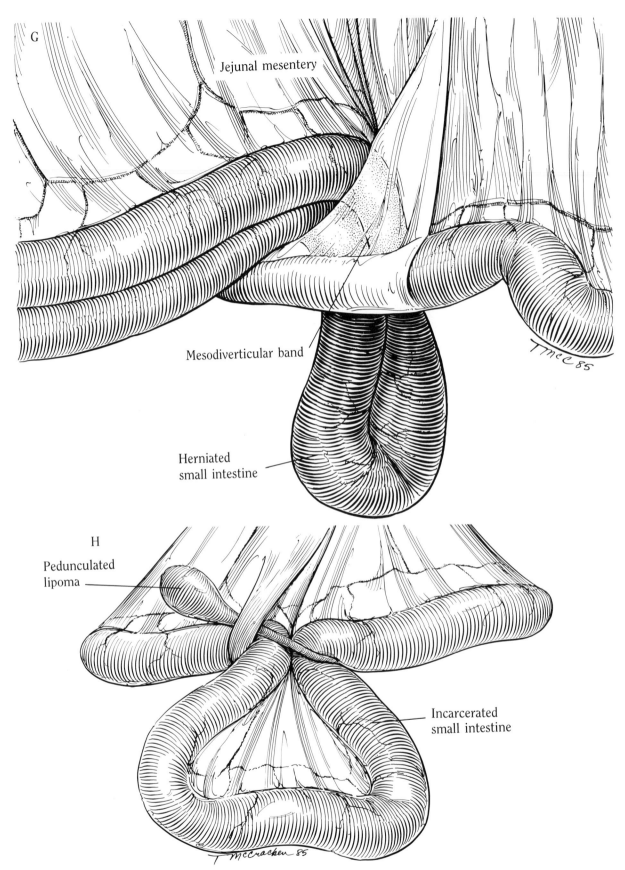

FIG. 7-3 (*Continued*). **G.** Mesenteric herniation in association with an anomalous mesodiverticular band. **H.** Strangulated obstruction of small intestine caused by a pedunculated lipoma.

reduction of the incarceration and volvulus and intestinal resection and anastomosis.

HERNIATION THROUGH OMENTAL DEFECTS

The small intestine may herniate through a rent in the greater omentum or a window formed by an omental adhesion.[14] It may also herniate through the gastrosplenic ligament[27] or through tears in the lesser omentum (hepatogastric and hepatoduodenal ligament).[8] Clinical signs and surgical management are similar to those for other internal hernias. Defects in the greater omentum are best handled by removal of the offending portion of the omentum. Obliteration of a defect in the lesser omentum is not feasible.

HERNIATION THROUGH THE BROAD LIGAMENT

Herniation of small intestine through the broad ligament has been reported but is uncommon.[1] Reduction (and resection and anastomosis if necessary) are performed. The defect in the mesometrium cannot be closed.

STRANGULATING HERNIA ASSOCIATED WITH A PEDUNCULATED LIPOMA

Simple obstruction associated with a pedunculated lipoma has been mentioned previously. Strangulating obstruction of the small intestine can occur when the pedicle of a pedunculated lipoma encircles a section of small intestine (Fig. 7-3H). Incarceration of intestine through a ring created by a pedicle of the lipoma can be considered as a form of internal hernia. Treatment involves severance of the pedicle, removal of the lipoma, and resection and anastomosis of the intestine.

External Hernias

An external hernia is a displacement of abdominal contents beyond the abdominal cavity. Examples include inguinal hernias, umbilical hernias, ventral abdominal hernias and diaphragmatic hernias.

INGUINAL OR SCROTAL HERNIA

The term *inguinal hernia* is usually used if hernial contents descend into the inguinal canal; if the contents descend into the scrotum, the term *scrotal hernia* is appropriate.[13] However, the term *inguinal hernia* is often used to mean either condition. Acquired inguinal hernia is a problem of stallions (there is apparently a predisposition in Standardbreds).[22] The condition is usually unilateral and almost always produces an acute strangulating obstruction of the jejunum or ileum. The vaginal ring forms the hernial orifice, and the tunica vaginalis forms the hernial sac (classified as *indirect* hernia). *Direct* herniation as it occurs in man, without involvement of the internal ring, has been reported rarely in the horse.[31] Clinical diagnosis of an inguinal hernia is confirmed with a combination of external palpation and rectal palpation of the inguinal rings.

For surgery, the horse is prepared for both an inguinal and a ventral midline laparotomy approach. An inguinal approach is made initially with a 15-cm skin incision over the involved testicle and extending through the subcutaneous fascia (this technique is described more fully in the section on repair of an inguinal hernia). Blunt dissection is used to separate the deep fascia from the common vaginal tunic, and the tunic is incised over the testicle, taking care to avoid herniated intestine. The incision is extended down to the internal ring, and the viability of the intestine is evaluated. Viable bowel can be returned to the abdomen through the inguinal ring. The intestine that has suffered severe vascular compromise is resected, and an end-to-end anastomosis is performed if this is feasible.

Commonly the compromised intestine will be in the caudal portion of the small intestine and cannot be exteriorized through the inguinal ring. In this instance the diseased bowel is returned to the abdominal cavity, and a resection and anastomosis (usually jejunocecal anastomosis) are performed through a ventral midline approach. In other cases, traction on the intestine is necessary from within the abdomen to reduce the hernia. Ventral midline laparotomy may also be indicated to evacuate distended intestine cranial to the obstruction. In one report of 24 operations, 14 patients required a ventral midline laparotomy in addition to the inguinal approach.[22]

Castration on the affected side and complete closure of the external inguinal ring are preferred to minimize the chance of recurrence of the hernia, as well as the possibility of an ischemic orchitis. With early diagnosis of the condition the prognosis should be good.

Surgical correction of inguinal hernias in foals is usually not necessary because most of them correct spontaneously as the foal grows. Occasionally, incarceration can result (the intestine can break through the common tunic and migrate subcutaneously in some cases) and surgical intervention is necessary.

UMBILICAL HERNIA

Incarceration of small intestine through an umbilical hernia is rare but occasionally occurs. Most umbilical hernias are reducible and produce no problems in their routine repair as discussed in our previous textbook.[28] If incarceration occurs, the hernia is reduced surgically, and resection and anastomosis are followed by umbilical herniorrhaphy.

VENTRAL HERNIA

Acquired hernias occur in the ventral or ventrolateral abdominal wall secondary to abdominal trauma, the stress of parturition, or previous abdominal surgery.[11] Acute incarceration is uncommon, but some abdominal discomfort can occur. Surgery is generally elective and delayed until acute inflammation and infection are under control and the hernial ring is sufficiently fibrosed. If intestinal incarceration occurs, immediate surgery is performed. Because the surrounding tissue is often very friable at this stage, hernial repair can be difficult.

The use of surgical mesh may be appropriate (see separate section for repair of hernia with mesh).

DIAPHRAGMATIC HERNIA

Diaphragmatic hernias are rare. Most cases are acquired,[3,17,33] but congenital hernias do occur.[25] The majority of the lesions occur in the tendinous portion of the diaphragm, most commonly where the centrum tendineum blends into the pars costalis. Congenital defects are infrequent, resulting from incomplete fusion of the pleuroperitoneal folds.[25]

The clinical signs associated with diaphragmatic hernia are variable and depend on the size of the hernial orifice and the amount of herniated viscera. Most cases of diaphragmatic hernia have been definitively diagnosed at laparotomy or necropsy. A definitive clinical diagnosis is possible by thoracic radiography. Successful surgical correction of nonstrangulating diaphragmatic hernia has been reported in one foal[25] and one mare.[23] A ventral midline laparotomy approach was used in each case, and a mesh implant was used to repair the diaphragmatic defect in the mare.[23] Generally, surgical repair in the adult horse is difficult due to an inaccessibility of the dorsal diaphragmatic rent, inability to retract the viscera, and the friability of the damaged diaphragmatic tissue. The first case of peritoneopericardial hernia into the pericardium of a horse was reported recently in a 3-year-old Standardbred stallion.[15] The problem was successfully repaired. The hernial defect was not closed, and the horse was normal one year later.[15]

References

1. Becht, J.L., and McIlwraith, C.W.: Jejunal displacement through the mesometrium in a pregnant mare. J. Am. Vet. Med. Assoc. 177:435, 1980.
2. Blackwell, R.B., and White, N.A.: Duodenitis-proximal jejunitis in the horse. Proceedings of the Equine Colic Research Symposium, Athens, Georgia. 1982, p. 106.
3. Crowhurst, R.C., Simpson, D.J., McEnery, R.J., et al.: Intestinal surgery in the horse. J. S. Afr. Vet. Assoc. 46:59, 1975.
4. Embertson, R.M., Colahan, P.T., Brown M.P., et al.: Ileal impaction in the horse. J. Am. Vet. Med. Assoc. 186:570, 1985.
5. Freeman, D.E., Koch, D.B., and Boles, C.L.: Mesodiverticular bands as a cause of small intestinal strangulation and volvulus in the horse. J. Am. Vet. Med. Assoc. 175:1089, 1979.
6. Horney, F.D., and Funk, K.A.: Ileal myotomy in the horse. Mod. Vet. Pract. 52:49, 1971.
7. Huskamp, B.: Diagnosis of gastroduodenojejunitis and its surgical treatment by a temporary duodenocaecostomy. Eq. Vet. J. 17:314, 1985.
8. Huskamp, B., Daniels, H., and Kopf, N.: Diseases of the stomach and intestine. In Diseases of the Horse. (O. Dietz and E. Wiesner, Eds.) Basel, S. Karger, 1984, p. 164.
9. Lindsay, W.A., Confer, A.W., and Ochoa, R.: Ileal smooth muscle hypertrophy and rupture in a horse. Eq. Vet. J. 13:66, 1981.
10. McIlwraith, C.W. (Ed.): Symposium on equine gastrointestinal surgery. Vet. Clin. North Am.: Large Anim. Pract., 4:1, 1982.
11. McIlwraith, C.W.: Equine digestive system. In The Practice of Large Animal Surgery. (Paul B. Jennings, Ed.) Philadelphia, W.B. Saunders, 1984, p. 554.
12. McIntosh, S.C., and Shupe, J.R.: Surgical correction of duodenal stenosis in the foal. Eq. Pract. 3:17, 1981.

13. Nieberle, K., and Cohrs, P.: Textbook of Special Pathological Anatomy of Domestic Animals. Oxford, Pergamon Press, 1967.
14. Norrie, R.D., and Heistand, D.L.: Chronic colic due to an omental adhesion in a mare. J. Am. Vet. Med. Assoc. 167:54, 1975.
15. Orsini, J.A., Koch, C., Stewart, B.: Peritoneopericardial hernia in a horse. J. Am. Vet. Med. Assoc. 179:907, 1981.
16. Owen, R. ap R., Physick-Sheard, P.W., Hilbert, B.J., et al.: Jejuno- or ileocecal anastomosis performed in seven horses exhibiting colic. Can. Vet. J. 165:164, 1975.
17. Pearson, H., Pinsent, P.J.N., Polley, L.R., et al.: Rupture of the diaphragm in the horse. Eq. Vet. J. 9:32, 1977.
18. Robertson, J.T.: Differential diagnosis and surgical management of surgical conditions of stomach and small intestine. Vet. Clin. North Am. Large Anim. Pract. 4:105, 1982.
19. Rooney, J.R.: Volvulus, strangulation and intussusception in the horse. Cornell Vet. 55:644, 1965.
20. Rooney, J.R., Sack, W.O., and Habel, R.E.: Guide to the Dissection of the Horse. Ann Arbor, MI, Edwards Brothers, 1967.
21. Rumbaugh, G.E., Smith, B.P., and Carlson, G.P.: Internal abdominal abscesses in the horse: A study of 25 cases. J. Am. Vet. Med. Assoc. 172:304, 1978.
22. Schneider, R.K., Milne, D.W., and Kohn, C.W.: Acquired inguinal hernia in the horse: A review of 27 cases. J. Am. Vet. Med. Assoc. 180:317, 1982.
23. Scott, E.A., and Fishback, W.A.: Surgical repair of diaphragmatic hernia in a horse. J. Am. Vet. Med. Assoc. 168:45, 1976.
24. Scott, E.A., and Todhunter, R.: Chronic intestinal intussusception in two horses. J. Am. Vet. Med. Assoc. 186:383, 1985.
25. Spiers, V.C., and Reynolds, W.T.: Surgical repair of a diaphragmatic hernia in a foal. Eq. Vet. J. 8:170, 1976.
26. Tate, L.P., Ralston, S.L., and Koch, C.M., et al.: Effects of extensive resection of the small intestine in the pony. Am. J. Vet. Res. 44:1187, 1983.
27. Tennant, B.: Intestinal obstruction in the horse: Some aspects of differential diagnosis in equine colic. Proceedings of the AAEP, 1976, p. 426.
28. Turner, A.S., and McIlwraith, C.W.: Techniques in Large Animal Surgery. Philadelphia, Lea & Febiger, 1982.
29. Turner, T.A., Adams, S.B., and White, N.A.: Small intestine incarceration through the epiploic foramen of the horse. J. Am. Vet. Med. Assoc. 184:731, 1984.
30. Valdez, H., McLaughlin, S.A., and Taylor, T.S.: A case of colic due to an abscess of the jejunum and its mesentery. J. Eq. Med. Surg. 3:36, 1979.
31. Vasey, J.R.: Simultaneous presence of a direct and an indirect inguinal hernia in a stallion. Aust. Vet. J. 57: 418, 1981.
32. Wagner, P.C., Grant, B.D., and Schmidt, J.M.: Duodenal stricture in a foal. Eq. Pract. 1:29, 1979.
33. Wimberley, H.C., Andrews, E.J., and Haschek, W.M.: Diaphragmatic hernias in the horse: A review of the literature and analysis of six additional cases. J. Am. Vet. Med. Assoc. 170:1404, 1977.

Surgical Correction of Displacements and Abnormalities of the Large Intestine

Simple Obstruction of the Large Intestine

Impaction with Ingesta

Impaction of the large intestine is a common cause of intestinal obstruction. It is commonly treated conservatively, but surgical intervention is appropriate when conservative methods fail to solve the problem. Impaction may involve the cecum, the large colon, or the small colon.

Impaction of the Cecum

Impaction of the cecum is normally insidious in onset, and the predisposing factors are vague.[8] It has been suggested, however, that the condition is more often secondary to a caudal obstruction or pathologic problem of the cecocolic orifice.[12] The course of the condition can be one of intermittent colic for a week or more. Because the cecum is a blind sac, fluid and some ingesta can bypass the obstruction. There are three forms of surgical therapy if the impaction is unresponsive to medical treatment.

Surgical intervention may be limited to a laparotomy (performed through a standing flank approach) with exposure of the cecum and injection of saline solution and the surfactant dioctyl sodium sulfosuccinate (DSS) directly into the impacted mass. Manual massage is performed to break up the impacted mass and distribute the injected fluids. In one recent report the results of such treatment were poor.[8]

Better results have been achieved with typhlotomy at the cecal apex and evacuation of the impacted contents (this evacuation is facilitated by the use of a hose)[8]. Early surgical intervention and evacuation of the cecum would seem appropriate based on recent findings regarding 12 cases of cecal impaction.[8] The duration of clinical signs before rupture ranged from 4 to 96 hours.[8] Failure of normal motility to return following cecal evacuation may also be a problem.

A third surgical procedure is a side-to-side anastomosis between an area of the cecum towards the apex and the right ventral colon to facilitate emptying of the cecum (see section on cecocolic anastomosis).

Impaction of the Large Colon

Impaction is a frequent cause of simple obstruction of the large colon. An impaction by ingesta usually occurs at the pelvic flexure or the right dorsal colon-transverse colon region where the large colon becomes narrow. The pelvic flexure has been identified as a region of resistance to aboral flow and is a probable pacemaker site.[23] Selective retention of large particles also occurs in the right dorsal colon, and the transverse colon provides more resistance to flow than the pelvic flexure.[3] Factors that may precipitate impaction include poor quality feed, decreased water intake and dehydration, and parasite damage. Sand impactions are a special problem that occur in the right dorsal or ventral colon. These are associated with the availability of sand or gravel in the feeding of horses off the ground.

Most impactions with ingesta respond to conservative medical management, which includes the administration of mineral oil and/or DSS together with oral and intravenous fluids if necessary. Medication is used for pain control. If the problem persists or if there is systemic deterioration or the development of refractory pain, surgical intervention is indicated. If surgery is delayed, devitalization of the large colon may occur.

The surgical manipulations for impactions of the large colon consist of evacuation accompanied by flushing of the large colon. Generally this is performed by exteriorization of the pelvic flexure, creation of an enterotomy, and flushing of warm water into the colon using a hose as illustrated in the section on enterotomy.[12] This technique is preferable to manually milking out dry ingesta, particularly for left dorsal-transverse colon impactions.

Sand impactions are more difficult to treat. Medical management may include the use of the natural fiber laxative psyllium hydrophylic mucilloid (Metamucil, Searle). Surgical intervention is indicated if there is no response to medical treatment and is the same as previously described for an ingesta impaction.

Impaction of the Small Colon

Ingesta impactions can also occur in the small colon, and a predisposition in ponies has been reported.[27] Methods of treatment of impactions of the small colon include injection into the bowel and massage, retrograde flushing and massage with a hose inserted per rectum,[26] or evacuation through an enterotomy.

As a final comment it should be remembered always that impaction can result secondarily whenever bowel stasis develops. Whenever an impaction is identified at surgery, a complete exploration should be performed to ensure that there is no other problem and that the impaction is indeed primary.

Foreign Body Impaction

A special form of impaction may occur in association with the ingestion of nondigestible foreign materials such as baling twine, braided materials, and rubber or nylon products. This situation is typically observed in foals and young horses,[7,13] and a particular problem has been experienced in association with ingestion of rubberized fencing material[7] or nylon cording from nylon-based products.[10] The impacting material consists of a firm concretion of ingesta surrounding the core of foreign fibrous strands. Long periods between exposure to the material and development of the clinical problem may occur, indicating that strands of cording may be present in the bowel lumen for a long time before amalgamating to cause an obstruction.[10]

The clinical signs are similar to those of impaction. However, owing to the nondegradable nature of the impacting mass, medical treatment is of no value or only palliative until the next attack. Surgical removal of the offending material is necessary, and enterotomy and removal are performed at an appropriate location in the bowel. The obstruction typically occurs in the small colon and/or transverse colon, but the material may extend into the right dorsal colon. Surgical exteriorization of the right dorsal colon-transverse colon or immediately adjacent to the small colon is not possible. Therefore, an enterotomy is made in a portion of the right dorsal colon that can be exteriorized or through the small colon distal to the obstruction. In some instances removal may not be possible, and bowel wall devitalization can also lead to rupture during surgical manipulation. The prognosis is fair if the bowel is healthy and if removal can be performed effectively without extensive contamination of the abdominal cavity. Formation of adhesions in the area is a potential complication.

Enteroliths

Enteroliths occur in the large intestine and can remain there for long periods unassociated with clinical signs until they become impacted in the narrow part of the digestive tract. They may cause obstruction in the right dorsal colon, transverse colon, or the proximal small colon (the latter site is the most common[5]). Large enteroliths are characteristic of the right dorsal colon.[11] The enteroliths are generally spherical or tetrahedral in shape. When multiple stones are present, they are usually tetrahedral.

The clinical symptoms will vary. Horses typically present with a recurrent mild colic. If the enterolith causes an incomplete blockage, the colic is similar to an impaction. Gas, fluid, and mineral oil can still be passed, but there is no solid fecal material. A complete obstruction will cause a colic that increases in intensity as tympany of the colon occurs.

Treatment is surgical removal. At surgery there will be distention of the colon cranial to the enterolith, and the small colon is empty caudal to the obstruction. If the enterolith is present in a portion of the bowel that can be exteriorized, an enterotomy is performed and the concretion removed. More often, the enterolith is in a segment of bowel that cannot be exteriorized (cranial small colon or caudal right dorsal colon). In this instance, the enterolith is moved retrograde until it is positioned in a portion of the dorsal colon that can be exteriorized for enterotomy. Alternatively, if it cannot be moved by external manipulation, an enterotomy is performed in the region of the diaphragmatic flexure (left dorsal colon), and an arm is inserted within the lumen of the bowel to grasp the enterolith (Fig. 7-4A). This can cause considerable contamination if care is not taken. Retrograde flushing with water using a hose inserted up the small colon is a useful

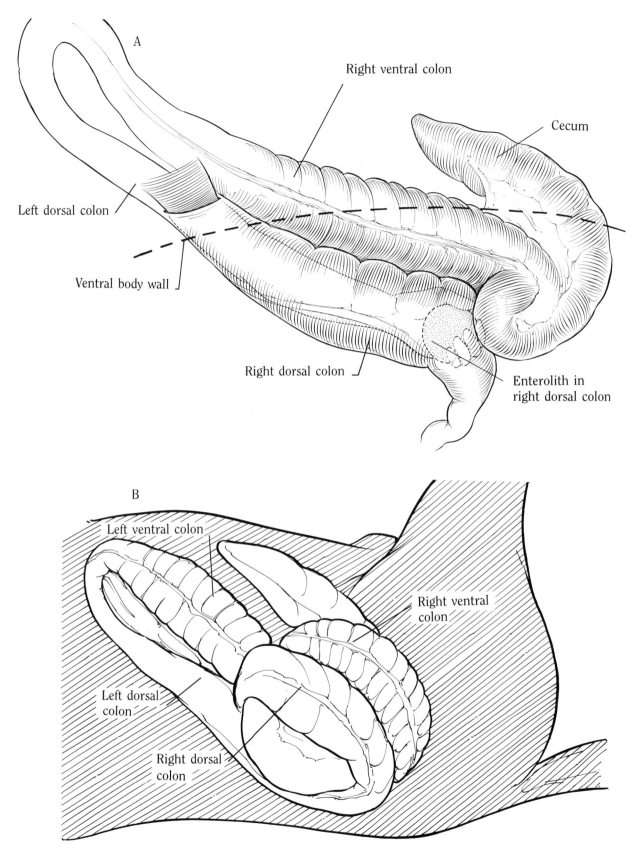

FIG. 7-4. Surgical correction of displacements and abnormalities of the large intestine (horse positioned in dorsal recumbency). **A.** Removal of enterolith from the right dorsal colon. **B.** Right dorsal displacement of the large colon.

adjunctive technique,[26] but caution should be exercised because of weakened ischemic bowel wall where the enterolith is lodged.

The prognosis is fair (47% success rate in one report of 30 cases).[5] Successful surgery depends on removal of the enterolith prior to bowel devitalization, as bowel rupture associated with removal of the enterolith is not uncommon. In addition, contamination of the abdominal cavity during removal can compromise the results.

Displacement or Nonstrangulating Torsion of the Large Colon

This category includes various conditions that have been generally classified as torsions but are characterized by an abnormal position of the large colon *without* strangulation of the blood supply. The normal flow of ingesta is arrested, but viability of the colon is not generally affected. These torsions are surgical conditions, but because of the lack of bowel strangulation, the patient experiences slow systemic deterioration and the success rate with timely surgical intervention is good. The clinical presentation is often acute because of tympany in the cecum and colon. Upon rectal examination, distention of the large colon will be palpated. Some patients will manifest a degree of colonic impaction.

A number of malpositions can occur. The most common displacement involves part or all of the large colon being displaced to the right and caudad, then winding back mediad and craniad around the fixed point formed by the cecum (Fig. 7-4B). The pelvic flexure is often displaced into the cranial aspect of the abdomen. This type of malposition may be complicated by torsion as well. European equine surgeons have classified such displacement as right dorsal displacement of the large colon.[16] In the surgical treatment, the surgeon first attempts to exteriorize the pelvic flexure, and gas and ingesta are then removed as necessary prior to correction. Ingesta is evacuated through an enterotomy at the pelvic flexure. Reduction is then effected by reversing the pathway in which the pelvic flexure has moved (moving pelvic flexure back around the right side of the base of the cecum and colon), and replacing the sternal and diaphragmatic segments of the colon in their normal cranial position with the pelvic flexure in its caudal position. Effective reduction is ascertained by being able to exteriorize the large colon normally and visualize the entire cecocolic fold. Such manipulations can be difficult and strenuous because they have to be performed in the depth of the abdomen. Tympany in the colon usually results in an early presentation of these cases, and with timely surgical intervention the prognosis is good.

In the other common form of nonstrangulating obstruction the pelvic flexure may be in a normal position, but the left dorsal and left ventral colon rotate 180 degrees around the sternal and diaphragmatic flexure (Fig. 7-4C). Although this is correctly considered as a torsion, it is generally nonstrangulating. It is also to be noted that rotations of 90 degrees or less are not clinical problems and are only incidental findings at surgery. The essential feature of the 180-degree

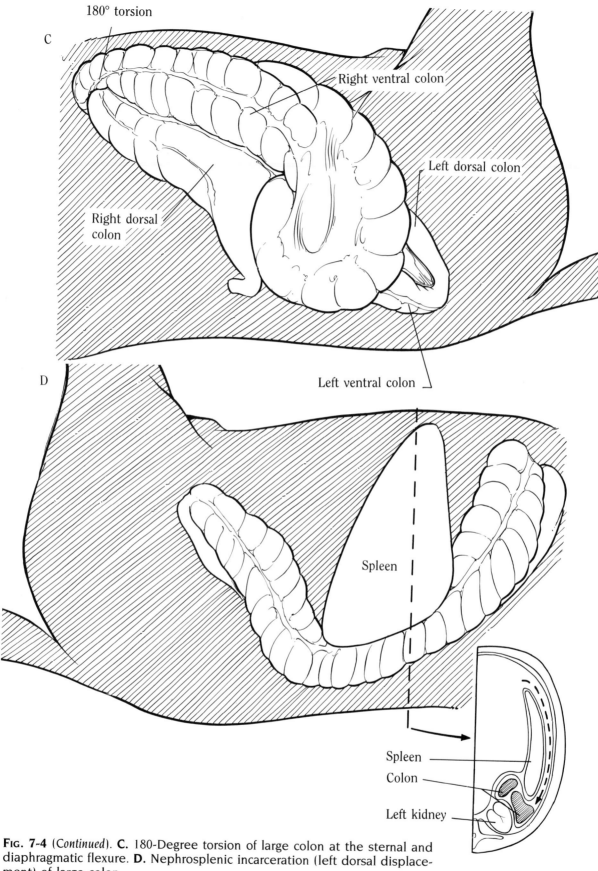

FIG. 7-4 (*Continued*). C. 180-Degree torsion of large colon at the sternal and diaphragmatic flexure. D. Nephrosplenic incarceration (left dorsal displacement) of large colon.

torsion is blockage to the passage of ingesta without compromise of vascularity. With progression of time or with more severe rotations the condition can become a strangulating one. These patients present with moderately painful colic due to large colon distention, and the distended large colon can be palpated on rectal examination. At surgery the malposition is identified. Edema of the mesentery implies an early vascular obstruction. If indicated, the colon is decompressed prior to detorsion. The prognosis is generally good in these cases because surgical intervention usually precedes any permanent changes in the intestinal wall or severe systemic deterioration.

Left Dorsal Displacement or Nephrosplenic Entrapment of the Large Colon

Left dorsal displacement involves the displacement of the large colon into a position between the dorsal body wall and the suspensory ligament of the spleen (nephrosplenic ligament)[18] (Fig. 7-4D). The colon becomes entrapped in a space formed by the left kidney, the nephrosplenic ligament, the dorsal edge of the spleen, and the dorsal abdominal wall. It is considered to occur either from a cranial direction or by slipping up laterally. The colon may become entrapped as far cranially as in the central regions of the right dorsal and ventral colon. Alternatively, it may involve only the left dorsal and ventral colon. The entrapment has been classified as complete or partial depending on whether the edge of the spleen is laterodorsal (complete) or ventral (partial) to the displaced bowel.[16] Commonly, the loop of colon that is entrapped over the nephrosplenic ligament is twisted 180 degrees about its long axis so that the ventral colon overlies the dorsal colon on the ligament.

The clinical presentations range from low grade intermittent colic to refractory unresponsive colic. Rectal findings will vary. They may include an impacted or gas-distended pelvic flexure, or in other instances the pelvic flexure is not palpable because it is displaced craniad. This is the usual situation if a larger segment of colon is incarcerated (such as incarceration involving the right dorsal and right ventral colons). It may be possible to palpate teniae of the colon extending up in a dorsocranial direction. Although the spleen may be displaced caudomediad, this is not a pathognomonic sign, since dilation of the stomach alone will cause splenic rotation.

These patients are generally treated surgically by midline laparotomy. If excessive distention or impaction of the colon is present, the left dorsal and left ventral colons are evacuated prior to any reduction. Following closure of the enterotomy and replacement of the left dorsal and left ventral colon in the abdomen, reduction can then be performed. Displacement is corrected by passing a hand between the spleen and body wall and retracting the spleen mediad as the colon is elevated. Following reduction, a check is made to ensure that the spleen is in its normal position against the left abdominal wall and that the reduced colon is free of twists. Generally, compromise to the colon is limited to a localized bruising and mild edema and is inconsequential. However, complications, including rupture of the large colon while reducing the displacement, recurrence of the displacement, degeneration of the bowel wall, and adhesions, can occur.

A treatment for left dorsal displacement of the colon without laparotomy has been developed and performed successfully in Europe.[6] This treatment necessitates a definitive clinical diagnosis per rectum. The horse is placed on its back with the hind limbs raised in hobbles by a winch. This causes the large colon to fall craniad. The horse is then lowered onto its left side and rotated manually onto its sternum and then over to its right side.[6] We have also successfully used this method.

Herniation of the left dorsal and left ventral colon through the gastrosplenic ligament can also occur. The signs are similar to those of left dorsal displacement, and the treatment involves reduction of the hernia.

Intramural Hematoma of the Small Colon

Hematoma is an uncommon cause of obstruction of the small colon.[19,25] It has been associated with chronic ulceration and iatrogenic rectal damage of unknown causes. The horse shows severe pain in excess of that normally seen with obstruction of the small colon. This has been associated with the distention of the intestinal wall associated with the hematoma. Treatment involves resection of the affected portion and an end-to-end anastomosis of the small colon.

Strangulating Obstruction of the Large Intestine
Intussusception of the Cecum

Intussusception of the cecum may occur either as a cecocecal or cecocolic intussusception.[2,9,19,20,24] Afflicted horses typically have subacute colic of several days' duration, but there is considerable variation. Cecocecal intussusception does not completely block the flow of ingesta from the small intestine, but cecocolic intussusception does. On surgical exploration absence of the cecum is noted, and the intussusception can be found by tracing the right ventral colon retrograde until the mass is found. Surgical treatment involves reduction of the intussusception (the colon may have to be opened) and surgical amputation of the apex of the cecum. This can be performed by resection and closure of the cecum with a double row of inverting sutures[22] or with the TA 90 stapling equipment.

Torsion of the Cecum

Torsion of the cecum alone is rare (this condition is most commonly associated with torsion of the colon). Incidental displacement of the cecum routinely encountered during surgery is commonly classified as torsion (usually 90 degrees) but is not considered to be a pathologic problem. If true cecal torsion occurs, it presents as an acute colic with a distended cecum, but a normal large colon. A discolored, distended cecal apex will be found on surgical exploration and the torsion located. Following decompression of the cecum the torsion is reduced. Resection will be indicated depending on the vascular compromise. The site of resection will depend on the degree of involvement of the cecum. Complete typhlectomy with ileocolic anastomosis has been described,[15] and this condition requires a flank laparotomy.

Torsion (Volvulus) of the Large Colon

The term *torsion* of the large colon implies compromise of the vascular supply, and this typically occurs with a 360-degree torsion of the entire large colon. This condition constitutes the most severe and rapidly fatal acute abdominal crisis in the horse. Most strangulating torsions are 360 degrees and occur either at the origin of the large colon and involve the cecum or just distal to the cecum in the right colon so that the cecum is not involved[17] (Fig. 7-4E). Because these

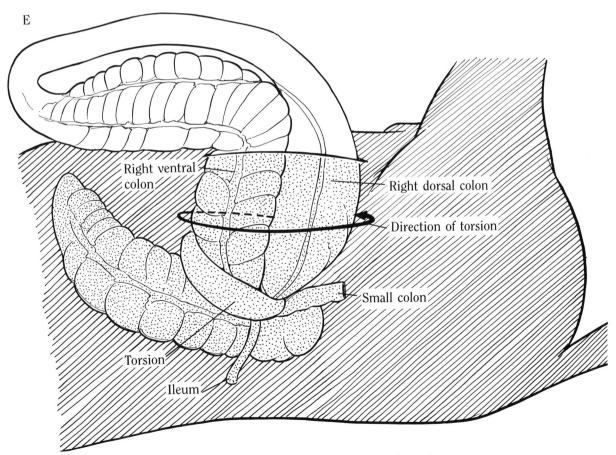

FIG. 7-4 (*Continued*). **E.** 360-Degree torsion (volvulus) of the large colon. The torsion is immediately distal to the cecocolic junction.

torsions occur near the origin of the large colon, strangulation of the blood supply results in a condition similar to strangulation of the mesenteric root in small intestinal volvulus; hence, this condition is commonly also referred to as volvulus of the large colon. In one report of 25 cases, the twist occurred at the base of the cecum or at the origin of the transverse colon.[4] Patients with strangulating torsions present with severe unrelenting abdominal pain, severe systemic signs, and marked abdominal distention.

Rapid surgical intervention is of paramount importance if these horses are to be saved. In general, the prognosis for torsions surgically corrected within 2 hours of occurring is good. With the typical 360-degree torsion seen at laparotomy the colon is grossly distended, but the pelvic flexure may appear in a normal position because of the complete 360-degree twist. The color of the serosa varies from white to blue to black, and the wall will be edematous. The large colon is evacuated prior to detorsion by an enterotomy at the pelvic flexure and flushing with warm water. This maneuver removes endotoxin that can be potentially absorbed following detorsion, and it also decreases distention prior to further manipulation of the bowel. At the time of enterotomy the stage of ischemic necrosis of the colon can be assessed based on the appearance of the mucosa. Dark bloody fluid contents at evacuation constitute another feature of necrosis of the mucosa. The direction of the torsion is then evaluated by palpation at the base of the colon. When the horse is viewed in the ventral surgical position, most torsions at the base of the colon are counterclockwise (Fig. 7-4E). With the twisted portion of the colon exteriorized, it is rotated in a clockwise direction to correct the torsion. Exteriorization and visualization of the cecocolic ligament running from the lateral band of the cecum to the right ventral colon is important to ensure that the torsion has been corrected.

The color of the serosal surface typically improves following detorsion, but mucosal evaluation is the more important criterion for assessing potential viability. The survival rate in these cases usually has been low because of the rapid development of bowel ischemia before surgical intervention. One needs to detorse a colon within 2 hours of its occurrence to anticipate a viable and complication-free case postoperatively. When the torsed colon is nonviable, resection is an option, except when the entire large colon is involved. Recently techniques have been developed for colon resection, and it is feasible to resect up to 90% of the large colon (see section on large colon resection). However, the surgeon must be able to surgically expose viable colon to perform the resection-anastamosis.

Intussusception of the Colon

Intussusception of the large colon is rare but has been reported.[21,28] In 2 cases the left dorsal colon was involved. In both cases the intussusception was resected. An end-to-end anastomosis was performed in one case,[28] and a side-to-side anastomosis performed in the other case.[21]

Incarceration and Volvulus of the Small Colon

Although the small colon has a long mesentery, both incarceration and volvulus are rare.[1,12] Incarceration can occur through a mesenteric rent or an association with a pedunculated lipoma. Treatment is the same as for a small intestinal incarceration.

References

1. Adams, S.B., and McIlwraith, C.W.: Abdominal crisis in the horse: A comparison of presurgical evaluation with surgical findings and results. Vet. Surg. 87:63, 1978.
2. Allison, C.J.: Invagination of the caecum into the colon in a Welsh pony. Eq. Vet. J. 9:84, 1977.
3. Argenzio, R.A.: Comparative physiology of the gastrointestinal system. In Veterinary Gastroenterology. (N.Y. Anderson, Ed.) Philadelphia, Lea & Febiger, 1980, pp. 172–198.
4. Barclay, W.P., Foerner, J.J., and Phillips, T.N.: Volvulus of the large colon in the horse. J. Am Vet. Med. Assoc. 177:629, 1980.
5. Blue, M.G.: Enteroliths in horses—a retrospective study of 30 cases. Eq. Vet. J. 111:76, 1979.
6. Boening, J.: Die Behandlung der "Milz-Nieren-Band"—Aufhangung beim Pferd durch Walzen in Allgemeinmarkose. Tierarztl. Umschau. 40:252, 1985.
7. Boles, C.L., and Kohn, C.W.: Fibrous foreign body impaction colic in young horses. J. Am. Vet. Med. Assoc. 179:193, 1981.
8. Campbell, M.L., Colahan, P.C., Brown, M.P., et al.: Cecal impaction in the horse. J. Am. Vet. Med. Assoc. 184:950, 1984.
9. Cowles, R.R. Jr., Bunch, S.E., and Flynn, D.V.: Cecal inversion in a horse. VM/SAC 72:1346, 1977.
10. DeGroot, A.: The significance of low packed cell volume in relation to the early diagnosis of intestinal obstruction in the horse; based on field observations. Proceedings of the AAEP 309, 1971.
11. Ferraro, G.L., Evans, D.R., Trunk, D.A. et al.: Medical and surgical management of enteroliths in Equidae. J. Am. Vet. Med. Assoc. 162:208, 1973.
12. Foerner, J.J.: Differential diagnosis and surgical management of diseases of the large intestine. Vet. Clin. North Am. Large Anim. Prac. 4:129, 1982.
13. Gay, C.C., Spiers, V.C., and Christie, B.A.: Foreign body obstruction of the small colon in six horses. Eq. Vet. J. 11:60, 1979.
14. Hackett, R.P.: Nonstrangulated colonic displacement in horses. J. Am. Vet. Med. Assoc. 182:235, 1983.
15. Huskamp, B.: Some problems associated with intestinal surgery in the horse. Eq. Vet. J. 9:111, 1977.
16. Huskamp, B., Daniels, H., and Kopf, N.: Diseases of the stomach and intestine. In Diseases of the Horse. (O. Dietz and E. Wiesner, Eds.) Basel, S. Karger GER., 1984, pp. 164.
17. Meagher, D.M.: Surgery of the large intestine in the horse. Arch. ACVS 3:9, 1974.
18. Milne, D.W., Tarr, M.J., and Lochner, F.K.: Left dorsal displacement of the colon in a horse. J. Eq. Med. Surg. 1:47, 1977.
19. Pearson, H., Messervy, A., and Pinsent, P.J.N.: Surgical treatment of abdominal disorders in the horse. J. Am. Vet. Med. Assoc. 159:1344, 1971.
20. Robertson, J.T., and Johnson, F.M.: Surgical correction of cecocolic intussusception in a horse. J. Am. Vet. Med. Assoc. 176:223, 1980.
21. Robertson, J.T., and Tate, L.P., Jr.: Resection of intussuscepted large colon in a horse. J. Am. Vet. Med. Assoc. 181:927, 1982.
22. Robertson, J.T.: Personal communication, 1985.
23. Sellers, A.F., Lowe, J.E., and Brondum, J.: Motor events in equine large colon. Am. J. Physiol. 237:E457, 1979.

24. Sembrad, S.D., and Moore, J.N.: Invagination of the cecal apex in a foal. Eq. Vet. J. 15:62, 1983.
25. Spiers, V.C., Van Veenendaal, J.C., Christie, B.A., et al.: Obstruction of the small colon by intramural haematoma in three horses. Aust. Vet. J. 57:88, 1981.
26. Taylor, T.S., Valdez, H., Norwood, G.W., et al.: Retrograde flushing for relief of obstruction in the transverse colon in the horse. Eq. Pract. 1:22, 1979.
27. Tennant, B.: Intestinal obstruction in the horse: Some aspects of differential diagnosis in equine colic. Proceedings AAEP, 1976, p. 426.
28. Wilson, D.G., and Wilson, W.D.: Intussusception of the left dorsal colon in a horse. J. Am. Vet. Med. Assoc. 183:464, 1983.

Enterotomy Techniques

Enterotomy is a basic procedure that plays a very important role in equine intestinal surgery. The selection of an enterotomy site in different parts of the intestinal tract is dependent on the surgeon's ability to exteriorize the viscus, the distribution of blood supply, the location of the lesion, and the anatomic site involved.[2]

Before performing an enterotomy, the viscus is isolated from the peritoneal cavity and other viscera by exteriorization and appropriate draping. Small enterotomies on the small intestine are performed on the long axis along the antimesenteric surface. For the colon, a longitudinal incision on the antimesenteric surface is selected. Enterotomies on the large colon are usually performed on the antimesenteric surface in the area of the pelvic flexure. There are some recent arguments against performing the enterotomy right at the pelvic flexure due to its identification as a pacemaker area. These areas lack teniae, are easily exteriorized, and provide relatively good access for evacuation. The pelvic flexure is the most commonly used area for evacuation of impactions, of both the pelvic flexure and the transverse colon, and the decompression of these cases is facilitated by flushing with a hose.[1] Hard masses in the lumen of the transverse colon, such as an enterolith, can be removed through an enterotomy in the right dorsal colon. This is a compromise because the enterotomy site is still some distance from the lesion, but it is a segment that can be exteriorized and "packed off" to maintain asepsis.

In the small colon enterotomy is also made parallel to the long axis and on the antimesenteric border. There is some debate as to whether the enterotomy should be made through the antimesenteric tenia or adjacent to it. While a longitudinal incision made adjacent to the tenia may risk alterations to the blood supply,[2] there is some question as to whether an incision through the muscular teniae is optimal for rapid wound healing.

We prefer the use of an assistant's hands to stabilize the bowel for enterotomy rather than using stay sutures or forceps. The enterotomy is made with a scalpel (Fig. 7-5A). In the case of the small intestine, excess intraluminal fluid can be aspirated with suction or induced to flow by extraluminal pressure applied with a gloved hand. Evacuation of small intestine through an enterotomy incision is difficult. Evacuation through a piece of intestine later to be discarded (if appropriate) is preferable in controlling contamination. Most evacuations of the large colon (those performed through the pelvic flexure) involve holding the pelvic flexure over a large container and evacuating fluid directly out through the enterotomy site. A hose is usually used to facilitate evacuation of the large colon[1] (Fig. 7-5B). An assistant inserts the hose through the enterotomy into the lumen of the dorsal or ventral colon. Water is flushed into the lumen, and the water is mixed with ingesta and then allowed to run out. By moving the hose further into the bowel and milking the mixture out, the large bowel can be almost completely emptied. The procedure can then be repeated on the

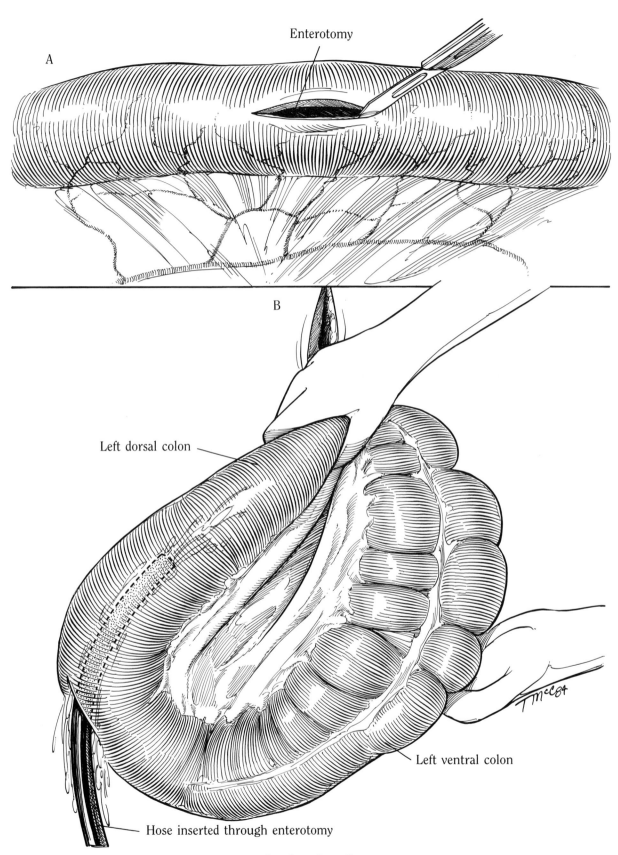

FIG. 7-5. Enterotomies. **A.** In antimesenteric border of small intestine. **B.** In area of pelvic flexure with irrigation hose in left dorsal colon.

opposite colon. This technique is particularly useful for the evacuation of ingesta or sand impactions where manual manipulation of rough, dry ingesta imposes considerable trauma to the wall of the colon.

When the evacuation of the bowel is complete, the bowel is prepared for closure by rinsing the enterotomy site with sterile polyionic fluid. Small intestinal enterotomies can be closed with a single continuous inverting layer (Cushing or Lembert pattern) using 2/0 absorbable suture, a two-layer inverting pattern, or one single interrupted layer using a Crushing or Gambee suture pattern of 2/0 absorbable suture material. Two-layer closures cause more inversion of tissue. Two-layer closures are more frequently utilized for large bowel enterotomies. Polyglactin 910 is preferred over catgut in the colon because of the relatively poor blood supply and an increased level of collagenase activity in this part of the bowel.[2]

Stomach enterotomy (gastrotomy) is rare but may be performed midway between the greater and lesser curvature with the incision placed parallel to the segmental gastric vessels. Since the stomach is relatively inaccessible and cannot be exteriorized, contamination is a problem. Decompression with a tube is preferred if possible. The stomach has a rich blood supply and heals rapidly, but because it secretes pepsin, a synthetic absorbable or nonabsorbable suture material has been recommended with a two-layer closure.[2]

References

1. Foerner, J.J.: Diseases of the large intestine: Differential diagnosis and surgical management. Vet. Clin. North Am. Large Anim. Pract., 4:129, 1982.
2. Stashak, T.S.: Techniques for enterotomy, decompression and intestinal resection—anastomosis. Vet. Clin. North Am. Large Anim. Pract., 4:147, 1982.

Intestinal Resection, Anastomosis, and Stapling— General Considerations

The initial problem with any intestinal resection is evaluation of intestinal integrity or viability and defining the margins of viability. Evaluation of the color of the intestines and mesentery, peristalsis, pulsation of the mesenteric vessels, and enterotomy to visualize mucosal color are still the most frequently used means to assess intestinal viability. Although newer, sophisticated means have been developed, including the use of intravenous infusion of fluorescein dye, the latter technique has not proved to be equal to its anticipated value in the horse.[10] Studies have shown bowel segments remaining viable after fluorescent patterns indicated a nonviable state. The situation is further complicated by the fact that, in the horse, unacceptable adhesion formation occurs after temporary ischemia despite the bowel remaining viable.[10] A general principle is that if the viability of a segment, particularly the ileum, is in question, resection is indicated. The principles of resection technique will be illustrated when discussing resection of the small intestine and end-to-end anastomosis.

Intestinal healing can be divided into three phases. Phase I, the lag phase, lasts from 0 to 4 days and is characterized by inflammatory edema. There is some tissue strength on day 1 and 2 because of the formation of fibrin clots, but by the third postoperative day the sutured intestine is functionally weakest because of the transition of fibrin breakdown (fibrinolysis) to the deposition of immature collagen.[9] Phase 2, the proliferative phase, lasts from 3 to 14 days and is characterized by formation of fibrous tissue and mucosal union. A rapid gain in tissue strength is associated with this phase. Phase 3, the remodeling phase, begins about day 10 and lasts to day 180. This period is characterized by a gradual increase in tissue strength as a result of collagen remodeling. It takes about 17 to 21 days for the anastomotic site to reach the tensile strength of normal adjacent bowel.

Rates and strengths of healing vary somewhat depending on the location of the intestinal anastomosis and the suture material selected. The small intestine provides the ideal set of circumstances, because it has an abundant blood supply, a strong mucosal layer, minimal intraluminal bacterial counts (compared to large bowel), semiliquid feces, and a mucosal layer capable of rapid regeneration.[9] In comparison, the colon has a relatively poor blood supply, high intraluminal bacterial counts, an increased level of collagenase, and more solid fecal material.

When considering anastomosis of the equine small intestine as a typical example, postoperative complications can result from anastomotic leakage, stenosis, or adhesions. Formation of an impervious seal, first intention healing with minimal fibrosis, and maintenance of an adequate luminal diameter are among the goals when trying to minimize the potential for such complications.[2]

Three general techniques of intestinal anastomosis are available: end-to-end, end-to-side, and side-to-side. End-to-end anastomosis is performed when sections of intestine of similar diameter are to be anastomosed. The technique is used for anastomosis of the small intestine and small colon and will be detailed here, using small intestine as an example. End-to-side anastomosis has been frequently utilized for ileal- or jejunal-cecal anastomosis. Side-to-side anastomosis is used in anastomosing the large colon and is an alternative technique for jejunal-cecal anastomosis. It is also used in gastrojejunostomy.

Suture Techniques

Various suture patterns can be used with these different anastomotic techniques. Suture placement is very important with regard to the strength and healing of an intestinal anastomosis in that suture placement should not compromise the vascular supply, and the submucosa must be engaged by each suture.[7] In order to minimize any vascular compromise, it has been proposed that sutures placed in an interrupted fashion perpendicular to the cut surface and parallel to the bowel's long axis are preferable.[9] Sutures placed in a continuous pattern with the bites parallel to the cut surface of the bowel and perpendicular to the long axis of the intestines (such as Cushing or Connell sutures) have a tendency to reduce the blood supply to the healing edge.[9] However, recent work indicates that while such interrupted suture patterns result in good histologic healing, adhesions develop in 50% of cases, whereas adhesions were not found in association with continuous inverting suture patterns.[2]

Intestinal anastomotic techniques can be classified according to whether they oppose, invert, or evert the incised edge of the bowel and as to whether they are performed in single or double rows.

OPPOSING SUTURES. End-to-end opposing sutures include the simple interrupted approximating suture that approximates all tunics of the intestine (Fig. 7-6A), a crushing suture that is placed in the same fashion as above but tied tightly enough to cut through the serosa, muscularis, and mucosa and snugly holds the submucosal tunics,[6] and the Gambee suture pattern placed so that the suture selectively picks up the mucosa and prevents its eversion (Fig. 7-6B). These sutures all provide good anatomic alignment of all intestinal layers, the lumen of the bowel is not compromised, minimal vascular compromise is noted, and the surgeon can be sure that the submucosa is engaged by the sutures. Also, rapid healing with mucosal union is noted, the techniques are simple to perform, distensibility is superior to other patterns, and there is early return to intestinal mobility.[8,9] The only detracting feature of such suture patterns is the potential for adhesion formation. Although one report found adhesions not to be a problem with the Gambee pattern,[8] a more recent study demonstrated adhesions associated with 50% of the Gambee and crushing anastomoses.[2]

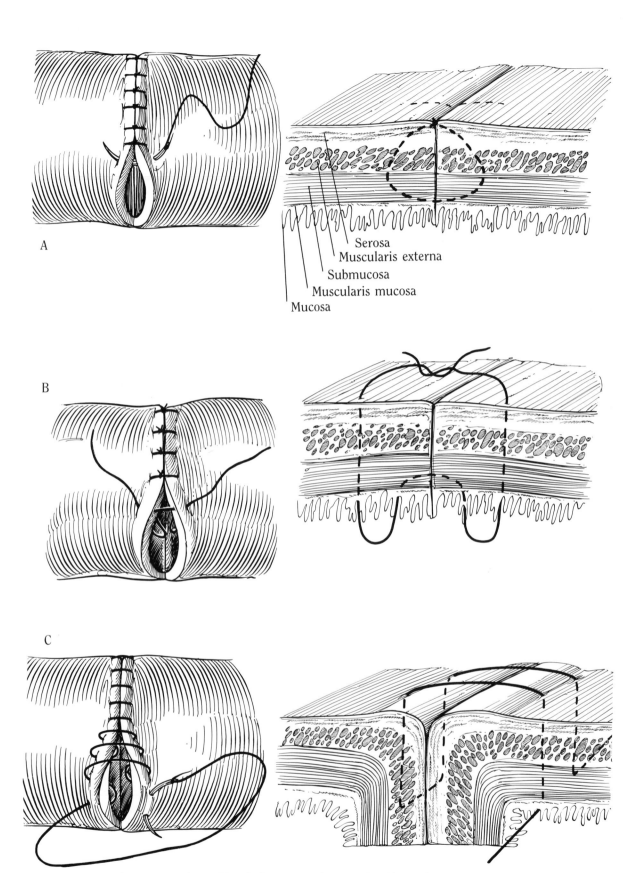

Serosa
Muscularis externa
Submucosa
Muscularis mucosa
Mucosa

Fig. 7-6. Intestinal anastomosis. **A.** Simple interrupted approximating suture.
B. Gambee suture (interrupted). **C.** Continuous inverting (Cushing) suture pattern.

INVERTING SUTURE PATTERNS. A double-layer inverting suture pattern still used by many surgeons includes the use of interrupted or continuous Cushing, Connell, Lembert, or Halsted techniques. Single-layer inverting suture patterns can also be performed in interrupted or continuous fashion, but the continuous is the most common (Fig. 7-6C). Two-layer inverting patterns have a high initial tensile and bursting strength. There are fewer adhesions, and because two layers are formed, the bowel can be adequately sealed and cleaned prior to placement of the second layer. However, internal cuff formation (from inverted tissues) may cause intraluminal obstruction. In addition, there is poor apposition of layers and kinking of the blood vessels, which will decrease blood flow causing retarded intestinal healing, delayed return to normal motility, and increased incidence of anatomic failure.[9] The ability of the intestine to distend is also reduced.[9] The one-layer inverting closure has similar problems but can be more rapidly applied and has less tissue reaction, earlier revascularization, and more rapid healing compared to the two-layer pattern.[9]

A two-layer inverting anastomosis composed of a simple continuous mucosal layer and a continuous Lembert seromuscular layer has been described for end-to-side jejunocecal anastomosis in the horse[4] and has been more recently studied with end-to-end anastomosis of the small intestine[2] (Fig. 7-6D). This technique eliminates some of the drawbacks of the conventional two-layer inverting patterns because the mucosa is opposed and only one layer is inverted, resulting in minimal reduction of luminal diameter. Recent comparative studies show that while fibrosis and suture tract inflammation are increased in

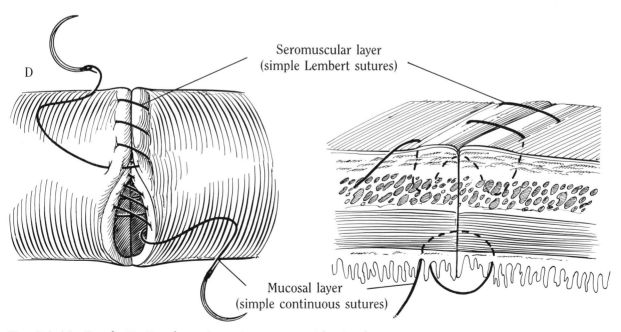

Seromuscular layer
(simple Lembert sutures)

Mucosal layer
(simple continuous sutures)

FIG. 7-6 (*Continued*). **D.** Two-layer inverting suture with simple continuous mucosal layer and continuous Lembert seromuscular layer.

this two-layer inverting technique, compared to Gambee and crushing patterns, no adhesions formed in 6 horses when the inverting technique was used, compared to 50% adhesion incidence with the other two techniques.[2]

In the same controlled study, the crushing anastomoses had the largest percentage of normal diameter (72% ± 15%) followed by the Gambee anastomoses (69% ± 19%). The two-layer inverting anastomoses had the smallest percentage of normal diameter (66% ± 16%); however, there was no significant difference in the mean percentage of normal diameter among the three techniques.[2] These authors concluded that the two-layer inverting technique of closure of the small intestine was superior to the single-layer techniques in that experiment because of its reduced incidence of adhesions and maintenance of adequate lumen diameter.[2]

Inverting patterns are still used with side-to-side anastomotic techniques using suture material.

EVERTING PATTERNS. We do not recommend everting patterns for intestinal anastomosis. The incidence of inflammation, adhesions, strictures, and peritonitis is higher than with the opposing and inverting techniques.[8,9] The everted bacteria-laden mucosa forms a nidus for infection and microabscesses.[8]

Obviously, the ideal suture pattern does not exist, but either the opposing or the modified inverting types, which are illustrated in Figure 7-6, are considered satisfactory. While it is acknowledged that, with tissue remodeling, the long-term result is probably the same, any interim problems such as stenosis or adhesion formation can be significant morbidity factors postoperatively because temporary bowel dysfunction can have marked clinical effects. The selection of suture material also merits consideration and is discussed below. With regard to suture patterns it should be recognized that suture material acts as a foreign body in the abdominal cavity and that more suture material is exposed to the peritoneum in single-layer interrupted patterns than in continuous patterns. It has also been shown in dogs that the crushing technique demonstrated greater avascular widths of tissue adjacent to the anastomosis than did a continuous approximating pattern.[5] This study also showed that there was less mucosal eversion and adhesion formation than with either crushing or approximating interrupted patterns. While it would seem that the opposing interrupted techniques offer the best apposition and healing, adhesion formation is of concern. It seems that a continuous approximating pattern may be an excellent compromise. Presently, the two-layer inverting technique with a continuous outer layer has the best results in terms of minimal adhesion formation.[2]

Suture material used for gastrointestinal anastomosis should have the qualities of easy handling with minimal tissue friction, reactivity, and capillarity. It is difficult to find one that fulfills all of these criteria. Until recently chromic catgut was the standard suture for gastrointestinal surgery, but the cellular inflammatory response and edema are undesirable, especially for circular closure of the intestine.[9] Polyglactin 910 (Vicryl), a synthetic multifilament absorbable suture, is now commonly used in the horse.[9] More recently, polydioxanone (PDS) offers the advantages of a monofilament suture without the intensive inflammatory response. It also retains strength longer and has a slower rate of absorption than the synthetic multifilament materials.[3] It is, however, somewhat more difficult to handle because it kinks.

A recent controlled study with the modified two-layer anastomotic technique demonstrates that suture pattern is a more critical factor than differences between monofilament and multifilament material.[3] Four different anastomoses were compared using combinations of polyglactin 910 and polydioxanone, with continuous and interrupted suture patterns in the seromuscular layer of a two-layer inverting technique. The mean diameter percentages following anastomoses were not significantly different between techniques. However, the pyogranulomatous suture tract inflammation previously reported with polyglactin 910 was reduced with polydioxanone. The major finding of significance was that the use of an interrupted suture pattern in the seromuscular layer resulted in a greater than 50% incidence of anastomotic adhesions, regardless of suture material, which is unacceptable for anastomosis of the small intestine in the horse.[3]

When anastomosis of the large colon is considered, the selection of a synthetic absorbable material over catgut is even more critical because of the slower healing rate of this section of the alimentary tract.

Intestinal Stapling Devices

The intestinal stapling instruments were originally developed in Russia and are now readily available. The staples are stainless steel and are nonreactive in the intestine. When inserted, the staple is shaped into the form of a "B" configuration, which allows capillary flow through the tissue clasped within the staple. The staple units also have a double row of staples, which alternates the staple placement. The intestinal staplers have the advantages of rapid execution of an anastomosis (which saves valuable surgical time), a nonreactive suture with less inflammation, and rapid healing of the incision. The units also can be used to reach relatively inaccessible regions with less chance of contamination compared to suturing. Disadvantages of the intestinal staplers are eversion of the tissue with the TA-55 and TA-90 units,* which will tend to promote adhesion formation, tearing or pulling of staples due to tension on the anastomotic site, and inadequate closure if the tissue is too thick. The expense of the staples also requires consideration.

There are several types of stapling devices. The two used for intestinal anastomosis are illustrated in the description of jejunocecal anastomosis. The first type goes under the designation of thoracoab-

---

*TA-55 or TA-90—Auto Suture, U.S. Surgical Corp., Norwalk, CT 06850.

dominal (TA-90 or TA-55, the number representing the length of the staple row). They are used to make a blind stump of intestine and also to close an enterotomy but produce an everted tissue apposition. The other instrument is called a gastrointestinal anastomosis instrument† or a GIA, and this produces two rows of double staples with a cutting blade between the rows. The two parts of the stapling apparatus are inserted into adjacent segments of bowel to produce a closure of the two bowel segments with a stoma within the closure. This results in inversion of the tissue edges. The GIA is routinely used for performing jejunocecal, ileocecal, cecocolic, or colic-colic anastomoses. The TA-90 is also used for creating a blind stump in the ileum with a jejunocecal anastomosis. These techniques are specifically demonstrated in the sections on jejunocecal anastomosis and large colon resection and anastomosis.

A third instrument called a ligator stapling device (LDS),* is used to ligate mesenteric vessels with two staples and cut between them to complete the removal. This device uses a crescent-shaped staple to close the vessel. It also can greatly decrease surgical time for bowel resections. When the mesentery is devitalized or there is excessive mesenteric fat, double ligation is recommended.[11] A fourth instrument, the EEA stapling device, is not currently used in the horse.

Some other rules that must be followed when using the stapling equipment include (1) use of tension-relieving sutures at each end of the suture line to prevent tension on the staples to avoid failure of the anastomoses and (2) making certain the tissue is thin enough to allow for proper staple penetration and staple closure in the completed "B" form.

Our experiences in the horse would generally agree with human studies reporting that, if the technical details of surgical stapling are mastered, the stapling technique appears to be as safe as suturing in the performance of anastomoses in the gastrointestinal tract. However, we also feel that the indications are *more limited* in the horse than in man, such as in the small intestine, where we consider the use of presently available stapling devices inappropriate for end-to-end anastomosis (the reasons are given in the next section). On the other hand, the stapling devices have increased our capabilities in colonic anastomoses and our speed in closing jejunocecal anastomoses.

References

1. Chassin, J.L., Rifkind, K.M., Sussman, B., et al.: The stapled gastrointestinal tract anastomosis: Incidence of postoperative complications compared with the sutured anastomosis. Ann. Surg. 188:689, 1978.
2. Dean, P.W., and Robertson, J.T.: Comparison of three suture techniques for anastomosis of the small intestine in the horse. Am. J. Vet. Res. 46:1282, 1985.
3. Dean, P.W., Robertson, J.T., and Jacobs, R.M.: A comparison of suture materials and suture patterns for inverting intestinal anastomosis in the horse. Am. J. Vet. Res. 46:2072, 1985.

†GIA—Auto Suture, U.S. Surgical Corp., Norwalk, CT 06850.
*LDS—Auto Suture, U.S. Surgical Corp., Norwalk, CT 06850.

4. Donawick, W.J., Christie, B.A., and Stewart, J.V.: Resection of diseased ileum in the horse. J. Am. Vet. Med. Assoc. 159:1146, 1971.

5. Ellison, G.W., Jokinen, M.P., and Park, R.D.: End-to-end approximating intestinal anastomosis in the dog: A comparative fluorescein dye angiographic and histopathologic evaluation. J. Am. Anim. Hosp. Assoc. 18:729, 1982.

6. Herthel, D.J.: Technique of intestinal anastomosis utilizing the crushing type suture. Proceedings of the Annual Convention of the American Association of Equine Practitioners in 1972. 1983, pp. 303–306.

7. Jansen, A., Becker, A.E., Brummelkamp, W.H., et al.: The importance of the apposition of the submucosal intestinal layers for primary wound healing of intestinal anastomosis. Surg. Gynec. Obstet. 152:51, 1981.

8. Reinertson, E.L.: Comparison of three techniques for intestinal anastomosis in Equidae. J. Am. Vet. Med. Assoc. 169:208, 1976.

9. Stashak, T.S.: Enterotomy, decompression, and intestinal anastomosis. In Vet. Clin. North. Am. Large Anim. Pract. 4:147, 1982.

10. Sullins, K.E., Stashak, T.S., and Mero, K.N.: Evaluation of fluorescein as an indicator of small intestinal viability in the horse. J. Am. Vet. Med. Assoc. 186:257, 1985.

11. White, N.A.: Intestinal stapling in the horse. ACVS Forum, 1984.

Resection and End-to-End Anastomosis of Small Intestine

Surgical Technique

The segment of intestine to be resected is exteriorized and isolated from the abdominal cavity and other normal viscera. The entire segment to be resected should include at least 10 to 20 cm of normal bowel at each end of the lesion to ensure normal vascularity at the anastomotic site. Impervious draping is used. Any exposed normal viscera are kept moist with saline or balanced electrolyte solution during this procedure. If possible, intestinal occlusion clamps should be placed across the borders of the fluid-filled ischemic bowel to prevent reflux of toxic fluids into normal adjacent intestines (Fig. 7-7A). The rationale for this is that toxic fluids can otherwise be absorbed through normal intestine and contribute to the endotoxemia of the patient. Following this, the contents in the normal bowel are hand stripped away from the occlusion clamps to a position approximately 20 cm beyond the proposed site of resection. A Penrose drain is placed through a small hole in the mesentery between segmental vessels to encircle the intestine and is pulled up snug and fixed with forceps to occlude the lumen (Fig. 7-7A). This procedure is repeated at the other resection location. Penrose drains are used rather than intestinal clamps because (1) they do not slip, (2) they do not interfere with bowel manipulations at the anastomotic site, (3) they effectively occlude the intestine, and (4) they do not cause the vascular compromise potentially possible with intestinal clamps. Having an assistant occlude the bowel lumen manually with a gauze sponge is an alternative.

Following placement of the Penrose drains, the resection site in the decompressed normal segment is selected based on its having a good segmental arterial supply to the antimesenteric surface. If possible, this site will be selected close to a major mesenteric artery. Intestinal clamps may then be placed across the bowel at the proposed line of resection (but on the discarded side of resection). These clamps are placed at an oblique angle of 60 degrees to the mesenteric surface. Such angulation of the line of resection ensures an adequate antimesenteric blood supply and a slightly increased luminal diameter at the anastomosis (Fig. 7-7A). Mesenteric vessels to the portion to be resected are bluntly dissected free of the mesentery with a hemostat, doubly ligated or stapled, and cut. The bowel is then resected immediately adjacent to the forceps and on the side that is being retained. No clamps are placed on the bowel that is to be retained and anastomosed. After transection of the bowel, the mesentery is incised, and the resected intestine is discarded.

With an assistant holding the ends of the intestine in apposition, anastomosis is performed (Fig. 7-7 B, C). The technique for the anastomosis will be based on personal preference. The choices of suture pattern and material have been discussed in the previous section. On

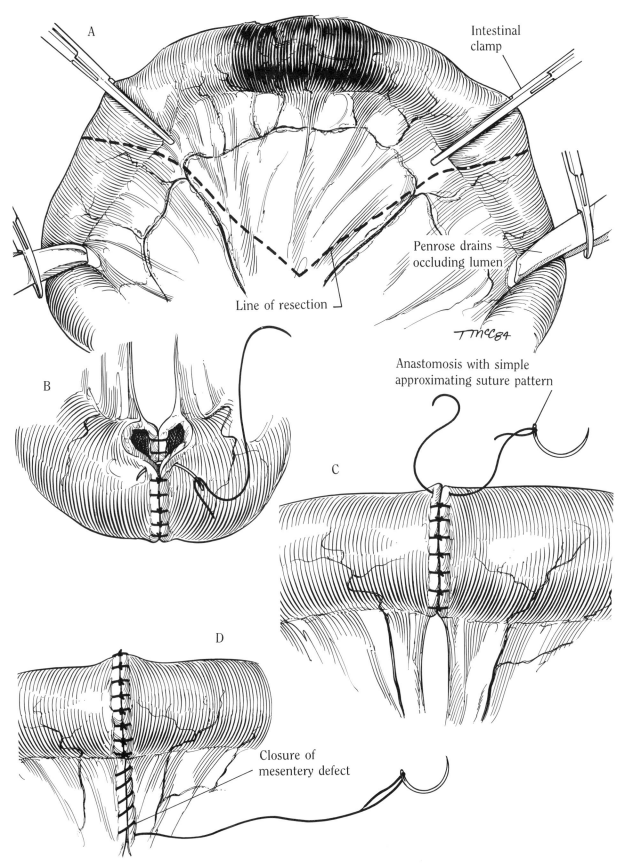

A

Intestinal clamp

Line of resection

Penrose drains occluding lumen

TMcC84

B

Anastomosis with simple approximating suture pattern

C

D

Closure of mesentery defect

FIG. 7-7. Resection and end-to-end anastomosis of small intestine.

the basis of current knowledge, an apposing anastomosis or a double-layered technique with *minimal inversion* should be used with synthetic absorbable suture material.[1,2] If the double-layered technique is used, the single continuous layer in the mucosa should be interrupted and tied at 180 degrees. It is important to make sure that normal alignment of the ends of the intestine is maintained so that there is no rotation of segments. Following completion of the intestinal anastomosis, the mesenteric defect is sutured in a simple continuous pattern. Care must be taken not to occlude vital mesenteric vessels (Fig. 7-7D).

Comments

The use of staples is not considered appropriate for end-to-end anastomosis of the small intestine. Although a triangulating technique using a TA-55 or TA-90 stapling device is apparently performed in man,[3] it results in undesirable mucosal eversion. Studies in the horse have confirmed that such a technique will result in extensive adhesion and stricture formation associated with the anastomoses and problems with colic postoperatively.[4] Another alternative would be to perform a side-to-side anastomosis of the small intestine with the two ends of the bowel stumped off. Such a technique could be performed with the GIA or TA staplers. However, in our experience, the use of such a side-to-side anastomosis can result in pocketing of intestinal contents and is not recommended.

Anastomosis of the small colon can be made using the same principles as described above for small intestine. However, the mesocolon contains considerable fat, making identification of the vessels difficult, and the procedure is consequently harder. Care also must be taken not to damage the blood supply to normal small colon, particularly if the margin for resection is adjacent to a segment that cannot be exteriorized and excessive tension could inflict permanent vascular damage.

References

1. Dean, P.W., and Robertson, J.T.: Comparison of three suture techniques for anastomosis of the small intestine in the horse. Am. J. Vet. Res. 46:1282, 1985.
2. Dean, P.W., Robertson, J.T., and Jacobs, R.M.: A comparison of suture materials and suture patterns for inverting intestinal anastomosis in the horse. Am. J. Vet. Res. 46:2072, 1985.
3. Reiling, R.B.: Staplers in gastrointestinal surgery. Surg. Clin. North Am. 60:381, 1981.
4. Sullins, K.E., Stashak, T.S., and Mero, K.M.: Evaluation of intestinal staples for end-to-end anastomosis of the small intestine in the horse. Vet. Surg. 14:87, 1985.

Jejunocecal Anastomosis

When any part of the ileum is to be resected, the jejunocecal anastomosis is recommended because the ileum has a single blood supply that would make any form of end-to-end anastomosis hazardous and, in addition, the ileocecal valve is inaccessible to surgery (the only possible exception to this statement is if the TA-90 is used in a blind fashion to resect ileum at the level of the ileocecal valve). Jejunocecal anastomosis was initially described in the English literature as an end-to-side anastomosis using suture material.[3] Its successful use has been subsequently documented by other authors.[6,8,10] The time-honored end-to-side technique using sutures as initially described by Donawick and his co-workers will be described and illustrated here.[3] Alternatives and the use of stapling equipment will also be addressed.

Surgical Technique

The technique is illustrated in Fig. 7-8. The basic principle is that a blind stump is made of the ileum, and viable small intestine (the site will vary depending on the amount of ileum and jejunum resected) is anastomosed into the cecum between its medial and dorsal bands in an end-to-side fashion. One author has reported better results with a side-to-side anastomosis,[4] and this technique will be illustrated also. The advantage of a side-to-side anastomosis is that the size of the stoma can be selected.

The cecum is brought out of the ventral midline incision, and the apex is pulled caudad to expose the dorsal band of the cecum. The dorsal band of the cecum is followed to the ileocecal fold and the ileum (Fig. 7-8A). Two intestinal clamps are then placed across the ileum close to the ileocecal junction but in an appropriately accessible place, and a scalpel is used to divide between them. The ileal stump is then closed with a Parker-Kerr oversew using 0 synthetic absorbable suture (Fig. 7-8B, C). Suturing can be very difficult if the ileum is edematous or swollen, and in this situation a two-layer inverting pattern is recommended. It is important to obtain as much inversion as possible with compromised ileum.

An alternative means of blind-stumping the ileum is provided by using the TA-90 as illustrated in Fig. 7-8D and E. The TA-90 is positioned and clamped shut. A bowel clamp is placed to prevent loss of bowel contents at the time of transection (Fig. 7-8D). The TA-90 is then fired, a scalpel is used to transect the bowel immediately proximal to the TA-90, and the TA-90 is then removed (Fig. 7-8E). The stapling device also provides a means of resecting ileum closer to the ileocecal junction, a definite advantage when the terminal ileum is considered nonviable. Once closure of the ileal stump has been completed, it is released back into the abdominal cavity.

The portion of bowel to be resected is then attended to. Prior to resection this portion of terminal small intestine is commonly used as a conduit to evacuate proximal bowel contents into a container after

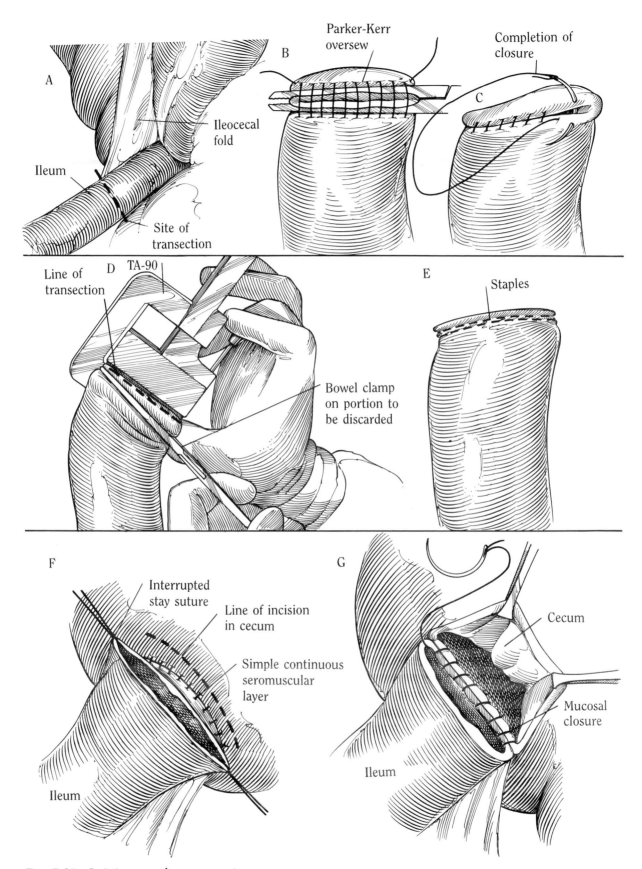

FIG. 7-8A–G. Jejunocecal anastomosis.

ligation of mesenteric vessels and division of the mesentery. Resection of the compromised piece of bowel is then completed in the same fashion as described in the previous section for end-to-end anastomosis of small intestine.

The portion of jejunum to be anastomosed to the cecum is occluded by Penrose drains and/or fingers rather than clamps and is placed in an accessible position distal (approximately 20 cm) to the ileocecal junction and between the medial and dorsal bands of the cecum. The long axis of the jejunum is perpendicular to the long axis of the cecum. Care is taken that the jejunum is not rotated 180 degrees, since this can occlude the jejunal lumen or compromise the mesentery. Interrupted stay sutures are then placed at the mesenteric and antimesenteric borders of the jejunum to fix the open end of the jejunum to the cecum in a stretched-out position with as wide a diameter as possible (Fig. 7-8F). The seromuscular layer of jejunum on the side adjacent to the cecum is then attached to the cecum in a simple continuous pattern using 2/0 suture material (Fig. 7-8F). An incision is then made in the cecum alongside the previous aligned suture line (Fig. 7-8F). The mucosa of the jejunum and cecum are then apposed in a simple continuous pattern around the entire circumference, interrupted with a knot at 180 degrees (Fig. 7-8G). The remaining sides of the seromuscular incisions in the cecum and jejunum are then closed in a continuous Lembert pattern (Fig. 7-8H).

It has been reported that better results might be obtained using a side-to-side anastomosis.[4] The advantage of a side-to-side anastomosis is that the size of the jejunocecal stoma can be selected and any risk of stomal edema and occlusion obviated. However, with careful attention to stretching of the jejunal end and not inverting mucosa, stomal occlusion does not seem to be a problem with the end-to-side technique.

The jejunocecal anastomosis can also be performed using stapling equipment in a side-to-side technique. The end of the jejunum to be anastomosed to the cecum is closed using the TA-90. The end of the jejunum is then placed on the cecum and tacked to the cecum using two stay sutures. Holes are then made in the jejunum and cecum, and the arm of the GIA instrument is inserted into one lumen and the anvil into the other (Fig. 7-8I). The instrument is then clamped together, the cartridge is fired, and the blade is pushed into position to create the stoma (Fig. 7-8I). The GIA is then unlocked and removed, and the holes are closed with an inverting suture (Fig. 7-8J). If a larger stoma is desired, the GIA can be applied twice. In a controlled study comparing the stapled side-to-side technique with the conventional sutured end-to-side anastomosis, the former was considered superior, based on both the postoperative course of the experimental animals as well as the necropsy findings.[1]

Opinion is divided whether the jejunal mesentery should be apposed to the cecum or left open completely. Proponents of the mesentery being left open completely consider that the chance of any postoperative incarceration is less with a large hole than with a small

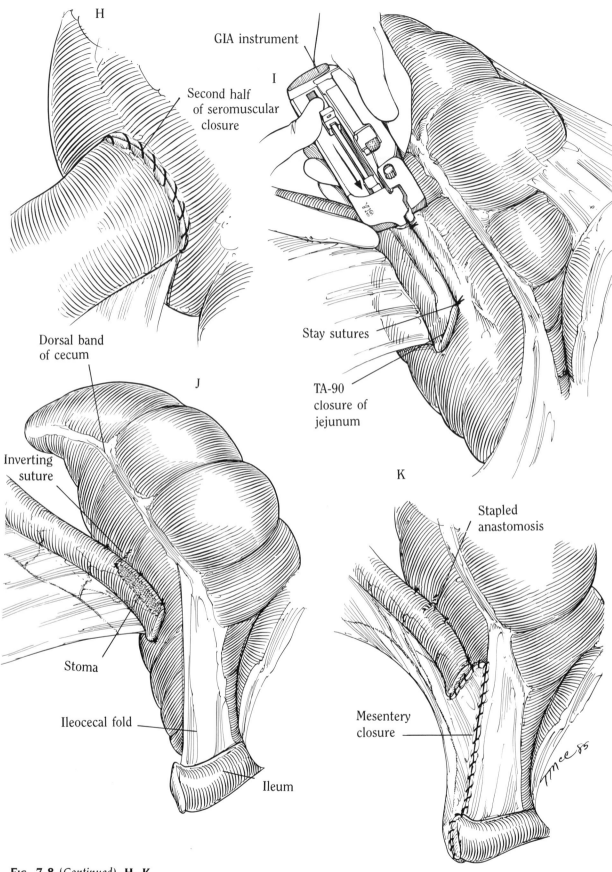

H

Second half
of seromuscular
closure

GIA instrument

I

Stay sutures

TA-90
closure of
jejunum

Dorsal band
of cecum

J

Inverting
suture

Stoma

Ileocecal fold

Ileum

K

Stapled
anastomosis

Mesentery
closure

Fig. 7-8 (*Continued*). **H–K.**

L

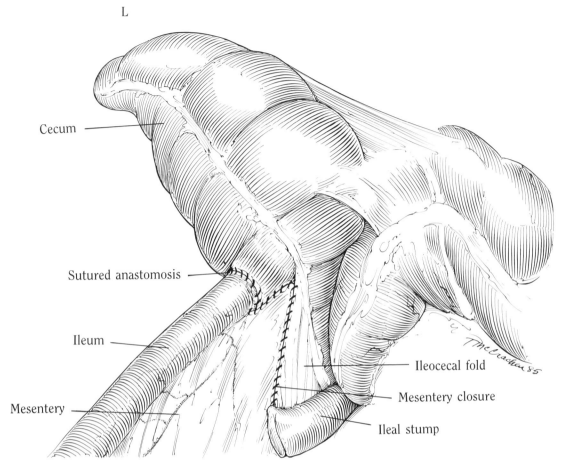

Cecum

Sutured anastomosis

Ileum

Mesentery

Ileocecal fold

Mesentery closure

Ileal stump

FIG. 7-8 (*Continued*). L.

hole that may develop with minor dehiscence of the mesenteric closure. Other authors have considered closure of the mesenteric defect to be essential.[5] The jejunal mesentery is sutured to the ileal stump, ileocecal fold, and dorsal band of the cecum. This closure is illustrated for a staple and a suture anastomosis in Fig. 7-8 K and L, respectively.

Comments

It should also be noted that there is a critical amount of small intestine that can be resected beyond which the patient can suffer permanent gastrointestinal compromise. These limits have been somewhat defined by the experimental work of Tate et al., which showed that at a point between resection of 40% and 60% of the small intestine, malabsorption, weight loss, and liver damage will develop.[11] An unexpected finding of this work was an altered d-xylose absorption curve when ileocecal bypass (without resection) was performed.

An alternative technique, jejunocecal bypass, can be performed when there is obstruction but viable bowel, such as in ileum impaction (obstipation),[5] ileal muscular hypertrophy,[5] or chronic ileal intussusception.[9] The bypass is created as a side-to-side anastomosis and leaves the normal ileal pathway open.[5]

References

1. Blackwell, R.B.: Jejunocecostomy in the horse: A comparison of two techniques. Proceedings Equine Colic Research Symposium, University of Georgia, 1982, pp. 288–289.
2. Dean, P.W., and Robertson, J.T.: Comparison of three suture techniques for anastomosis of the small intestine in the horse. Am. J. Vet. Res. 46:1282, 1985.
3. Donawick, W.J., Christie, B.A., and Stewart, J.V.: Resection of diseased ileum in the horse. J. Am. Vet. Med. Assoc. 159:1145, 1971.
4. Huskamp, B.: The various types and frequency as seen in the Animal Hospital in Hochmoor. In Proceedings Equine Colic Research Symposium, University of Georgia, 1982, pp. 261–272.
5. Kersjes, A.W., Nemeth, F., and Rutgers, L.J.E.: Atlas of Large Animal Surgery. Baltimore, Williams & Wilkins, 1985.
6. Owen, R. ap R., Physick-Sheard, P.W., Hilbert, B.J., et al.: Jejuno- or ileocecal anastomosis performed in seven horses exhibiting colic. Can. Vet. J. 165: 164, 1975.
7. Peterson, F.M., and Stewart, J.V.: Experimental ileocecal anastomosis in the horse. J. Eq. Med. Surg. 2:461, 1978.
8. Robertson, J.T.: Conditions of the stomach and small intestine. Vet. Clin. North Am. Large Anim. Pract. 4:105, 1982.
9. Scott, E.A., and Todhunter, R.: Chronic intestinal intussusception in two horses. J. Am. Vet. Med. Assoc. 186:383, 1985.
10. Stashak, T.S.: Techniques for enterotomy, decompression and intestinal resection-anastomosis. Vet. Clin. North Am. Large Anim. Pract. 4:147, 1982.
11. Tate, L.P., Ralston, S.L., and Koch, C.M., et al.: Effects of extensive resection of the small intestine in the pony. Am. J. Vet. Res. 44:1187, 1983.

Large Colon Resection and Anastomosis

Resection and anastomosis of the large colon has not been a commonly performed procedure in the past.[5] Considerable progress has been made recently, however, and the indications for colon resection are significant in number (including strangulation obstruction of the mobile portions of the large colon, large intramural lesions, focal stricture, and mural devitalization due to long-standing obstructions).

Resection of the dorsal and ventral large colon at the sternal and diaphragmatic flexures has been performed successfully in clinical cases without long term nutritional compromise.[8] More extensive resections can also be accomplished.[1,2] Resection of the entire large colon is not practical at this time due to the inability to surgically expose it. Localized lesions such as a focal stricture or an infarcted area may be amenable to selective resection and end-to-end anastomosis with sutures.[1,4,7] When greater amounts of bowel (left dorsal and ventral colon or parts of the right dorsal and ventral colon as well) require resection, a side-to-side anastomosis with closure of the ends of each colon is performed.

Closure and transection of adjacent colons followed by a side-to-side colocolostomy can be performed with suturing or stapling equipment. Both techniques are described.

Additional Instrumentation

If stapling techniques are used, both the TA-90 and GIA instruments are necessary. In a typical case of 60% colon resection with closure and resection of the adjacent colons and their side-to-side anastomosis, 4 to 6 cartridges of staples for the TA-90 and 4 cartridges for the GIA will be used.

Surgical Techniques

FOCAL RESECTION WITH END-TO-END ANASTOMOSIS. This technique is only used for focal lesions as illustrated in Figure 7-9A.[9] Contents are milked out of the region of bowel to be resected. The artery and vein at either end of the segment to be removed are doubly ligated and transected. The mesocolon adjacent to the segment of colon to be removed is separated from the colon. Intestinal clamps are placed on the colon to be removed as illustrated in simple end-to-end anastomosis of the small intestine. The colon is transected with a scalpel at either end of the lesion and removed. An end-to-end anastomosis is then performed using a suture pattern of the surgeon's preference. A double-layer (simple-continuous oversewn with a continuous Lembert) pattern is illustrated in Figure 7-9B. The anastomotic site is rinsed off thoroughly, and the colon is returned to the abdomen.

When a focal resection is performed but the ends of the bowel are disparate in size, a tapering procedure is used as illustrated in Figure 7-9C and D.[1,7] An example of such a situation would be the removal of the pelvic flexure when the left ventral colon has a larger diameter than the left dorsal colon.

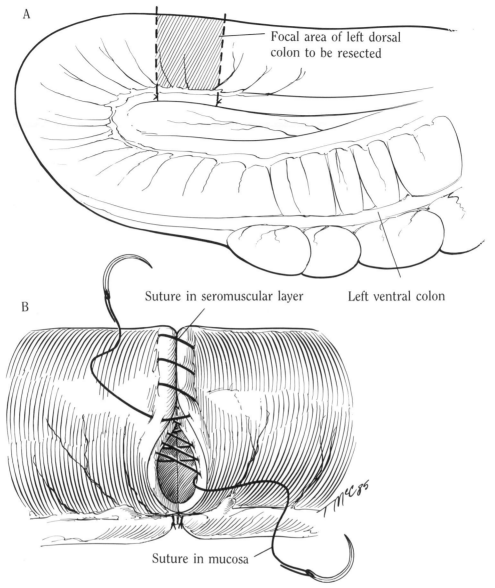

A

Focal area of left dorsal colon to be resected

Suture in seromuscular layer   Left ventral colon

B

Suture in mucosa

FIG. 7-9. Large colon resection and anastomosis. **A, B.** Focal resection and anastomosis.

RESECTION OF ADJACENT ARMS OF COLON AND SIDE-TO-SIDE ANASTOMOSIS USING SUTURES. If a significant amount of colon is to be resected and stapling equipment is unavailable, the following technique can be used. Resection of the left dorsal and left ventral colon at the level of the sternal and diaphragmatic flexure is used as an example. Both the left ventral and dorsal colons are sectioned transversely with a scalpel and sutured closed with a double inverting suture pattern (Fig. 7-9E). Occlusion of the left ventral colon and the right ventral colon is important during this procedure. A 15- to 20-cm length of adjacent left ventral and left dorsal colon is then apposed using a simple continuous seromuscular suture and linear incisions are then made in the adja-

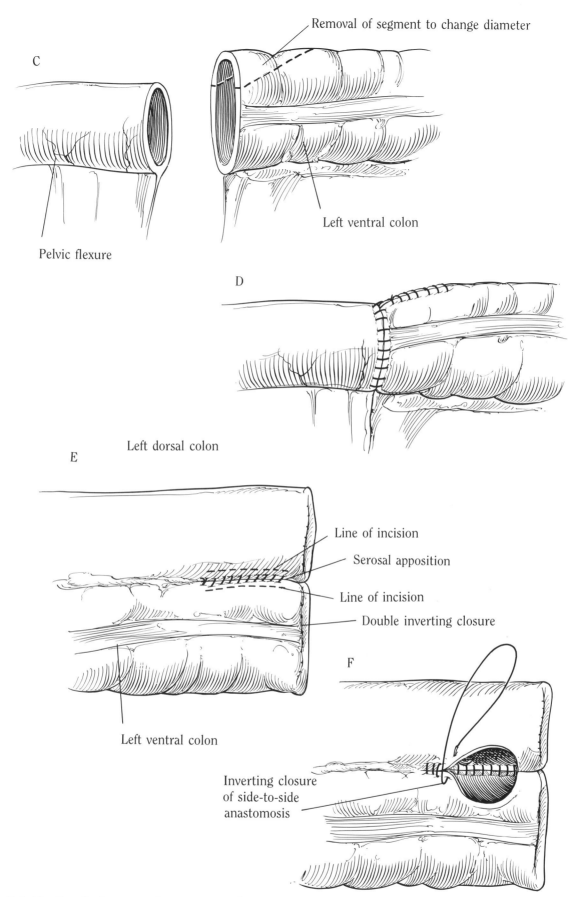

C

Removal of segment to change diameter

Left ventral colon

Pelvic flexure

D

Left dorsal colon

E

Line of incision

Serosal apposition

Line of incision

Double inverting closure

Left ventral colon

F

Inverting closure
of side-to-side
anastomosis

FIG. 7-9 (*Continued*). **C, D.** Focal resection and anastomosis with ends of disparate diameter. **E, F.** Resection of adjacent arms of colon and side-to-side anastomosis.

cent portions of the ventral and dorsal colons (Fig. 7-9E). A continuous suture is then used to oppose adjacent portions of the dorsal and ventral colons (which creates the stoma) (Fig. 7-9F). Side-to-side anastomosis has also been performed prior to closure of the ends, but the potential for contamination is increased.[3]

RESECTION AND SIDE-TO SIDE ANASTOMOSIS WITH STAPLING EQUIPMENT. This technique for large colon resection and anastomosis was developed by Sullins and Stashak.[8] Transection at the level of the sternal and diaphragmatic flexure (approximately 60% resection) will be illustrated (Fig. 7-9G). The dorsal and ventral colons are occluded with bowel clamps to prevent ingesta from reaching the anastomotic sites. These clamps are placed directly opposite each other and distal to a prominent intramural vessel (Fig. 7-9H). The dorsal and ventral colic vessels (right colic vessel and colic branches of the ileocolic vessels, respectively) are dissected from the mesentery and doubly ligated. The TA-90 stapler is then used to place a double staggered row of stainless steel staples across the dorsal and ventral colon between the point of vessel ligation and the intestinal clamps (Fig. 7-9H). Because the TA-90 staple line is only 9 cm in length, several applications are required to close the colons in the adult horse. Care is also taken to make each sequential staple row overlap the end of the previously applied row to ensure a complete seal. Then the resected portion of intestine is transected with a scalpel (Fig. 7-9I).

A side-to-side anastomosis between the right dorsal and right ventral colons is then performed commencing 1.5 cm from the distal extremity of the stapled intestinal stumps. The stoma is placed on the juxtaparietal side of the colons and parallel to their longitudinal axes. Five simple interrupted sutures of no. 2-0 polyglactin 910 are placed 5 cm apart to appose the dorsal and ventral colons so that the distal and proximal sutures are 20 cm apart (Fig. 7-9J). A 1-cm stab incision is then made into the lumina of both colons 5 cm from the distal stay suture. The GIA stapler is then inserted along this line between the two stay sutures and closed, and the staples are applied (Fig. 7-9J). This procedure is performed both cranial and caudal to the stab incision and is repeated through a second stab incision 5 cm from the cranial stay suture. In this way the instrument applications effect a continuous 20-cm side-to-side anastomosis (Fig. 7-9K). (A smaller stoma, effected through a single stab incision with two placements of the GIA proximad and one distad has also been used successfully.) The two incisions used for entry of the GIA instrument are closed with a double inverting layer of continuous sutures in a Lembert pattern using no. 2-0 polyglactin 910 (Fig. 7-9L). Reinforcing sutures of the same material are also placed at the cranial and caudal limits of the stapled anastomosis. The resection-anastomosis site is then cleansed by rinsing and returned to the abdomen. A ¼-inch fenestrated drain is placed in the abdomen prior to closure.

If cost is of some concern, the side-to-side anastomosis can be performed with sutures after the transection with the TA-90 stapler.[7] A

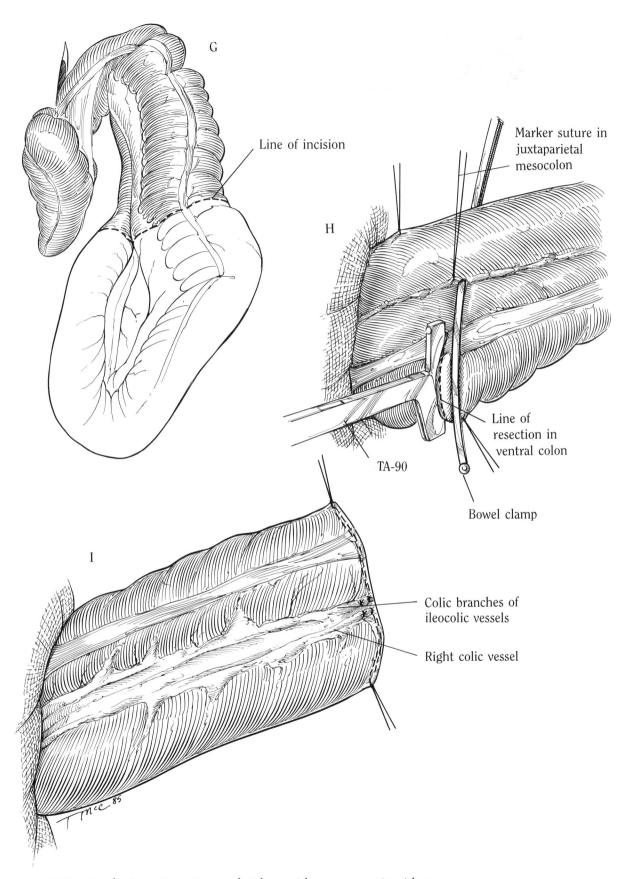

G

Line of incision

Marker suture in
juxtaparietal
mesocolon

H

Line of
resection in
ventral colon

TA-90

Bowel clamp

I

Colic branches of
ileocolic vessels

Right colic vessel

Fig. 7-9 (*Continued*). **G–I.** Resection and side-to-side anastomosis with stapling equipment.

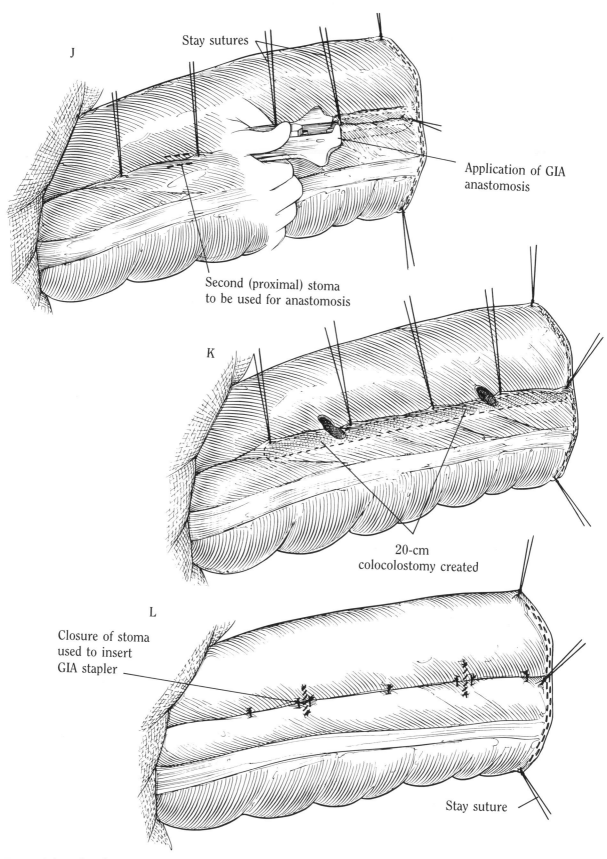

Stay sutures

J

Application of GIA anastomosis

Second (proximal) stoma to be used for anastomosis

K

20-cm colocolostomy created

L

Closure of stoma used to insert GIA stapler

Stay suture

FIG. 7-9 (Continued). **J–L.**

20-cm continuous Cushing pattern using no. 2-0 polyglactin 910 is placed to appose the dorsal and ventral colons approximately 1 cm from their attachments to the mesocolon and starting 1.5 cm from the distal extremity of the stapled intestinal stumps. The lumens of the colon are opened adjacent to the suture line, and a continuous Connell suture pattern is used to appose the mucosa in a stoma. The original Cushing pattern is then continued to complete a second anastomotic layer.

Postoperative Management

Feed is withheld overnight and one gallon of mineral oil is administered by nasogastric tube before access to feed is allowed. The horses are placed on antibiotics.

Comments

In an experimental study using this technique it took approximately 20 minutes to perform the staple anastomosis with a normal large colon.[8] In another group of animals, a sutured anastomosis (double inverting anastomosis, Cushing-Connell) was used, and this took approximately 45 minutes and also resulted in significantly more contamination of the surgical field. For these reasons the authors felt that the stapling technique was the procedure of choice.[8] Omental adhesions formed over the everted stapled stumps of the dorsal and ventral colons in all horses but did not apparently cause any problems. The proximity of the stumps to the origin of the greater omentum may make these adhesions inconsequential. While it is possible to invert the edges of the colons with a suture line, it was felt by the originators of this technique that this would bury contaminated mucosa and could potentially result in abscessation along the stumps. An alternative technique to staple instrumentation is to use a double inverting suture pattern to close off the ends of the colon; however, this method is more time-consuming and also results in more contamination of the surgical field. The originators of the stapled anastomosis considered the stapled stumps to be acceptable in the large colon.[8]

More extensive large colon resection can also be performed in the horse at the cecocolic junction. The use of this technique removing approximately 95% of the length of the large colon as measured from the cecocolic orifice and transverse colon to the pelvic flexure has been described in 10 normal horses.[2] Four horses died and three of these had failure or contamination of the transection staple line. Although experience has resolved some of these problems, it cannot be considered a routine technique for clinical cases at the present time.

References

1. Bertone, A.L., Stashak, T.S., and Sullins, K.E.: Large colon resection and anastomosis in horses. J. Am. Vet. Med. Assoc. 188:612, 1985.
2. Bertone, A.L., Stashak, T.S, and Sullins, K.E.: Experimental large colon resection at the cecocolic ligament in the horse. Vet. Surg. In press.
3. Boening, K.J.: Personal Communication, 1985.

4. Embertson, R.M., Schneider, R.K., and Granstedt, M.: Partial resection and anastomosis of the large colon in a horse. J. Am. Vet. Med. Assoc. 180:1230, 1982.
5. Huskamp, B.: Some problems associated with intestinal surgery in the horse. Eq. Vet. J. 9:111, 1977.
6. Robertson, J.T., and Tate, L.P. Jr.: Resection of intussuscepted large colon in a horse. J. Am. Vet. Med. Assoc. 181:927, 1982.
7. Stashak, T.S.: Techniques for enterotomy, decompression and intestinal resection/anastomosis. Vet. Clin. North Am. Large Anim. Pract. 4:147, 1982.
8. Sullins, K.E., and Stashak, T.S.: Evaluation of large intestinal resection in the horse at the sternal and diaphragmatic flexure. Submitted. Vet. Surg.
9. Wilson, D.G., and Wilson, W.D.: Intussusception of the left dorsal colon in a horse. J. Am. Vet. Med. Assoc. 183:464, 1983.

Cecocolic Anastomosis

A side-to-side anastomosis is sometimes indicated in cases of severe cecal impaction where continued function of the cecum following its evacuation is of concern. In these instances we have performed a side-to-side anastomosis between an area towards the apex of the cecum and adjacent to the right ventral colon.

Anesthesia and Surgical Preparation

The surgery is performed under general anesthesia using a conventional ventral midline laparotomy. As in most cases of intestinal anastomosis, the decision to perform this surgical technique is an intraoperative one.

Additional Instrumentation

The stapling procedure requires the GIA instrument and 2 cartridges of staples.

Surgical Technique

The cecum is evacuated through an enterotomy initially (between the lateral and ventral cecal tenia is a convenient site). A side-to-side anastomosis using the GIA instrument is performed in a fashion similar to that previously described for resection and anastomosis of the large colon.

The cecocolic anastomosis is performed between the lateral and ventral bands of the colon and the lateral and dorsal bands of the cecum (Fig. 7-10A). The cecum and right ventral colon are attached with three stay sutures placed at 5-cm intervals, and a central 1-cm stab incision is made to allow placement of the GIA stapler. The GIA instrument is inserted initially proximad, placed in position, and fixed to create a stoma (Fig. 7-10B). The instrument is then placed distad to create an additional 5 cm of stoma. The incision used for entry of the GIA instrument is then closed with a double inverting layer of continuous sutures in a Lembert pattern using no. 2-0 synthetic absorbable material (Fig. 7-10C). If a larger stoma is desired, a 20-cm stoma can be created with two stab incisions and four applications of the GIA stapler as described for the side-to-side anastomotic technique for the large colon. Since the illustration and description of this technique were prepared for this text, the technique has been documented in the literature, and a seromuscular suture closure to support the GIA anastomosis was recommended.[2]

Comments

The cecocolic anastomosis is recommended for cases of cecal impaction when compromise of normal cecal function or emptying is anticipated (or has already been encountered). It is an inappropriate technique if the viability of the cecum has been compromised. In these latter cases, a partial or complete typhlectomy is required. Partial typhlectomy (of the apex) can be efficiently performed with the

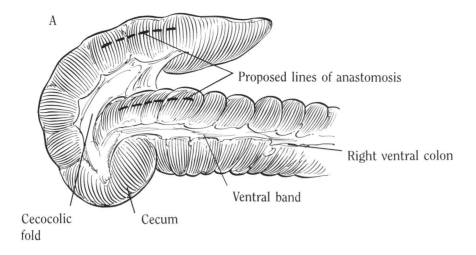

A

Proposed lines of anastomosis

Right ventral colon

Ventral band

Cecum

Cecocolic
fold

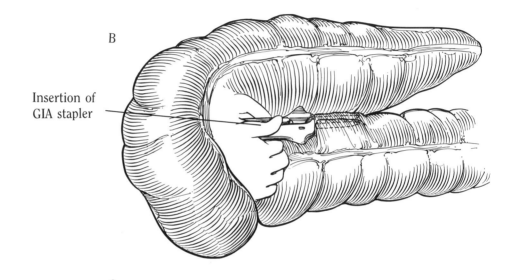

B

Insertion of
GIA stapler

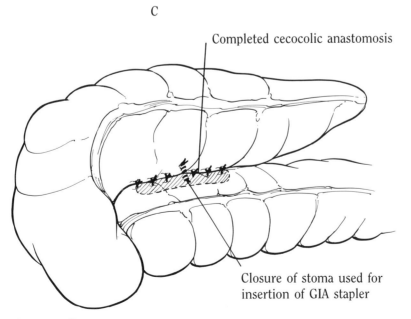

C

Completed cecocolic anastomosis

Closure of stoma used for
insertion of GIA stapler

Fig. 7-10. Cecocolic anastomosis.

TA-90 stapling device. Total typhlectomy and ileocolostomy have been described, but they are not a routine procedure. It requires a right flank approach to the abdomen and rib resection.[1] Because of the infrequent demand for this technique, it is not illustrated here and interested readers should consult the original reference.

References

1. Huskamp, B.: Some problems associated with intestinal surgery in the horse. Eq. Vet. J. 9:111, 1977.
2. Ross, M.W., Tate, L.D., and Donawick, W.J.: Cecocolic anastomosis for the surgical management of cecal impaction in horses. Vet. Surg., 15:85, 1986.

Temporary Diverting Colostomy for the Management of Rectal Tears

Rectal tears are a relatively common accident and are typically iatrogenic in association with rectal examination.[10] The consequences of a rectal tear depend on its size and position, the tissue layers penetrated, and the time between injury and the initiation of treatment. Rectal tears have been classified according to the tissue layers penetrated at the time of injury.[1] An attempt is made to manage most partial rectal tears by medical means. Very few significant tears are directly repairable, but methods of direct repair have been described for certain situations.[2] When there is a significant rectal tear, the technique of temporary diverting colostomy is necessary to divert fecal material from the rectal tear until it has healed sufficiently. The technique has been used with moderate success.[3,7,9,11] Recently, more consistent results have been described, and with experience the complications can be decreased.[4,8] For severe rectal tears, colostomy is the only technique that offers a chance for survival. In addition, with experience, the technique has been improved to obviate some of the complications.

Both end colostomies (transection of the small colon with closure of the distal segment)[4,7,9,11] and loop colostomies (continuity of colon maintained with diversion through a stoma on the antimesenteric aspect of the small colon)[3,8,9] have been used. End colostomy had been proposed as the better technique in that it ensures *complete* diversion of feces from the caudal colon.[1] The one drawback that has been noted in earlier reports, that of marked atrophy of the distal segment of the colon, which required special techniques for reanastomosis, has been obviated by earlier reanastomosis of the colon.[4,5] However, a diverting colostomy has been used successfully and will be illustrated in this sequence. Both techniques will be illustrated. A "low flank" approach is used for the colostomy. This approach is preferable to a ventral abdominal approach in the prevention of herniation of the small colon out through the colostomy site and also stricturing of the lumen by tight fascial bands ventrally.

If management of the tear is medically attempted, feed is withheld and a laxative agent is given until the feces are soft. Enemas in the initial period are indicated. Tears are often compounded by the animal straining to defecate, and there is a tendency for fecal material to lodge in the tissue defect. Periodic cleaning of the area of the rectal defect can be indicated and is a good opportunity to assess an additional tearing or separation. If in three to four days the wound margins are thickened and granulating without progression of the tear, medical management will probably be adequate. When there is any tendency for walling off of an abscess, the region must be kept open to drain. Periodic evaluation of peritoneal fluid samples is also helpful in monitoring the condition. If a complete tear is present or if a partial tear is approaching complete penetration, a diverting colostomy should be performed.

Anesthesia and Surgical Preparation

Palpation of the rectal tear itself should be done only after the animal is sedated and restrained to minimize any additional damage. A lidocaine enema may be beneficial, and a fiberoptic endoscope will sometimes allow direct visualization. With the flank technique, most colostomies can be created under local analgesia with the sedated animal standing. If the patient is not appropriate for standing surgery or contamination of the peritoneal cavity is considered to be a problem and the peritoneum is going to be irrigated, then general anesthesia with the patient in lateral recumbency is appropriate. The patient should be placed on broad-spectrum antibiotics as soon as the problem is ascertained and the decision to operate has been made.

Surgical Technique

END COLOSTOMY. A low paralumbar flank incision is made through the skin, incising the external abdominal oblique fascia in the same direction (Fig. 7-11A). The internal abdominal oblique muscle, transversus abdominis aponeurosis, and peritoneum are bluntly perforated. The small colon is exteriorized, and the area of rectal damage may be evaluated more directly at this stage with palpation. The small colon should be transected at least 1 meter cranial to the area of the tear to allow adequate manipulation of the small colon at the time of repair (Fig. 7-11B). The mesentery of the small colon is divided for half its distance to allow mobility of the two ends. The transected portion of the caudal segment of small colon is evacuated, and the end is oversewn with a double inverting layer of suture material using no. 2-0 polyglactin 910 (Vicryl) (Fig. 7-11C). At this stage, the surgeon has the choice of placing the transected end of the cranial segment in the ventral portion of the flank incision or positioning it through a *separate* stoma located ventrally to the laparotomy incision. If a separate stoma is made, the transected end of the cranial segment of small colon is oversewn prior to its being pulled through the stoma. The stoma is created by making a circular incision of slightly smaller diameter than that of in the small colon through skin and fascia of the external abdominal oblique muscle. The muscle layers of the internal abdominal oblique, and transversus abdominis are separated along the fiber planes, but short perpendicular incisions are made in these two layers to reduce the constricting effect of the muscles.[11]

Prior to final positioning of the transected end of the proximal cranial portion of the small colon, the transected end is prepared into a cuff. The mucosa of the transected end (stoma) is folded back and sutured to the serosa in a simple continuous pattern with two to three ties (Fig. 7-11D). The cut stoma is placed in position so the cuff is outside of the skin (Fig. 7-11E), and four to five simple interrupted sutures are placed between the transversus abdominis muscle and the serosa of the small colon to tack it in place. Similarly, other simple interrupted sutures are placed between the internal abdominal oblique muscle and the small colon, and these layers are closed dor-

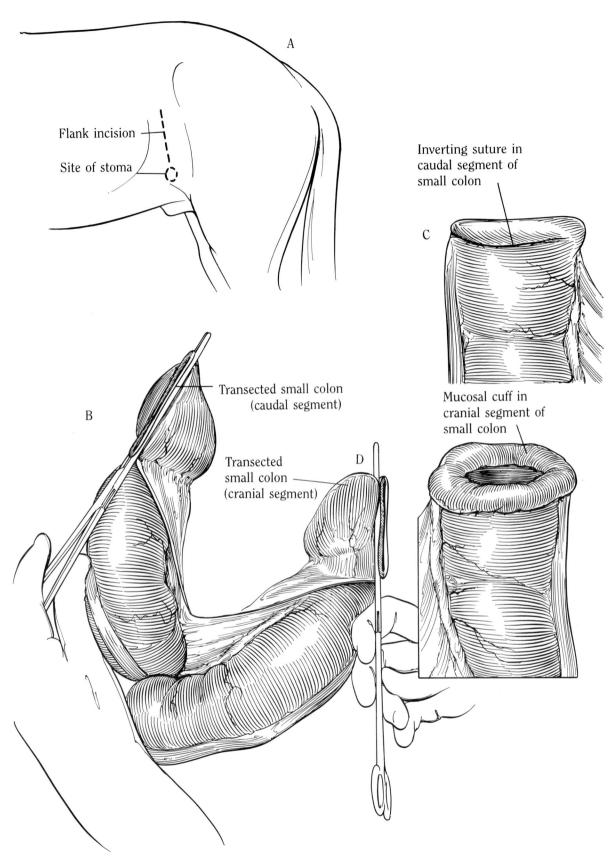

Fig. 7-11. Colostomy for managment of rectal tears. **A–D.** End colostomy.

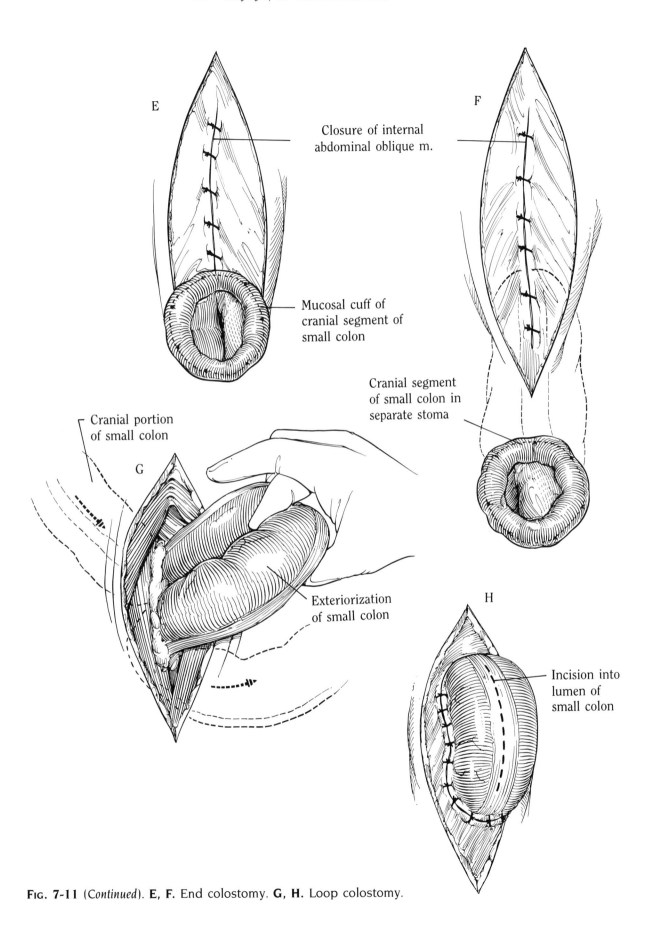

Closure of internal abdominal oblique m.

Mucosal cuff of cranial segment of small colon

Cranial segment of small colon in separate stoma

Cranial portion of small colon

Exteriorization of small colon

Incision into lumen of small colon

FIG. 7-11 (*Continued*). **E, F.** End colostomy. **G, H.** Loop colostomy.

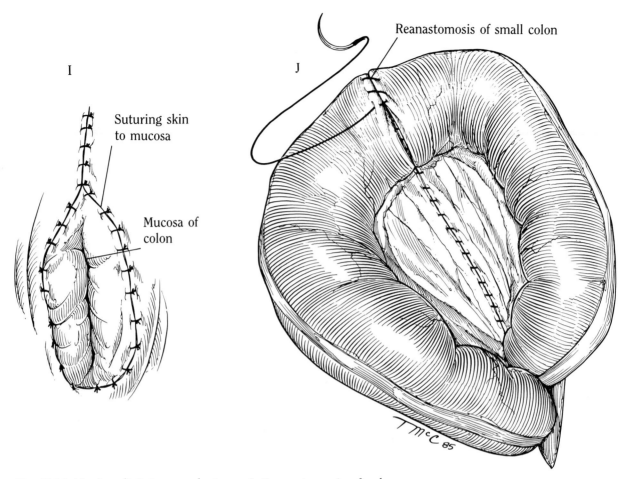

I

Suturing skin
to mucosa

Mucosa of
colon

J

Reanastomosis of small colon

FIG. 7-11 (*Continued*). I. Loop colostomy. J. Reanastomosis of colon.

sally to the colostomy stoma if the colostomy is being placed within the initial laparotomy incision (Fig. 7-11E).[4] If sutures are at 1 and 3 o'clock in one layer, they are placed at 2 and 4 o'clock in the next layer. Simple interrupted sutures are then placed between the external abdominal oblique fascia and the small colon (this is the principal stabilizing layer), and the dorsal aspects of the laparotomy incision are closed. Subcutaneous tissue is then pulled in immediately behind and adjacent to the margins of the reflected mucosal cuff and sutured to the small colon. The skin is not sutured to the small colon at the stoma but is closed dorsally to the stoma.

If the cranial small colon is placed through a separate stoma, it is tacked in place in the deeper layers and positioned in the same fashion relative to the skin as previously described (Fig. 7-11F). The flank laparotomy incision is closed routinely. One surgeon has also performed a colostomy by creating a circular stoma alone of sufficient size to place a hand through and grasp the small colon. This technique is appropriate only when there is no contamination of the peritoneal cavity to deal with and therefore limited surgical exposure is required.[5] In the contaminated situation the operation will be performed under general anesthesia, and an open laparotomy will be performed with extensive lavage of the peritoneum and placement of ventral abdominal drains for the postoperative period.

LOOP COLOSTOMY. The principle behind the loop colostomy is to retain the caudal segment of small colon at the surgical site and through regular gentle retroflushing of the caudal segment retain its size and partial function. At the same time the fecal material is diverted. A left flank incision is made in the same fashion as previously described using a modified "grid" approach with a vertical incision in the external abdominal oblique muscle layer. The colon is exteriorized (Fig. 7-11G) and placed vertically (cranial side of small colon at the dorsal part of the incision so fecal flow is ventrad) in the ventral aspect of the incision with the antimesenteric band placed laterally (Fig. 7-11H). The loop of small colon is sutured to the edges of the external abdominal oblique fascia with no. 0 polyglactin 910 (Vicryl) in a simple interrupted or continuous pattern with the sutures not penetrating the lumen of the colon (Fig. 7-11H). The laparotomy incision dorsal to the colostomy site is closed routinely. A 6-cm incision is then made into the lumen of the small colon along the antimesenteric band, and the mucosa is sutured to the skin incision using nonabsorbable suture material in a simple interrupted or mattress pattern (Fig. 7-11I). Skin to mucosa closure is initially performed ventrally, and the musculature is loosely closed dorsally before completion of the colostomy closure.

POSTOPERATIVE MANAGEMENT. Petrolatum is applied ventral to the colostomy to prevent scalding. In the case of the loop colostomy the rectum and caudal segment of small colon are flushed daily to help maintain function of the caudal segment (this procedure is not essential). With the end colostomy no catheters are placed postoperatively within the bowel lumen. Broad-spectrum systemic antibiotics are used in the initial stages in either type, and the horse is maintained on a laxative diet (fresh green grass is ideal). The colostomy site is kept clean. In the case of the end colostomy the mucosal cuff will swell and then slough in 3 to 7 days.[4] Periodic examination of the region of rectal damage will determine when the caudal segment is adequately healed. It is sometimes appropriate to put a finger in the tear hole daily to prevent an abscess or to keep an abscess open.[5] Generally on clinical cases, reanastomosis can be performed 12 to 14 days following the initial surgery. If the surgeon waits 30 days, problems with atrophy of the caudal segment of small colon will be experienced.

REANASTOMOSIS OF SMALL COLON. In the case of the end colostomy, if reanastomosis is performed 12 to 14 days after the colostomy, end-to-end anastomosis is feasible. The left flank laparotomy is repeated and the cranial portion of small colon is removed from the incision and the end is transected. The oversewn stump of the caudal end is similarly transected and an end-to-end anastomosis is performed using a simple continuous pattern in the mucosa followed by a continuous inverting Lembert pattern in the seromuscular layers (Fig. 7-11J). If reanastomosis is performed at a later time and atrophy of the caudal segment is significant, an end-to-side anastomosis is necessary.

If a loop colostomy has been performed, the temporary colostomy is separated from its attachment to the skin incision at around 14 days, the enterotomy is closed, and the small colon is replaced in the abdomen. The laparotomy incision is then closed routinely in the appropriate layers.

In either case the animal is maintained on a slightly laxative diet after reanastomosis. Normal diet can be resumed gradually over the following two weeks. It is to be noted that with the loop colostomy, relaparotomy is not necessary, as the colostomy can be closed using the previously created stoma. Should the enterotomy site be traumatized, it is still possible to exteriorize the descending colon sufficiently to perform an end-to-end anastomosis without making another abdominal incision.

Comments

Possible complications to this colostomy procedure include detachment of the small colon, prolapse, herniation,[6] retraction, and stenosis.[7] These can be obviated by good technique and positioning of the colostomy site in the ventral part of the flank. Reanastomosis in two weeks (which is generally sufficient for most tears) obviates some of the complications.

The use of temporary rectal liners placed within the involved rectum with an anchoring attachment craniad to the tear has been described.[12] These have been suggested as an alternative method of managing rectal tears but are yet to be perfected.

References

1. Arnold, J.S., and Meagher, D.M.: Management of rectal tears in the horse. J. Eq. Med. Surg. 2:64, 1978.
2. Arnold, J.S., Meagher, D.M., and Lohse, C.L.: Rectal tears in the horse. J. Eq. Med. Surg. 2:55, 1978.
3. Azzie, M.A.J.: Temporary colostomy in the management of rectal tumors in the horse. J. Afr. Vet. Assoc. 46:121, 1975.
4. Boles, C.L.: Rectal tears and colostomies. American College of Veterinary Surgeons Annual Forum, 1984.
5. Boles, C.L., and Herthel, D.J.: Alamo Pintado Equine Clinic: Personal communication, 1975.
6. Brown, M.: Rectal tears. L.A. Pract., 4:185, 1982.
7. Herthel, D.J.: Colostomy in the mare. Proceedings of the 20th Annual Convention of the AAEP, 1974. 1975, p. 187.
8. Shires, M.: The temporary loop colostomy—another choice. Proceedings of the Equine Colic Research Symposium, University of Georgia 1982, p. 293.
9. Spiers, V.C., Christie, B.A., and Van Veenendaal, J.C.: The management of rectal tears in horses. Aust. Vet. J. 56:313, 1980.
10. Stanffer, V.D.: Equine rectal tears—a malpractice problem. J. Am. Vet. Med. Assoc. 178:798, 1981.
11. Stashak, T.S., and Knight, A.P.: Temporary diverting colostomy of the management of small colon tears in the horse: A case report. J. Eq. Med. Surg. 2:196, 1978.
12. Taylor, T.: Temporary indwelling liner as an aid to treatment of equine rectal tears. American College of Veterinary Surgeons Annual Meeting, 1981.

Inguinal Herniorrhaphy

Inguinal and scrotal hernias usually occur in two situations in the horse. They are seen in the adult stallion and in the newborn colt. As in most domestic animals inguinal hernias in the horse are usually *indirect* whereby viscera (usually jejunum or ileum) pass through the vaginal ring into the vaginal process or tunica vaginalis, which forms the hernial sac.[2,4] The adult stallion frequently has signs of colic shortly after breeding a mare or some other strenuous activity such as jumping a fence.[1,2,4,5] Such activities presumably result in stretching of the inguinal rings, as well as an increase in intraabdominal pressure and the occurrence of the hernia.[1,4] Rectal examination of such a patient will reveal intestine descending into the ring, confirming the diagnosis. The testicle and scrotum on that side may feel enlarged and tense. The hernia must be differentiated from torsion of the testicle and thrombosis of the testicular artery, which are rare.[2]

Shortly after its occurrence, an inguinal hernia in a stallion sometimes can be manually reduced per rectum. This technique of reduction should be discouraged because of the risk of tearing the intestine or rectum and the chance of recurrence of the hernia. In addition, the entrapped bowel may have undergone irreversible morphologic changes requiring resection that will not be evident, clinically, for several days. Inguinal or scrotal hernia in the mature horse is therefore best thought of as a surgical emergency, even if the horse is not showing signs of abdominal distress.

In the young colt, inguinal and scrotal hernias occur at birth or shortly thereafter. Descent of the testicle occurs at or near birth; thereafter the relatively large ring begins to close and becomes relatively smaller. Many of these hernias in foals can be treated conservatively by manually reducing the hernia ("buying time" for the ring to become smaller). Many spontaneously reduce by three to six months of age.[2] On the other hand, surgery is indicated if manual reduction becomes impossible or the foal begins to show signs of colic, an indication of incarceration of bowel. In very large hernias where the external inguinal ring is greater than 10 to 12 cm, spontaneous closure is unlikely and immediate elective surgery is indicated.

Although reduction per rectum is not possible in the foal, surgical treatment is almost identical to that for the colt. Both are described in this chapter.

Anesthesia and Surgical Preparation

Attention must be given to the overall hydration and acid base status of the stallion or colt before surgery. If the animal has an acute intestinal obstruction, then the horse must be given the appropriate supportive treatment.

Safe anesthetic regimens are essential to the successful outcome of the case. Intravenous anesthetics that severely compromise the already compromised patient have no place in modern equine surgery.

The herniorraphy is performed under general anesthesia with the patient in dorsal recumbency. It is of some help to have the animal slightly tilted to one side during reduction of the hernia. The scrotal and inguinal areas usually require some clipping, although hair in this region is usually scant. In the mature stallion, massive swellings and edema of the incarcerated bowel may make manual reduction impossible. The surgeon needs to be prepared for a *supplementary midline laparotomy incision*. A paramedian or midline approach can be used. We prefer the ventral midline approach, cranial to the prepuce and directed through the linea alba. Therefore *both* the scrotal region and the ventral midline region always should be simultaneously prepared for sterile surgery in a routine manner. These regions are draped in anticipation of using both procedures, so that the surgeon can use them without risking a break in aseptic technique.

Additional Instrumentation

Malleable or Balfour retractors and a blunt teat bistoury.

Surgical Technique

A straight incision (approximately 10 cm long in foals and 15 cm long in adults) is made directly over the external inguinal ring, in a location similar to what would be made with an inguinal approach to cryptorchidism (Fig. 7-12A). Larger hernias may require even longer incisions. The incision must be made cautiously, because the loops of intestine may be located quite superficially. The incision is made only through the skin, subcutaneous tissues, and fascia over the inguinal ring. Two methods are currently available for management of the hernia from this point. In the first method (only applicable for a nonincarcerated hernia in a foal), the common vaginal tunic is freed from surrounding tissues by blunt dissection (Fig. 7-12B). The contents of the hernia are then milked into the abdominal cavity while steady traction is exerted on the testis, tunics, and spermatic cord. The freed vaginal hernia is not incised. The entire structure is then twisted several times on its long axis, aiding in the passage of the herniated intestine into the peritoneal cavity. The spermatic cord is transfixed with a ligature just distal to the inguinal ring, using no. 1 or no. 2 synthetic absorbable suture material of the surgeon's choice, and then emasculated distal to the ligature. This technique resembles the method used to correct an inguinal hernia in a piglet.[3] The superficial inguinal ring is then sutured with 3 or 4 preplaced simple interrupted sutures by the method outlined below. It is obviously important to see that all the intestine has been replaced into the abdominal cavity when using this method.

The other variation of this technique is the one preferred by us and most other surgeons. The incision is made through the skin and subcutaneous tissues, directly over the testicle if it is palpable, or directly over the external inguinal ring. As the incision is carried deeper through the common vaginal tunic and its overlying fascia, care must be taken not to incise through underlying intestine. When the incision is complete, bowel will be immediately visible (Fig.

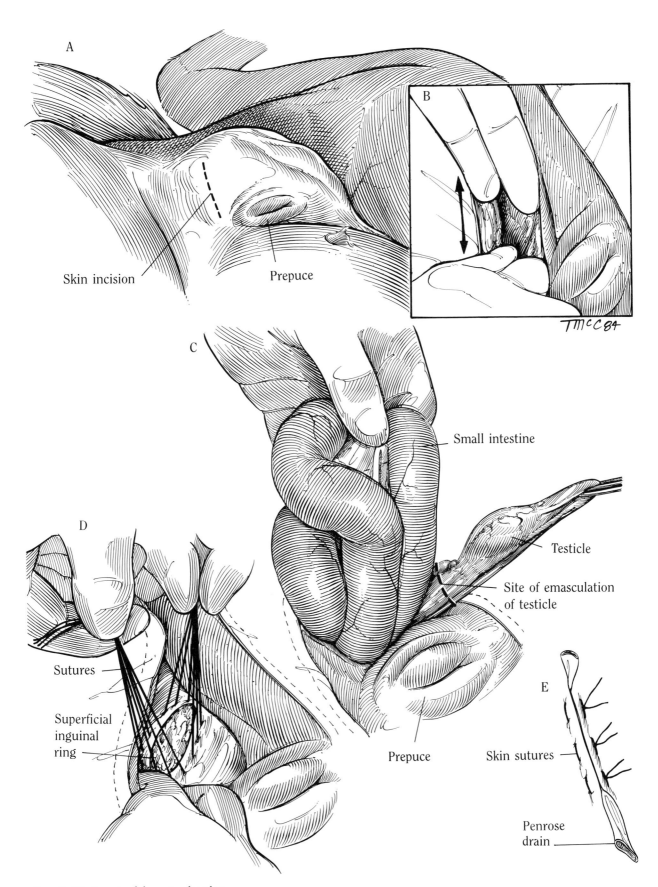

FIG. 7-12. Inguinal herniorrhaphy.

7-12C). In very large scrotal hernias in foals, the common vaginal tunic may have been ruptured, allowing intestine to become localized subcutaneously. Since intestine may dissect toward the stifle, one must be careful when incising over the skin to avoid serious damage to the bowel. The bowel should be adequately exteriorized and inspected. Any necrotic bowel, or bowel of questionable viability, should be resected and an end-to-end anastomosis performed using methods outlined elsewhere in this book. If the bowel has become invested in a layer of fibrin, it is our feeling that resection and anastomosis are required because of the high susceptibility of such bowel to adhesions. If the intestine appears viable, it is replaced into the abdomen. Decompression at several sites with the aid of suction and an 18-gauge needle may be necessary.

At this point in the procedure, the testis involved in the hernia is transfixed just proximal to the inguinal ring, emasculated distal to the ligature, and removed. The ability to confidently close the ring is compromised unless the testis is removed. If the *viability* of the testicle is questionable, then there should be no argument whether to remove it because of the risk of an ischemic orchitis. The testicle is frequently edematous due to impairment of venous return.

It is generally felt that a hernia occurring following breeding is probably due to a predisposing weakness since birth and that castration is the most ethical thing to do because of the heritability of the condition.[5] A higher than normal incidence of scrotal hernia has been reported in certain breeds such as the Standardbred than in other breeds.[2] If the stallion is not valued for breeding, then the opposite testicle *as well* should be removed.

The inguinal canal on the opposite site should always be checked for size, and this inguinal ring should be sutured closed if castration is performed.

If the internal inguinal ring is too small to allow the safe replacement of bowel into the abdomen, then it can be enlarged. To do this safely without damaging the bowel one of us (AST) has used a blunt teat bistoury inserted into the abdomen protected by an index finger. When the cutting edge of the knife is against the internal ring free of interposing bowel, the ring can be enlarged slightly by a gentle sawing motion. This appears to be safer than trying to cut the ring with scissors.

Following reduction of the hernia, the superficial (external) inguinal ring is closed. The superficial inguinal ring is a slit in the aponeurosis of the external abdominal oblique muscle. Its medial border is usually well defined and easily identified. Its lateral border is made up of dense fascia on the medial side of the thigh. Anywhere from 3 to 6 or 7 preplaced simple interrupted sutures are used to close the ring. The closure should be initiated beyond the cranial end of the ring and ended beyond the caudal end, taking bites at different distances from the edge (thereby not weakening the ring along a common plane[3]) (Figure 7-12D). The suture material is usually a synthetic absorbable material of the surgeon's choice and U.S.P. no. 2 (Metric no. 5) in size.

It can be inserted as a double strand in very large horses, such as the draft breeds. Care is taken to avoid the external pudendal artery and vein. Slight adduction of the limb as the sutures are tied, reduces the distances between the edges of the ring, and facilitates closure.

A layer of inguinal fascia is usually available and should be sutured over the external inguinal ring to provide further strength to the closure. A Penrose drain can be placed in the wound but must exit from the most ventral aspect of the hernia pocket. The skin can be partially closed to facilitate rapid healing. The sutures in the skin should not be tied too tightly, as swelling rapidly ensues, making removal difficult. The ends of the skin sutures should be long to facilitate their retrieval at the time of removal.

In the mature stallion it is an option to pack the subcutaneous area with a length of sterile cotton gauze. This is used in lieu of a Penrose drain. The gauze should not be forced down the inguinal canal but merely placed in the subcutaneous space in an accordion-like fashion, and allowed to exit through the most ventral aspect of the incision. The first author (C.W.M.) does not use drains or gauze packing routinely.

If a ventral midline incision has been used, it should be closed using a synthetic absorbable suture material of the surgeon's choice and of the appropriate size. The subcutaneous fascia and skin of this wound should also be closed.

Postoperative Management

Attention must be paid to the fluid, electrolyte, and acid base balance of the horse. Careful postoperative monitoring in those critical cases is essential for a successful outcome.

Antibiotics are recommended especially if there was a break in aseptic technique or there was an intestinal anastomosis. Antibiotics with a good gram-negative spectrum will be necessary in some instances. Tetanus immunization is essential. The horse (or mare and foal) should be confined alone for three to four weeks following surgery.

Immediately following surgery, horses that are large enough to permit rectal examination should be examined to see that there has been complete reduction of the hernia. The surgeon should also check to see if the hernia ring is still closed. A violent recovery from anesthesia can potentially disrupt the sutures in the external inguinal ring. One should also check to see that bowel is not adhered to the inguinal ring as a result of fibrin exudation from the surgery site or that a suture has not inadvertently hooked a piece of intestine.

If a Penrose drain has been placed, it should be gently manipulated to encourage drainage. It should be removed three to four days after surgery. If gauze packing has been used, it is removed over a two to three day period, or all at once, depending on the surgeon's preference. It should not be removed unless a rectal examination reveals that the inguinal rings are free of bowel.

Following removal of the gauze or Penrose drain, the horse should be hand-walked to help minimize postoperative swelling. Hand-walking should be done twice daily and gradually increased as the animal becomes more comfortable. The normal playful physical activities of foals will provide sufficient exercise themselves to minimize swelling.

At no stage during the first three to four weeks after surgery should the animal be turned out with other horses. Excessive activity is likely to disrupt the suture line and lead to recurrence of the hernia.

Comments

The open technique of inguinal herniorrhaphy allows visualization of the incarcerated intestine, testicle, and spermatic cord, and a more accurate assessment of their viability or the presence of adhesions. This method is essential if the bowel has become strangulated and resection and end-to-end anastomosis are required. It also facilitates enlargement of the inguinal ring to enable reduction of the hernia. As discussed previously, a second incision (through the linea alba, cranial to the prepuce) is frequently necessary if difficulty is encountered in returning the bowel to the abdomen. The operator can insert a gloved hand and suitably protected arm through this more cranial incision, reach caudad to the affected inguinal ring, and by applying judicious traction on the affected bowel, help reduce the hernia. Both diseased and adjacent normal bowel can be exteriorized through this incision without the tension needed to exteriorize it through the inguinal canal. The midline incision is also essential if a jejunal-cecal anastomosis is necessary due to vascular compromise of the ileum.

References

1. Goetz, T. E., Boulton, C.H., and Coffman, J.R.: Inguinal and scrotal hernias in colts and stallions. Compend. Contin. Educ. Pract. Vet. 3:272, 1981.
2. Schneider, R.K., Milne, D.W., and Kohn, C.W.: Acquired inguinal hernia in the horse: A review of 27 cases. J. Am. Vet. Med. Assoc. 180:317, 1982.
3. Turner, A.S., and McIlwraith, C.W.: Inguinal herniorrhapy in the piglet. In Techniques in Large Animal Surgery. Philadelphia, Lea & Febiger, 1982, p. 312.
4. Vasey, J.R.: Simultaneous presence of a direct and indirect inguinal hernia in a stallion. Aust. Vet. J. 57:481, 1981.
5. Vaughan, J.T.: Surgery of the male equine reproductive system. In Textbook of Large Animal Surgery. (P. Jennings, Ed.) Philadelphia, W.B. Saunders, 1984.

Herniorrhaphy Using Synthetic Mesh and a Fascial Overlay

An abdominal hernia requiring a synthetic mesh is usually acquired, and may be the result of previous abdominal surgery, an unusual case of a failed umbilical herniorrhapy, or trauma to the lower flank area. In our experience, incisional hernias are most likely to occur if the laparotomy incision becomes infected or if the horse is afflicted with a concurrent infection in another organ system. A concurrent peritonitis resulting in a hypoproteinemia frequently produces "delayed" wound healing. Complications such as postoperative diarrhea (e.g., salmonellosis) or pneumonia may exacerbate weight loss and what is termed as a "catabolic state."[6]

Because herniorrhaphy with mesh implantation can usually be done on an elective basis, the horse should be in the best physical condition obtainable, that is, an anabolic state prior to the commencement of surgery. Horses that are thin and recovering from a protracted postoperative convalescence following intestinal surgery should receive the appropriate nutritional therapy before surgery of this magnitude is attempted. Certainly a horse that is coughing because of pneumonia would be a poor risk for mesh implantation because of the tension placed on the suture line during coughing episodes.

Candidates for herniorrhaphy with mesh implantation frequently have suture abscesses and fistulae as a result of previous surgery. Sepsis and edema at the surgical site *must* be attended to before mesh implantation. The surgeon should be prepared to remove offending suture material to resolve this condition in a separate operation. Ideally, a well-defined fibrous ring should be palpable. Frequently, the edges of the hernia are indistinct, and rather than being one continuous defect, there exists a series of smaller holes in the linea alba.

Whether to repair the hernia routinely with a suture closure or to use a synthetic mesh is clearly a matter of surgical judgment. Incisional hernias have been referred to us for mesh implantation when it has been feasible to close the defect with standard techniques. Sometimes in these situations we would advise that the abdominal wall be closed using a meticulously applied Mayo overlap (vest-over-pants) or a near-far-far-near suture pattern with heavy (e.g., no. 2) synthetic absorbable suture material. If the surgeon is absolutely confident that sepsis has been eliminated from the surgical site, then one of the braided synthetics may be used.

Anesthesia and Surgical Preparation

The herniorraphy must be performed under as ideal facilities as available and under strict aseptic techniques. Because the procedure is time-consuming and tedious, general anesthesia using inhalation agents such as halothane is mandatory. Because of the long surgery time and the fact that surgery involves implantation of a large foreign body that may potentiate infection, in our opinion, perioperative antibiotics are indicated. Even though the surgery is performed under aseptic conditions, tissue handling and its subsequent devitalization are more than for most operations. This, combined with the prospect of having undetectable sepsis at the surgical site from previous surgery, indicates that antibiotic coverage is appropriate.

Prior to induction of anesthesia, the ventral midline and hernial sac are clipped. Following induction of anesthesia, the horse is placed in dorsal recumbency, and any areas that were not clipped while the horse was standing are now attended to. The area is shaved and prepared for surgery in a routine manner. The method described was first applied to the horse by Scott and termed a "fascial overlay" technique.[5]

Additional Instrumentation

Several synthetic meshes are available for herniorrhaphy in both people and domestic animals. Metallic meshes (e.g., tantalum and stainless steel) were used initially, but these tended to fragment and better alternatives now exist.[5] The most frequently used material (and used by us) is knitted polypropylene mesh.* This mesh is easily handled, does not fragment with time, has low reactivity (inertness), and has a high tensile strength.[3,5,6] It is also tolerated well in the face of infection.[1,4] The cut edges resist fraying, and capillaries can grow through the mesh.[6] Woven plastic (nylon)† mesh has the same desirable characteristics as polypropylene. Since it is woven rather than knitted, there is less sagging, but it does fray when cut.[6] Its main advantage is its cost relative to polypropylene, and for this reason it has become the implant of choice for some surgeons, especially in food animals where cost is a factor.[6] Teflon (polytetrafluoroethylene, PTFE) has been used experimentally in rabbits, but there are no reports of its use in the horse. It was concluded in one study that PTFE was superior to polypropylene.[1]

Also available to the surgeon should be an unlimited supply of a compatible suture material with an atraumatic noncutting needle (so as not to lacerate the mesh) to anchor the mesh to the body wall. Preferably, this suture should be monofilament (e.g., nylon or polypropylene). There are, however, numerous reports of successful herniorrhaphy using braided synthetic materials such as Mersilene to anchor the mesh.

Surgical Technique

Following draping, the extent of the hernia (including any smaller holes in the linea alba) is palpated. A semielliptical incision extending beyond the cranial and caudal margins of the hernia is made (Fig. 7-13A). The skin border is grasped with Backhaus towel clamps, and

---

* Marlex Mesh #1266, Dowd Inc., Providence, RI.
† Proxplast, Goshen Laboratory, Goshen, NY.

the skin flap and subcutaneous tissue are reflected to one side (Fig. 7-13B). Hemostasis should be attended to at this point. The hernial sac is incised carefully along the fascial margins of the hernia, except at the base, which is left attached (Fig. 7-13B). The hernial sac (fibrous sac and peritoneum) is then reflected toward its opposite attached base (Fig. 7-13C). A moistened hand towel is inserted in the abdomen to keep the bowel from interfering with the placement of the mesh.

A double layer of the synthetic mesh, which has been trimmed to shape, is placed deep to the exposed fascial margin of the hernia but superficial to the retroperitoneal fat and peritoneum. Folding the edge of the mesh to the outside should be attempted. This prevents the viscera from contact with the rough edge of the mesh and possible bowel perforation. If the mesh is not folded, it should be absolutely flat.[2] The mesh is initially anchored on the side of the hernia that corresponds to the attached edge of the fascial flap. An incision is initiated *from the peritoneal side* of the flap, and dissection is continued until the fascial margin of the hernial sac is encountered.

The mesh is then anchored to this fascial border by simple interrupted mattress sutures. The sutures should be preplaced (using hemostats to secure the free ends) around one half of the fascial border, using nonabsorbable synthetic suture material. Each suture passes from exterior to interior, is looped longitudinally through the mesh, then exits from interior to exterior. The bites through the fascial ring should be placed at right angles to the edge of the hernia, and each suture should be to 1 to 2 cm apart. The suture should enter the fascial ring approximately 3 to 4 cm from the edge of the hernia and enter the mesh an equal distance from the hernia's edge. Tension on the mesh will be dispersed through the use of multiple sutures, thereby reducing the potential necrosing effect of the sutures. The surgeon should attempt to place the anchoring sutures in as dense and mature fibrous tissue as can be found along the hernia margins. The preplaced sutures along this side of the hernia are now tied, and the mesh is trimmed further to fit the opposite margin of the hernia. The mesh should be 2 to 3 cm larger than the defect.

The mesh is anchored in the remaining side of the hernia in an identical fashion as the first side. Peritoneum and retroperitoneal fat are dissected away from the fascia that comprises the hernia border, and preplacement of the sutures is begun. The location of these sutures should be such that when tightened simultaneously the mesh should be drawn tightly across the defect forming a *flat* diaphragm, without folds or wrinkles. Some sutures may have to be removed and repositioned to achieve this effect (Fig. 7-13C).

Excess tissue from the fascial flap is trimmed off, and the flap is then sutured to the free hernia margin, using nonabsorbable suture material in a simple interrupted pattern (Fig. 7-13D). The mesh now lies deep to the fascial margins and is covered by the fascial tissues that once comprised the hernial sac. By keeping the hernial sac attached at one edge and suturing it over the implant, tension on the mesh is reduced and drainage of abdominal fluid and subsequent seroma formation are virtually eliminated.

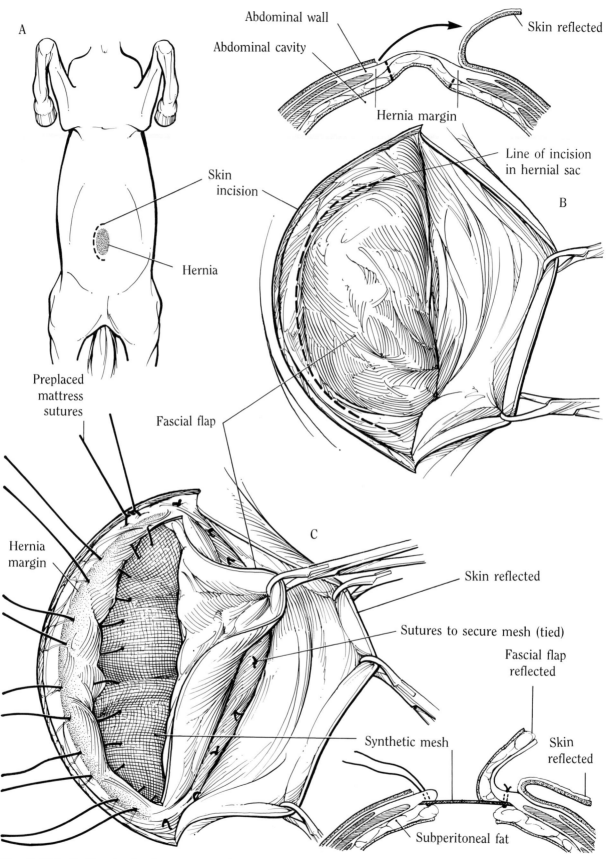

A

Skin
incision

Hernia

Preplaced
mattress
sutures

Fascial flap

Abdominal wall

Abdominal cavity

Skin reflected

Hernia margin

Line of incision
in hernial sac

B

C

Hernia
margin

Skin reflected

Sutures to secure mesh (tied)

Fascial flap
reflected

Skin
reflected

Synthetic mesh

Subperitoneal fat

Fig. 7-13A–C. Herniorrhaphy using synthetic mesh.

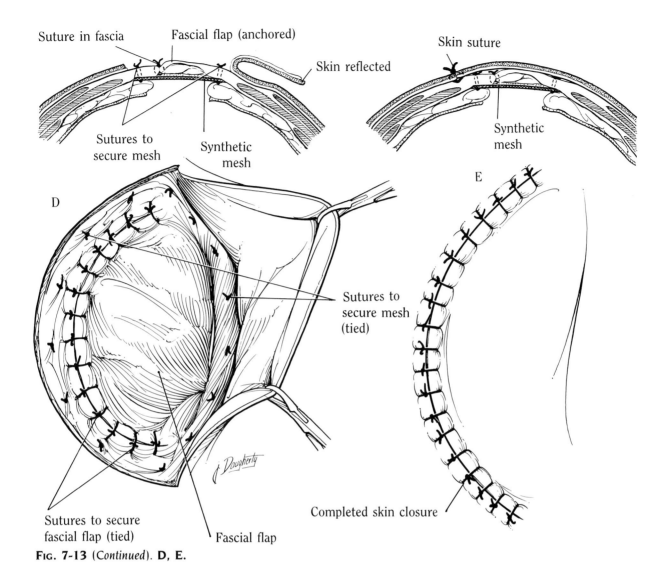

FIG. 7-13 (*Continued*). **D, E.**

Subcutaneous tissues are approximated with absorbable sutures in a simple continuous pattern. Any excess skin (found in the more pendulous hernias) is resected. The skin is either sutured with nonabsorbable monofilament suture in a simple interrupted pattern or apposed with stainless steel staples (Fig. 7-13E).

Postoperative Management

Antibiotics are continued for three days. We administer nonsteroidal antiinflammatory drugs such as phenylbutazone for the first two days to reduce incisional pain and minimize swelling.[7]

Some surgeons advocate a "belly bandage" or corset arrangement to help support the surgical repair. Another benefit of these devices is their ability to keep the surgical site free of dirt, straw, urine, and feces if the horse decides to lie down. Another method of protection is to secure a stent bandage such as a folded hand towel over the incision.

Comments

The fascial overlay method has been previously described for use in the horse.[5] It offers some obvious advantages to earlier methods that involved removal of the hernial sac. By preserving the flap and suturing it over the mesh, tension, drainage, and seroma formation are reduced.[5] Equally as important, the technique provides a very substantial additional layer of tissue between the implant and the external environment. This decreases the chances of infection gaining access to the mesh by way of the skin incision and establishing infection. Nevertheless, attention must still be paid to asepsis, gentle tissue handling, and hemostasis. Although it has been stated that synthetic meshes tolerate infection remarkably well, we strongly advocate that all evidence of sepsis be controlled before mesh implantation. Since monofilament suture materials are the best material to use in the face of sepsis, we advocate their use over the braided synthetic materials (Mersilene, Tevdek, Polydek). Attention must be given to proper knotting techniques when monofilament sutures are used.

When the abdomen is entered, care must be taken to avoid incising bowel that may be adhered to the abdominal wall. This would result in inadvertent spillage of bowel contents, with a risk of fatal peritonitis. If this were to happen, the offending bowel should be repaired, and extensive lavage of the abdomen be performed. The mesh implantation would have to be abandoned until the horse has made complete recovery.

Other authors have reported using a double application of a mesh for herniorrhaphy.[3] One layer is placed deep to the hernia ring, and the other is placed superficial to it. With this method it is technically more difficult to suture the meshes to the hernia margins, either independently or together. Also with this method, one of the mesh layers is much closer to the external environment, making infection a greater risk. In addition, it has been observed that adhesions of bowel to the mesh are more likely to form with the mesh placed intraperitoneally. Adhesions seem to occur more frequently when the mesh is placed on the abdominal floor in contrast to the use of the mesh for flank herniorrhaphy.

The use of synthetic meshes for hernias in other locations in horses is well established.[6] Hernias of the flank of the horse are usually large, and primary apposition of the edges of the hernia is usually accompanied by excessive tension. With flank hernias in horses, the use of a neatly constructed fascial flap as described previously is impossible. However, the principles of mesh implantation are the same. As much soft tissue as possible should be placed between the mesh and subcutaneous and skin layers to minimize the possibility of infection becoming established around the mesh.

It has been demonstrated in human surgery that synthetic meshes such as polypropylene tolerate infection well. They are sometimes used to provide a scaffolding for granulation tissue ingrowth in patients with massive abdominal wall defects (e.g., extensive trauma with tissue loss or resection of malignant tumors). As the granulation tissue grows into the mesh, it cleans the mesh of bacteria even when there is gross purulence and allows the mesh to remain intact rather than requiring removal.[7] However, managing such a case of open granulation over mesh is much more difficult in the equine patient than in humans. We cannot overemphasize the need to avoid infection around the implant. If drainage and fistulation begin, several options are available. In some cases drainage can be traced to one or two offending anchoring sutures that can be manually removed without necessitating removal of the entire implant. If the entire implant requires removal, then the surgeon has no choice but to remove it and wait till the infection has resolved before implanting another mesh. All signs of drainage must be eliminated before a second surgical procedure is considered.

Adhesions and subsequent intestinal obstruction have been observed with mesh implantation in horses,[6] although the polypropylene mesh used by the authors is as well tolerated intraperitoneally as any material currently available. Adhesions are treated by laparotomy and intestinal resection as appropriate.

References

1. Elliot, M.P., and Julev, G.L.: Comparison of Marlex mesh and microporous Teflon sheets when used for hernia repair in the experimental animal. Am. J. Surg. 137:342, 1979.
2. Gilsdor in discussion of McCarthy, J.D., and Twiest, M.W.: Intraperitoneal polypropylene mesh support of incisional herniorrhaphy. Am. J. Surg. 142:707, 1981.
3. Hilbert, B.J., Slatter, D.H., and McDermott, J.D.: Repair of a massive abdominal hernia in a horse using polypropylene mesh. Aust. Vet. J. 54:588, 1978.
4. McCarthy, J.D., and Twiest, M.W.: Intraperitoneal polypropylene mesh support of incisional herniorrhaphy. Am. J. Surg. 142:707, 1981.
5. Scott, E.A.: Repair of incisional hernias on the horse. J. Am. Vet. Med. Assoc. 175:1203, 1979.
6. Tulleners, E.P., and Fretz, P.B.: Prosthetic repair of large abdominal wall defects in horses and food animals. J. Am. Vet. Med. Assoc. 182:258, 1983.
7. Voyles, C.R., Richardson, J.D., Bland, K.I. et al.: Emergency abdominal wall reconstruction with polypropylene mesh. Ann. Surg. 194:219, 1981.

8

Surgery of the Urogenital System

Ovariectomy (Tumor Removal)

One or both ovaries have been removed in the mare for surgical correction of various ovarian conditions.[2,3,4,9] The most frequent indication for removal of a pathologic ovary is a granulosa cell tumor. Other ovarian tumors (teratoma, cystadenoma, adenocarcinoma, dysgerminoma, arrhenoblastoma, and ovarian lymphosarcoma) occur in mares but are much less common.[5] The surgical removal would be handled in the same fashion as discussed here for an ovary with a granulosa cell tumor. Less common indications for ovariectomy include ovarian abscess and hematoma, ovarian cysts, nymphomania, and prevention of estrus.[8,9] Bilateral ovariectomy is more commonly done to alter the mare physiologically rather than to remove a pathologic ovary. The prognosis following ovariectomy in cases of severe nymphomania is unpredictable, as the problem may not be attributable to ovarian dysfunction.[9]

For the removal of normal sized ovaries a number of surgical approaches are available, including colpotomy (removal *per vaginum*), flank with the mare standing, or flank, ventral midline, or paramedian with the animal under general anesthesia. The surgical situation of greatest clinical importance and the one that presents special problems and potential complications is removal of an enlarged tumorous ovary (with granulosa cell tumor being the usual problem). This is the surgical technique that will be described. It is the authors' opinion that the midline or paramedian approach is the most versatile one, not only for removal of a tumorous ovary but also for a bilateral ovariectomy. Although a tumorous ovary can be removed and transfixion ligation performed through a flank approach, exposure can be difficult with a severely enlarged ovary due to the limitations in size of the paralumbar fossa. In these situations, the ventral midline approach provides improved access, and the size of the incision is flexible. It is also the logical approach when the ovarian size cannot be completely determined on rectal palpation.[1] Any previous misgivings about disadvantages of a ventral midline approach in terms of healing or potential dehiscence or herniation are no longer tenable. The technique using a ventral midline incision located just cranial to the mammary glands will be described.

Mares afflicted with a granulosa cell tumor of the ovary can have different clinical signs varying from anestrus, masculine or stallion-like behavior and continuous estrus to asymptomatic, with the tumor being found on a routine rectal examination. Usually the uninvolved ovary is suppressed in its activity and palpates as small and firm.[3,7] It is felt that the clinical signs can be related to abnormal hormone production within the ovary. In three cases studied the tumor fluid generally contained higher levels of progesterone and testosterone than of estrogen.[7]

While removal of a granulosa cell tumor may be considered as an elective procedure, it is one that carries a number of potential complications that have been experienced by the authors and recognized by other surgeons.[2,3,6] These complications are discussed later and the technique presented here is intended to minimize these potential complications as much as possible.

Anesthesia and Surgical Preparation

An ovariectomy is performed under inhalation anesthesia. Flunixin meglumine and procaine penicillin are administered preoperatively. Hypotensive premedicants should be particularly avoided with this operation due to concerns with low blood pressure and postoperative rhabdomyolysis and nerve paresis.[3] During the surgical procedure, careful attention should be paid to blood pressure monitoring, as well as other routine monitoring devices. If low pressures are recorded when indirect techniques are used, a direct arterial catheter should be placed. The horse is prepared for aseptic surgery, with an incision directed craniad from the mammary gland.

Surgical Technique

A ventral midline incision is made, beginning immediately cranial to the mammary gland and extending a variable distance beyond the umbilicus depending on the size of the ovary. The incision is continued through the linea alba and peritoneum in a routine fashion. Some mares have considerable subcutaneous fat immediately cranial to the mammary gland. The affected ovary is located and exteriorized as much as possible (Fig. 8-1A). Exteriorization can be difficult with a large ovary, owing to the short nature of the pedicle and the breadth of the attachments. Balfour or Finochietto retractors may be helpful with small ovaries, but not with large ovaries where manual retraction and pressure on the body wall adjacent to the incision are necessary.

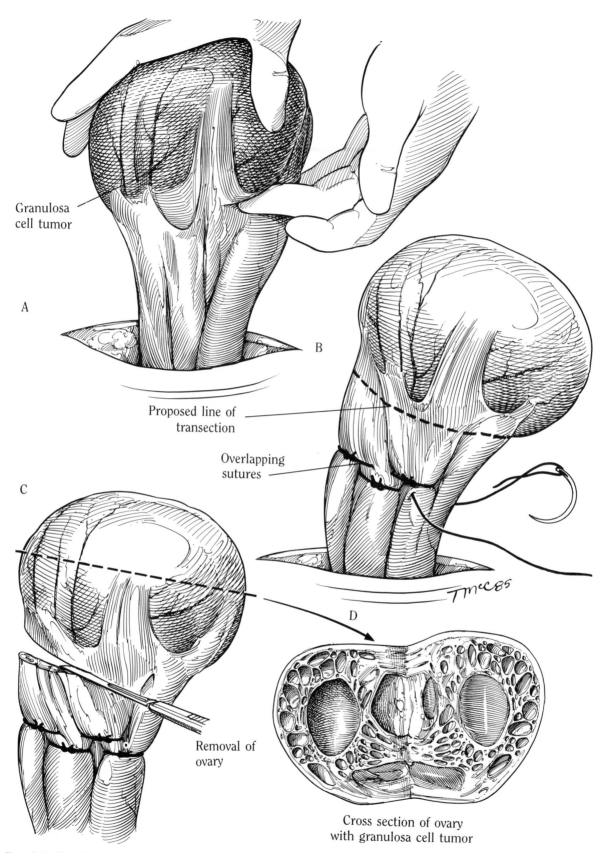

Granulosa
cell tumor

A

B

Proposed line of
transection

Overlapping
sutures

C

D

Removal of
ovary

Cross section of ovary
with granulosa cell tumor

Fig. 8-1. Ovariectomy (tumor removal).

Prior to ligation of the ovary, 8 ml of 2% lidocaine are injected into the pedicle using a 20-gauge needle attached to an intravenous set. The pedicle is then relaxed for a few minutes before commencing ligation. This procedure is done in an attempt to minimize intraoperative as well as postoperative complications. Since performing this technique on clinical cases, we have not seen the marked drop in blood pressure associated with traction or ligation that was our finding in previous cases.[2,3,10]

Transfixion ligation of segments of the pedicle is performed in the fashion illustrated in Figure 8-1B, using no. 2 catgut or synthetic absorbable suture material. These sutures are also overlapped so that no vessels escape ligation. All portions of the pedicle are ligated, and following ligation of a portion, the ovary can be severed from that portion of the pedicle. This maneuver can help provide increased exposure to the remaining pedicle. The extensive blood supply in pathologic ovaries provides the greatest surgical challenge with this technique. It is important to remember the effect of tension and relaxation when placing ligatures. A ligature that may seem to be secure and tight on a stretched pedicle may loosen and slip after release. While tension is usually necessary for placement of the individual sutures, it is important to relax this tension on the pedicle when the knot is actually tied. Failure to do so probably accounts for the considerable postoperative hemorrhage that has been experienced in some cases. Our experience with removal of a teratomatous ovary has been that fibrosis around the vessels can make effective ligation particularly difficult. When ligation is completed, the ovary is severed (Fig. 8-1C), and the stump is carefully evaluated for hemorrhage. Some authors consider that the cut edge should be oversewn at this stage to prevent formation of adhesions.[2,5] This can be performed with an inverting suture pattern using no. 00 suture material.

An alternative technique for large tumors that are difficult to exteriorize is to use the TA-90 surgical stapling equipment for ligation across the pedicle. The use of this instrument is described in the section on gastrointestinal surgery.

After the ovary has been removed and carefully checked to ensure that no hemorrhage is occurring, the ventral midline incision is closed with interrupted or far-near, near-far sutures of no. 2 synthetic absorbable material in the linea alba, or a simple continuous suture using no. 2 polyglycolic acid suture. A simple continuous suture of no. 0 synthetic absorbable material is used in the subcutaneous tissue, and the skin is closed with a continuous lock stitch. If surgical staples are used in the skin, they can be difficult to remove postoperatively.

Postoperative Management and Complications

Patients are maintained on postoperative antibiotics for 3 days and flunixin meglumine also for 3 days. Intensive care, including fluid therapy and close monitoring, may be important depending on the status of the animal postoperatively. Ovariectomy is attended by various degrees of pain, and the routine use of analgesics during the first

24 to 48 hours after surgery will enhance postsurgical recovery. Severe intractable abdominal pain is suggestive of a more serious problem. Ileus can develop in some of these patients and will require appropriate management. It has been suggested by one group that very large hematomas of the right ovary or ovarian pedicle may place extramural pressure on the terminal ileum or proximal jejunum, interrupt the flow of ingesta, and produce signs of colic.[6] We have observed a clinical syndrome comparable to this. The pain often seen in these cases may be associated with some degree of hemorrhage postoperatively. Major hemorrhage requiring surgical reintervention should not occur. Formation of adhesions and hematoma around the pedicle are all potential developments that should be minimized by good technique. Manual massage per rectum to break down adhesions has been described,[6] but is not routinely performed by us.

In one report of 78 cases, complications were experienced in 19 mares.[3] These included formation of seroma or hematoma at the incision site, superficial infection at the incision site, nerve paresis following recovery from anesthesia (including femoral, peroneal, or radial nerves), generalized rhabdomyolysis following recovery from anesthesia, postoperative shock, wound dehiscence, herniation, and peritonitis, and postsurgical diarrhea. Six mares died in this study.[3] It has been suggested that this high incidence of postanesthetic complications is related to a decrease in arterial pressure when tension is placed on the ovarian pedicle, but this has not been proven.[2,3] Any degree of peritonitis is generally localized to adhesions around the pedicle site.

Comments

Given that no immediate complications develop, ovariectomy is associated with a reasonably high percentage of mares resuming normal reproductive activity.[1,3] In one report, regular estrus returned in 42 of 57 mares that were followed up, and the time from surgery to the return of the regular estrous cycle ranged from 2 to 16 months.[3] In another report there was a 64% resumption of normal reproductive activity.[1]

References

1. Bosu, W.T.K., Van Camp, S.C., Miller, R.B., and Owen, R. ap R.: Ovarian disorders: Clinical and morphological observations in 30 mares. Can. Vet. J. 23:6,1982.
2. Colahan, P.T.: Female urogenital surgery. In Equine Medicine and Surgery, 3rd ed. (R.A. Mansmann, E.S. McAllister, and P.W. Pratt, Eds.) Santa Barbara, CA, American Veterinary Publications, 1982, p. 1367.
3. Meagher, D.M., Wheat, J.D., Hughes, J.P., et al.: Granulosa cell tumors of mares—a review of 78 cases. Proceedings 1977 Meeting of the American Association of Equine Practitioners, p. 133.
4. Pearson, H., Pinsent, P.J.N., Denny, H.R., and Waterman, A.: The indications for equine laparotomy—analysis of 140 cases. Eq. Vet. J. 7:131, 1975.
5. Pugh, D.G., and Bowen, J.M.: Equine ovarian tumors. Compend. Cont. Educ. 12:5710, 1985.
6. Scott, E.A., and Kunze, D.J.: Ovariectomy in the mare: Presurgical, surgical and postsurgical considerations. Eq. Med. Surg. 1:5, 1977.

7. Stickle, R.L., Erb, R.E., Fessler, J.F., and Runnels, L.J.: Equine granulosa cell tumors. J. Am. Vet. Med. Assoc. 167:148, 1975.
8. Vaughan, J.T.: Equine urogenital system. In The Practice of Large Animal Surgery. (P.B. Jennings, Ed.) Philadelphia, W.B. Saunders, 1984, p. 1122.
9. Walker, D.F., and Vaughan, J.T.: Bovine and Equine Urogenital Surgery. Philadelphia, Lea & Febiger, 1980.
10. Wright, M., McIlwraith, C.W., and Stashak, T.S.: Unpublished data, 1980.

Urethroplasty (Urethral Extension)

Urethroplasty is a surgical technique that provides caudal extension of the urethra. It is performed in mares that have retention of voided urine in the vaginal fornix (and consequent cervicitis and endometritis). These mares are generally barren multiparous mares, and the condition results from poor vaginal muscle tone and elongated ligamentous support allowing the vagina to fall below the level of the pelvic floor.[1,2,5] Sloping of the cranial pelvis ventrad, prominent ischiatic tuberosities, poor physical condition, a sunken perineum, and pneumovagina may be associated with the syndrome.[1,3]

Urethroplasty is designed to create surgically a mucosal shelf from the urethra to the mucocutaneous junction so that urine is voided to the exterior rather than into the vestibule. It is an alternative technique to that previously developed by Monin,[3] whereby the transverse fold over the external urethral orifice is used to provide a caudal extension. Monin's technique has been described in our previous textbook.[4] The technique described here is considered to be preferred for urine pooling in the vagina, and in one study was successful in 16 of 18 mares.[1] The correction of the problem should be attempted early rather than late, since in prolonged cases permanent endometrial degeneration with persistent infertility can occur.

Anesthesia and Surgical Preparation

Prior to surgery, the mare's reproductive capability should be evaluated using a uterine biopsy to help determine the extent of degenerative uterine changes that may have occurred.[1] A tranquilizer should be administered preoperatively.

Surgery is performed with the mare standing and restrained in the stocks. Epidural anesthesia using 2% lidocaine hydrochloride usually provides adequate anesthesia for the procedure. However when previous epidural anesthesia has been given, supplemental local analgesia may be necessary. Fecal material in the rectum is manually evacuated, and the tail is wrapped and tied out of the way. The perineal area is prepared surgically and a no. 30 French Foley catheter (Bardex, American Hospital, San Francisco, CA) is placed in the bladder to prevent urine contamination of the surgical field during the procedure (Fig. 8-2A). Retraction of the vulvar lips is provided by Balfour retractors or stay sutures in the vulva.

Surgical Technique

The transverse fold overlying the external urethral orifice is grasped with thumb forceps, and the thin caudal edge of the fold is split into dorsal and ventral layers with a scalpel (Fig. 8-2B). This incision is continued caudad along the left and right ventrolateral walls of the vestibule to approximately 2 cm from the mucocutaneous junction of the vulvar labia. The mucosa along the incision is then undermined dorsad and ventrad to create two mucosal layers. This submucosal dissection is continued until the edges of the mucosal shelves can be

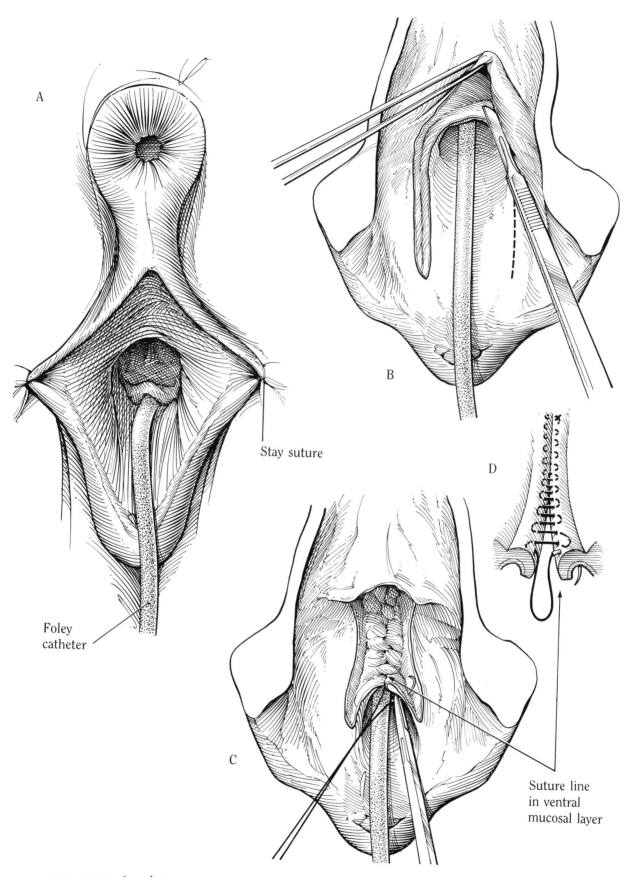

A

Stay suture

Foley
catheter

B

C

D

Suture line
in ventral
mucosal layer

FIG. 8-2A–D. Urethroplasty.

readily apposed in the midline. The mucosal layers are then apposed right side to left side with three layers of suture.

The right ventral mucosal layer is apposed to the left ventral mucosal layer by a continuous horizontal mattress pattern of no. 2-0 nylon or polypropylene (Prolene Ethicon, Summerville, NJ). The suture line is kept tight to ensure apposition throughout its entire length, and the mucosal surface is thus everted ventrad (Fig. 8-2C, D). The submucosal tissue between the two mucosal shelves is then apposed, using a simple continuous suture pattern of no. 2-0 nylon polypropylene (Fig. 8-2E). (This suture line is optional and can be omitted.) The right dorsal mucosal shelf is then apposed to the left dorsal mucosal shelf with no. 2-0 nylon or polypropylene sutures in a continuous horizontal mattress pattern such that the mucosal surface is everted dorsad (Fig. 8-2F, G). Synthetic absorbable monofilament suture material may be substituted in all layers.

The Foley catheter is removed after completion of the procedure.

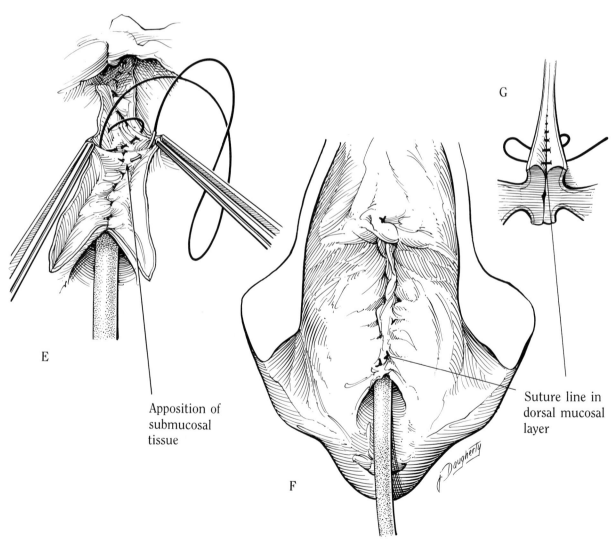

E

Apposition of submucosal tissue

Suture line in dorsal mucosal layer

F

FIG. 8-2 (*Continued*). **E–G.**

Postoperative Management

Tetanus prophylaxis and procaine penicillin (10,000 units/lb b.i.d.) are administered postoperatively. Antiinflammatory medication may help minimize local irritation. Sutures are not removed, but their retention has not been associated with adverse consequences.

Comments

In the initial report of this technique, urine pooling was no longer observed in 16 (89%) of the 18 mares in which urethroplasty was performed. Failure in the remaining 2 cases was due to formation of a fistula in the cranial extremity of the suture line. Of the 16 successful cases, 11 mares were known to have been rebred and 7 (64%) conceived (determined by rectal palpation or delivery of a live foal). In most mares, the mucosa and submucosa of the vaginal walls have sufficient elasticity and lend themselves well to surgical manipulation and satisfactory postoperative healing. When vaginal atrophy or scarring of the vaginal wall (due to advanced age, dystocia, or previously unsuccessful attempts at urethral extension) are present, these patients are poor candidates for the procedure. This was the situation in the 2 cases reported by Brown et al. where fistulas had formed (both mares had had unsuccessful urethral extensions previously).[1]

The second submucosal suture line can be omitted.[1] It has been suggested that it may be used when there is excessive tension on the suture line in an attempt to decrease the likelihood of fistula formation. Local anesthesia should be infiltrated into the vaginal wall only if absolutely necessary, as it can potentially delay healing. The polypropylene sutures were not removed in any of the mares reported by Brown et al., and no complications have been seen as a result.[1] It is recommended that mares be bred by artificial insemination to prevent trauma to the urethral extension on insertion of the penis.[1] However, mares have been bred naturally with no reported problems.

References

1. Brown, M.P., Colahan, P.T., and Hawkins, D.L.: Urethral extension for treatment of urine pooling in mares. J. Am. Vet. Med. Assoc. 173:1005, 1978.
2. Colahan, P.T.: Female urogenital surgery. In Equine Medicine and Surgery, 3rd ed. (R.A. Mansmann, E.S. McAllister, and P.W. Pratt, Eds.) Santa Barbara, CA, American Veterinary Publications, 1982, p. 1367.
3. Monin, T.: Vaginoplasty: A Surgical Treatment for Urine Pooling in the Mare. Proceedings 19th Meeting American Association of Equine Practitioners, 1972, pp. 99–102.
4. Turner, A.S., and McIlwraith, C.W.: Techniques in Large Animal Surgery. Philadelphia, Lea & Febiger, 1982.
5. Vaughan: Equine urogenital system. In The Practice of Large Animal Surgery. (P.B. Jennings, Jr., Ed.) Philadelphia, W.B. Saunders, 1984, p. 1122.

Episioplasty (Perineal Body Reconstruction)

Episioplasty is an extension of the concept of Caslick's operation and was initially introduced as a means of reducing the size of the vulva to prevent aspiration of air associated with ascending reproductive tract infections. The Caslick's technique has been described in our previous textbook.[3] Episioplasty provides a method of repairing compromised function of the constrictor muscles of the vulva and vestibule, which serve, together with the labia, as a defense against environmental contamination of the reproductive tract. The general situation is represented by a case of chronic pneumovagina where no effective valvular action remains in the vestibule. This situation is in contrast to that in the normal mare where, after parting the labia (overriding the constrictor vulvae muscle), the constrictor vestibule muscle still provides closure of the vestibule. The vulvar and vestibular sphincters can become incompetent due to repeated stretching during foalings or second degree lacerations.[1,4] The circular muscles that form the sphincters of the anus, vulva, and vestibule intersect in the perineal body, and any disruption in this region will cause loss of function.

Such advanced cases of pneumovagina are more of a problem of the aged rather than of the young animal. In some situations, sagging viscera (splanchnoptosis) associated with gradual stretching of the mesometrium and enlargement of the abdominal cavity also can be present. It may be necessary to perform urethroplasty (separately described) for vesicovaginal reflux of urine along with the episioplasty.[4] The technique described requires special dissection and reconstruction of the perineal body and ceiling of the vestibule, as well as the dorsal commissure of the vulva.

Anesthesia and Surgical Preparation

The episioplasty is performed on the standing animal restrained in stocks. Some degree of tranquilization is usually necessary (the combined use of xylazine and butorphanol has been useful). Epidural anesthesia using 2% lidocaine will provide analgesia to the level of the transverse fold over the external urethral orifice. If any additional anesthesia in the deeper tissues is required, local infiltration of the ischiorectal region can be performed. The tail is bandaged and tied out of the way, and the rectum is manually evacuated prior to surgery. The perineum and vulva are surgically prepared and the surgical field draped.

Surgical Technique

The labia are retracted, using stay sutures in the vulva, or long-jawed Balfour retractors. An incision is made along the mucocutaneous junction of the labia in a dorsoventral direction and extended craniad along the dorsal commissure of the vestibule to the vicinity of the vaginovestibular junction (approximately 15 cm craniad from the edge of the labium) (Fig. 8-3A). The lines of incision are best demonstrated on the sagittal view represented diagramatically in Figure 8-3B and are in the shape of a triangle. This triangular section of mucosa is then dissected submucosally from the dorsum and dorsolateral aspect of the vestibule and removed (Fig. 8-3C). Care is used in the submucosal dissection to ensure that the rectum is not penetrated. The incised edge of the mucosa of the right side of the vestibule is then sutured to the incised edge of the left side of the vestibule using a simple continuous pattern of no. 0 polydioxanone (PDS) (Fig. 8-3D). The raw triangular surface dorsal to this suture line is apposed with simple interrupted sutures of no. 0 PDS (Fig. 8-3E). Both layers are sutured from the cranial to the caudal aspects of the incision. In some cases having deep cranial dissection, the continuous suture line in the mucosa may need to be alternated with the "quilting" sutures above. These suture lines are brought out to the skin, and the skin of the perineum and vulva is then closed as for the Caslick's procedure (Fig. 8-3F). Some deeper horizontal mattress sutures are then placed across the reconstructed perineal body (Fig. 8-3G).

Postoperative Management

Tetanus prophylaxis is administered and systemic antibiotic therapy (procaine penicillin 10,000 units b.i.d.) is maintained for three days. The skin sutures are removed at 10 to 12 days, but complete healing of the deeper tissues will take 4 to 8 weeks. Complete sexual rest is essential at this time.[1] Any return to natural breeding will also be related to the resolution of any uterine infection.[2]

References

1. Colahan, P.T.: Female urogenital surgery. In Equine Medicine and Surgery. (R.A. Mansmann, E.S. McAllister, and P.W. Pratt, Eds.) Santa Barbara, CA, American Veterinary Publications, 1982, pp. 1367–1384.
2. Gadd, J.D.: The relationship of bacterial cultures, microscopic smear examination and medical treatment to surgical correction of barren mares. Proceedings 21st Meeting American Association of Equine Practitioners, 1975, pp. 362–368.
3. Turner, A.S., and McIlwraith, C.W.: Textbook of Large Animal Surgery. Philadelphia, Lea & Febiger, 1982.
4. Vaughan, J.T.: Equine urogenital system. In The Practice of Large Animal Surgery. (P.B. Jennings, Ed.) Philadelphia, W.B. Saunders, 1984, pp. 1122–1150.

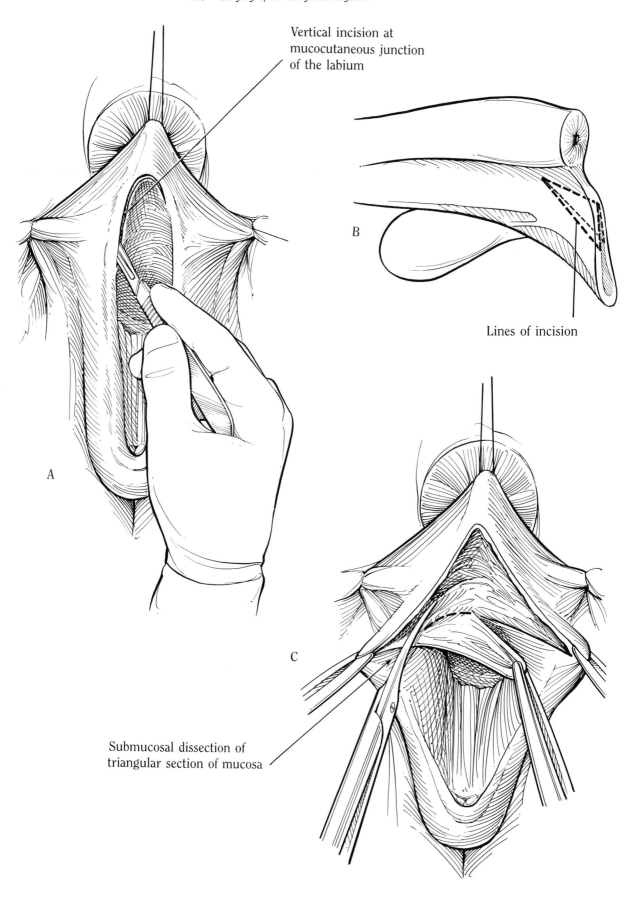

Vertical incision at
mucocutaneous junction
of the labium

A

B

Lines of incision

C

Submucosal dissection of
triangular section of mucosa

FIG. 8-3A–C. Episioplasty.

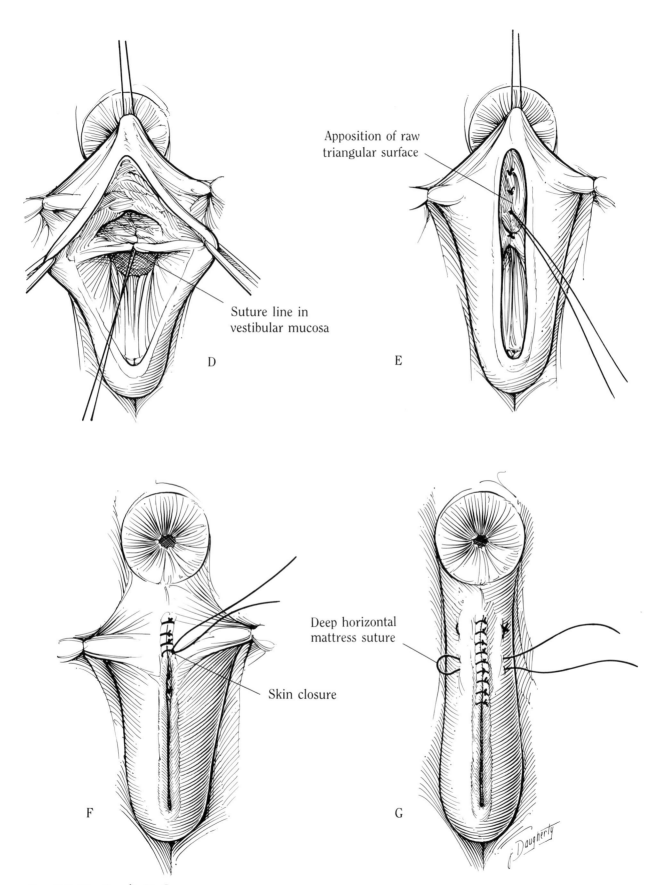

Apposition of raw
triangular surface

Suture line in
vestibular mucosa

D

E

Deep horizontal
mattress suture

Skin closure

F

G

Daugherty

Fig. 8-3 (Continued). **D–G.**

Removal of Cystic Calculi (Laparocystotomy)

Cystic calculi in the horse are caused by precipitation of urine salts upon a nidus. Such calculi are usually solitary. The nidi for calculi formation include fibrin, leukocytes, whole blood, albumin, or urinary mucoproteins. Two types of calculi are seen in horses. One type is rough and spiculated, relatively soft (they can be fragmented), and very abrasive to the wall of the bladder, often producing traumatic cystitis. The other type is a smooth, hard, whitish appearing calculus. Both types are similar chemically, consisting of calcium carbonate with magnesium, ammonium, and phosphate making up other constituents.[1]

A horse with a cystic calculus will exhibit dysuria, stranguria, pollalkiuria, and hematuria. Less common signs include mild colic, loss of condition, and a stilted gait. The horse will adopt the urinating stance for sometime before and after micturition. Soiling and scalding of the perineum and between the legs may also be seen.

The condition is suspected on the basis of clinical signs, and a more definitive diagnosis is based on rectal examination. Since cystic calculi usually do not produce clinical signs until they have reached a certain size, they are fairly obvious on rectal palpation. Their presence can be confirmed by cystoscopy using a flexible endoscope.[1] Urinalysis will show a concurrent cystitis with crystalluria, red blood cells, white blood cells, and bacteria.

Various surgical approaches are available for removal of cystic calculi. Other than laparocystotomy described here, urethrostomy, pararectal cystotomy (Goekel's operation) in males, and urethral sphincterotomy in mares have all been described.[1] Laparocystotomy is the approach that is most widely applicable, is less traumatic, and is the most commonly used for larger calculi.

Anesthesia and Surgical Preparation

Prior to surgery the horse should be placed on preoperative antibiotics. This will minimize the risk of postoperative peritonitis, since spillage of some urine into the abdominal cavity is frequently unavoidable as the stone is being manipulated out of the bladder. The operation is performed under general anesthesia with the horse in dorsal recumbency. The horse should be off feed for at least 24 hours to allow as much emptying of the intestinal tract (particularly the cecum and colon) as possible. This will reduce the interference by bowel during exteriorization of the bladder.

After the horse is positioned for surgery (with slight elevation of the hindquarters), the prepuce should be packed with dry cotton gauzes and held closed with 2 or 3 Backhaus towel clamps. The caudal ventral abdomen, prepuce, and vaginal area are prepared for aseptic surgery.

Additional Instrumentation

Laparocystotomy requires suitable suction apparatus to remove urine, abdominal surgery suction tip (e.g., Yankauer), narrow umbilical tape (e.g., ⅛-inch), and Balfour retractors.

Surgical Technique

A ventral paramedian incision is used in the male and a ventral midline incision in the female. For the paramedian approach, a 20-cm incision is made between the midline (prepuce) and the inguinal ring. The incision is carried through the superficial and deep abdominal fascia, rectus abdominis muscle, and peritoneum. The large pudendal and superficial abdominal vessels are ligated. In the mare the midline incision should extend from the umbilicus, caudal to the prepubic tendon. Considerable fat and aereolar tissue will be encountered as the incision is extended between the mammary glands. When the abdomen is entered, a large Balfour retractor is inserted to help keep the incision apart and facilitate exteriorization of the bladder edges.

When performing this operation for the first time the neophyte surgeon is always impressed at just how far caudally in the pelvic cavity the bladder is located. It will feel small and contracted. The bladder is located by inserting a hand into the abdomen caudad and dorsad into the pelvic canal. The contracted bladder and calculus are grasped behind the calculus, as with a clenched fist.[2] Steady traction is begun in an attempt to fatigue the musculature of the bladder. Eventually, relaxation will occur, but it may take several minutes. When the bladder and stone are exteriorized as much as possible, the bladder will occupy a good proportion of the incision, and this will help prevent exposure of the bowel (Fig. 8-4A).[4] The bladder is then isolated with moist towels. Two stay sutures of narrow cotton umbilical tape are placed through the bladder wall at each end of the proposed incision (Fig. 8-4A). The length of the incision will be somewhat variable, depending upon the size of the calculus. The incision is made directly onto the stone. The edges of the incision are then grasped with Allis tissue forceps at its midpoint. Additional points of fixation such as this will help manipulate the wound edges and prevent spillage of any residual urine into the abdominal cavity. It is frequently difficult to extract the stone (especially the rough-surfaced type) because the bladder mucosa is firmly adhered and interdigitates with the rough surface of the stone. To remove the stone, the bladder mucosa must be peeled slowly away from the mucosa much as the bovine placental caruncle and uterine cotyledon are separated.[2] When the stone has been removed, any debris (sand) that remains in the bladder must be removed. Dry gauzes are useful for manual removal of the larger fragments, and saline lavage and suction can be used to get smaller fragments and any blood clots.

The closure of the bladder should be in two layers, using a synthetic absorbable suture material (2/0 or 0 gauge) such as polyglycolic

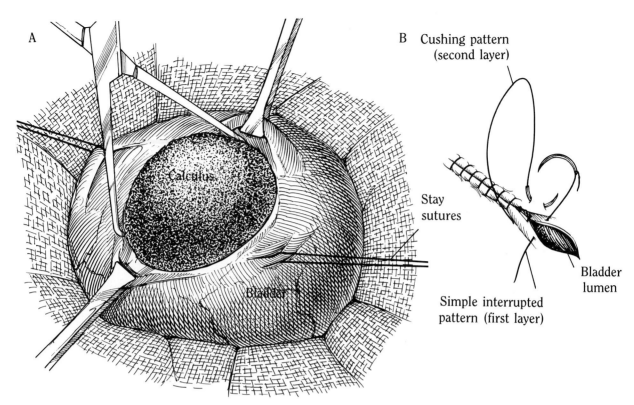

FIG. 8-4. Laparocystotomy for removal of cystic calculus.

acid (Dexon), polyglactin 910 (Vicryl), or polydioxanone (PDS). The first layer of sutures can be a simple interrupted or simple continuous pattern, but the second layer should be one of the inverting patterns, such as a continuous Lembert or Cushing pattern (Fig. 8-4B). Any towels used to pack off the bladder are now removed, and a new pair of outer gloves are donned by the surgeon. The abdomen should now be copiously lavaged with warm balanced electrolyte solution and as much retrieved by suction as possible.

Closure of the midline incision on the mare is routinely performed in three or four layers, depending on the surgeon's choice. Closure of the paramedian incision is usually a little more tedious. Here the superficial and deep rectus sheaths of the rectus abdominis muscle are closed separately (the superficial rectus sheath is the critical layer).

Postoperative Management

Postoperative antibiotics are continued for several days following surgery. Penicillin is a good choice because it is excreted in the urine in an active form. No real studies have shown just how long such coverage should continue because there are so many variables. These include the degree of cystitis present and the amount of spillage of urine into the abdominal cavity during surgery. A rectal examination should be performed several times during the first 36 hours to "brush off" any bowel that may be beginning to adhere to the incision in the bladder. Obviously this should be done with some caution, but it can prevent adhesions of bowel to the bladder from forming postoperatively if done several times during the first 36 hours postoperatively. We do not use urinary acidifiers or catheters.

Comments

The main advantage of laparocystotomy over other approaches for stone removal is that it is possible to ensure that all fragments of calculus have been removed.[3] Any fragments remaining can act as a potential nidus for future stone formation or potentially move down the urinary tract and cause urethral obstruction. Subischial urethrostomy and crushing the stone with a lithotrite has been advocated in the past because it did not require general anesthesia. With safer anesthetic techniques now available, this method should be used only for horses that are extremely poor anesthetic risks (e.g., advanced debilitation) or possibly for economic reasons. This method also requires adequate restraint, and there is a much greater chance of leaving debris in the bladder. The long-range prognosis following removal of cystic calculi should always be guarded because these horses are probably prone to stone formation.

References

1. DeBowes, R.M., Nyrop, K.A., and Boulton, C.H.: Cystic calculi in the horse. Symp. Cont. Educ. 6:5268, 1984.
2. Hackett, R.P., Vaughan, J.T., and Tennant, B.C.: Diseases of the Urinary Bladder in Equine Medicine and Surgery, 3rd ed. (R.A. Mansmann, E.S. McAllister, and P.W. Pratt, Eds.) Santa Barbara, CA, American Veterinary Publications, 1983, p. 912.
3. Lowe, J.E.: Suprapubic cystotomy in a gelding. Cornell Vet. 50:510, 1960.
4. Reed, D.G.: Suprapubic cystotomy in a stallion. Can. J. Comp. Med. Vet. Sci. 28:95, 1964.

Resection of the Diseased Urachus in Foals

In utero the urachus is a connection between the urinary bladder and the allantoic cavity.[3] Normally the urachus closes at, or soon after, birth and is eventually reduced to a scar at the apex of the bladder. The urachus may persist as a fistula between the umbilicus and the urinary bladder, allowing urine to escape. More importantly, it can act as an avenue for bacterial infection and lead to infections elsewhere in the foal's body.[1-6] It has been suggested also that infection of the umbilicus can lead to a reopening of the urachus, rather than infection being the result of a patent urachus.[3] Abscessation of the umbilical vein or umbilical arteries can also occur, and this can act as a nidus of infection.

The sequelae to an unattended infection in this area are well documented and can be devastating to the health of the animal. These include retrograde cystitis, osteomyelitis, infectious arthritis, meningitis, and hypopyon and have been termed the "polyarthritis-septicemia complex."[1] For these reasons, early extensive resection of the urachus and a portion of the bladder is indicated. Resection is indicated in cases that have not responded to the more conservative methods of treatment, which usually include cauterization with silver nitrate or strong iodine solutions. Evans advocates exploration of the umbilicus in foals showing signs of polyarthritis that have not responded quickly to antibiotics.[1] These foals may have abscessation of the umbilical vein or arteries requiring en bloc resection.[1] In rare instances, a urachal diverticulum is encountered.[4]

Anesthesia and Surgical Preparation

Perioperative treatment of the foal with broad-spectrum antibiotics is always indicated to minimize the chances of bacteremia at the time of surgical manipulation. They are indicated if the area is abscessed and septic contents spill into the abdomen during surgery. Foals that are bacteremic/septicemic may require more aggressive therapy such as intravenous antibiotics and intravenous electrolytes before risking general anesthesia.

Inhalation anesthesia such as halothane induced by mask, followed by endotracheal intubation is the preferred technique. We do not advocate the intravenous anesthesias, such as pentobarbitone or chloral hydrate, because they are too depressing for poor-risk patients that may be septicemic.

The foal is positioned in dorsal recumbency, and a soft rubber urinary catheter is inserted into the bladder to evacuate it. In male foals, the penis should be clamped to one side with the catheter in place, to prevent urine spilling into the surgical site. The preputial area should be packed with a few gauze sponges and sealed with towel clamps to help keep this area out of the surgical field. The urachal area is frequently moist and should be cleaned when the hair in this area has been clipped. If pus is actively draining from the urachal stump, the stump should be ligated.[2] An alternative is to invert the umbilicus with Lembert sutures placed in the skin.[3] The ventral abdomen is then clipped and prepared for aseptic surgery in a routine manner.

Surgical Technique

A narrow fusiform incision is made, centered over the umbilicus (Fig. 8-5A). The skin and the subcutaneous tissue are then dissected free of the body wall, leaving the umbilicus still attached (Fig. 8-5B).

Incision into the body wall, and subsequently into the abdomen, is made by incising the linea alba cranial to the umbilicus. When the abdominal cavity is entered, the surgeon will be able to insert an index finger and feel the dimensions of the urachus and the fusiform-shaped bladder. A second such incision can be made caudal to the umbilicus, and the umbilical arteries palpated. The incision in the linea alba is continued around either side of the urachus allowing complete en bloc resection (Fig. 8-5B).

The skin, umbilicus, urachus, and apex of the bladder are freed completely of the body wall in preparation for amputation. If the urachus is patent and there is no evidence of abscessation and fibrosis, it will palpate as a cord of tissue approximately 1 cm thick. Such cases can be managed by double ligation and transection of the urachus. Frequently it is difficult to distinguish the bladder from the urachus. The structure will be enlarged and inflamed because of fibrosis, and amputation must be made further caudad, along with a portion of the apex of the bladder.[2]

The diseased urachus can be amputated in several ways (Fig. 8-5C). Stay sutures can be placed in the bladder, and the urachus can be transected. If an abscess is suspected, Doyen forceps can be used to minimize spillage of septic contents. It is wise to pack off the remainder of the abdominal cavity with moist towels should contamination occur.

The bladder should be transected through healthy-appearing wall and closed in two layers. We prefer an initial simple interrupted layer of sutures (Fig. 8-5D) followed by an inverting layer using a Cushing or continuous Lembert pattern that ensures a watertight seal. Synthetic, absorbable suture material such as 2/0 polyglycolic acid or polyglactin 910 (Dexon, Vicryl) is recommended. Nonabsorbable suture material is contraindicated because of its predisposition to calculus formation when exposed to urine.

The umbilical vein and umbilical arteries should always be inspected.[3] If abscessation of either the umbilical vein (extending craniad to the liver) or the arteries (extending caudad to the iliac arteries) is discovered, then the entire abscessed vessel must be resected.[1] The umbilical vein should be double ligated. Otherwise, it will bleed because there are no valves. We have encountered foals where this vein was thickened to 2 cm in diameter, full of pus, and extending craniad to the liver. In such cases resection as close to the liver as possible must be attempted, but the risks of spillage or uncontrollable hermorrhage are high.

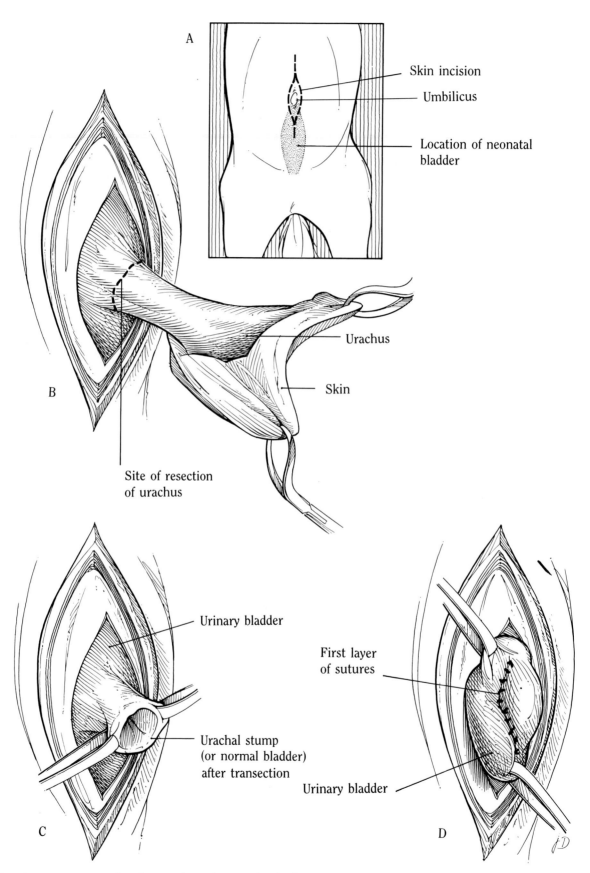

A

Skin incision

Umbilicus

Location of neonatal bladder

B

Urachus

Skin

Site of resection of urachus

C

Urinary bladder

Urachal stump (or normal bladder) after transection

D

First layer of sutures

Urinary bladder

FIG. 8-5. Resection of a diseased urachus in the foal.

Following the resection of the diseased urachus, the entire abdomen should be rinsed with warm balanced polyionic solution that is then removed by suction. This procedure should be performed several times if septic abscess contents have spilled during dissection. The abdominal wall should be closed in three layers. A simple continuous or simple interrupted layer of one of the synthetic absorbable suture materials (no. 1 or no. 2) is used to close the linea alba. A simple continuous layer of a similar suture material (no. 2/0) is used in the subcutaneous tissues. The skin can be closed with skin staples or nonabsorbable suture material of the surgeon's choice.

Postoperative Management

Postoperative fluid therapy is indicated in foals that are compromised. These include foals that are febrile or toxemic prior to surgery. Intravenous antibiotics may be indicated as well. Antibiotic therapy (intramuscular route) should be maintained for up to five to seven days following surgery.

Since this condition is part of a "complex," the clinician must pay attention to signs of metastatic bacterial localization. This means aggressive ancillary treatment for cases of infectious arthritis and meningitis. Any signs of acute lameness should be investigated immediately and treated as an emergency situation. The surgical treatment for infectious arthritis is discussed elsewhere in this book (see pages 171–175).

References

1. Evans, L.H.: Surgical treatment for the polyarthritis-septicemia complex in young foals. Arch. Am. Coll. Vet. Surg. 6:44, 1977.
2. Hackett, R.P., Vaughan, J.T., and Tennant, B.C.: The Urinary System in Equine Medicine and Surgery. (R.A. Mansmann and E.S. McAllister Eds.) Santa Barbara, CA, American Veterinary Publications, 1982.
3. Richardson, D.W.: Urogenital problems in the neonatal foal. Equine Practice Symposium on Neonatal Equine Disease. Vet. Clin. North Am. 1:179, 1985.
4. Robertson, J.T.: In Proceedings of the Equine General Surgery Seminar. 12th Annual Surgical Forum, Chicago, IL, p. 93, 1984.
5. Robertson, J.T.: Personal Communication, The Ohio State University, 1984.
6. Vaughan, J.T., Walker, D.F., and Williams, D.J.: The genital system. In Textbook of Large Animal Surgery. (F.W. Oehme, and J.E. Prier, Eds.) Baltimore, Williams & Wilkins, 1974.

Cystorrhapy for Ruptured Bladder in Foals

Rupture of the urinary bladder occurs most frequently in newborn male foals. It is rarely seen in adults.[1-6] The cause of the condition is unknown, although it is believed that strong forceful abdominal contractions at the time of parturition are the major contributing factor.[5] Occasionally defects of the bladder wall, rather than traumatic ruptures, are seen.[6]

The clinical signs of ruptured bladder in a foal may be quite subtle in the initial stages. This leads to a delay in diagnosis which may be life threatening because of the associated electrolyte abnormalities that ensue. For this reason most are referred to our clinic at 3 to 7 days of age. The foals will be depressed and anorexic and have an increased heart rate and respiratory rate. They will strain intermittently and attempt unsuccessfully to urinate. The abdomen will be distended, and ballottement produces a fluid wave. Abdominal paracentesis will reveal a clear odorless fluid (usually voluminous) that froths when shaken and emits an ammonia odor when heated.[5] To obtain additional confirmation of the diagnosis, a suitable dye such as methylene blue or an axosulfamide (e.g. Neoprontosil*) can be injected through a urinary catheter and then checked to see if it readily flows out an indwelling abdominocentesis catheter. Positive contrast cystography as an aid to diagnosis is popular with other species such as the dog but is not used routinely at our clinic. We resort to this method only when all other methods of diagnosis are inconclusive. The differential diagnosis of ruptured bladder in a foal includes retained meconium, colic due to impending enteritis, ureteral defects, rupture of the urachus, and the rare case of atresia of portions of the intestinal tract.

Anesthesia and Surgical Preparation

Anesthesia should not be induced until the severe electrolyte abnormalities that occur with this condition have been corrected. Typically these foals are hyponatremic and perhaps hypochloremic due to an inability to excrete urine. More significantly, they are hyperkalemic because of failure to effectively excrete potassium.[1-4] There may also be a slight to moderate metabolic acidosis. This array of metabolic derangements can lead to life-threatening cardiac arrhythmias, including premature ventricular contractions, ventricular fibrillation, third degree A-V block, and cardiac arrest, because of potentiation of the cardiotoxicity of the general anesthesia.[3,4]

Although surgery should be scheduled as soon as possible, it is highly recommended that some degree of preoperative stabilization be achieved. Intravenous catheterization and administration of 0.9% saline solution should be performed. Bicarbonate should be administered in 5% dextrose if metabolic acidosis exists. It has also been suggested that dextrose and insulin be given because of their hypo-

---

*Neoprontosil. Winthrop Laboratories, New York, NY.

kalemic effect.[3,4] The dose is 0.5 g of dextrose/kg bwt and 0.1 unit of crystalline insulin/kg bwt intravenously.[3,4] This can also be administered during anesthesia if arrhythmias occur. Care should be taken to see that the foal does not become hypothermic. For this reason, the judicious use of heating pads is indicated. We place the foal on a waterbed filled with warm water. Body heat can also be lost by using cold saline solutions to flush the abdomen. Tilting the animal toward the hindquarters will minimize the pressure on the diaphragm from the fluid in the abdomen.

Decompression of the abdomen prior to inducing anesthesia is also of benefit. As well as removing toxic metabolites, it will minimize the respiratory embarrassment caused by the distention. The midline should be clipped and scrubbed. A suitable catheter of the surgeon's choice should be inserted after the appropriate local skin analgesic has been applied. Suitable catheters include Foley, Sump, or de Pezzer types although a blunt teat cannula can be used for short-term drainage.

Foals with severe metabolic changes can be peritoneally dialyzed for as long as 12 hours preoperatively to make them a safer anesthetic risk.[2] Anesthesia is induced by mask, using halothane. A soft rubber catheter is inserted aseptically through the penis into the bladder and directed to one side. The preputial area should be sealed with towel clamps to exclude this potentially contaminated area from the surgical site. The foal is placed in dorsal recumbency, and the ventral midline is prepared for aseptic surgery in a routine manner.

Additional Instrumentation

Balfour retractors, soft rubber urinary catheters, warmed normal (0.9%) saline solution.

Surgical Technique

A narrow elliptical skin incision that is pointed at both ends is made around the urachus. The incision is extended back to the anterior margin of the prepuce as illustrated in the approach for the diseased urachus (Fig. 8-5A). This approach will allow adequate access to the torn bladder and allows the urachus itself to be freed and attended to if the need arises.

The urachal stump is then dissected free by continuing the elliptical incision through the abdominal wall at its midline. The incision in the linea alba should be extended caudad several centimeters in the direction of the prepuce as necessary. The urachus should be freed from the ventral body wall (where it is still attached at this age) using sharp dissection as illustrated previously (Fig. 8-5B). It can be used to maintain traction on the bladder as it is repaired. Later the urachus will be removed completely from the bladder and either ligated or transected and oversewn, since this area may be a potential source of leakage during the postoperative period. Some surgeons prefer a paramedian approach beside the prepuce.

The incision is made through the skin and extended caudad to the prepubic tendon. In the male foal the incision is made through the skin and the rectus abdominis muscle and the aponeurosis from the internal and external abdominal oblique muscles. The incision is carried deeper through transverse fascia to the peritoneum. Hemostasis is more likely to be a problem with this approach than for the incision in the linea alba.

The craniodorsal wall of the bladder should be inspected first, because this is where the smaller traumatic tears are most often found.[4] The ventral aspect of the bladder should be examined also, since larger defects have been reported in this region. These more ventral tears frequently extend far into the pelvic canal, making it difficult to locate the caudal end of the defect (Fig. 8-6). To assist exploration, a Balfour retractor can be inserted and the intestines packed off with moist towels.

When the tear has been found, the edges should be examined. If they are excessively necrotic, debridement with a good sharp pair of Metzenbaum scissors is recommended. A variety of suture patterns can be used for closure. We use a simple interrupted pattern in the

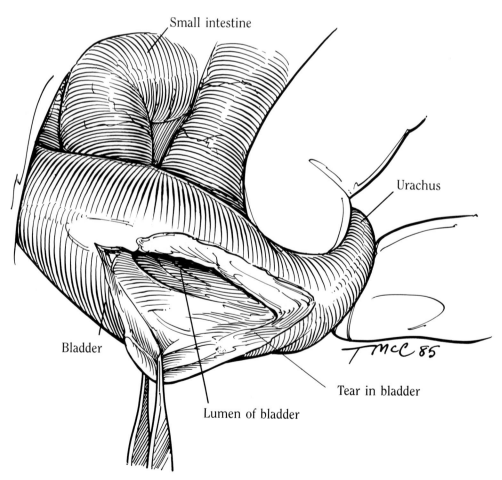

FIG. 8-6. Cystorrhaphy for ruptured bladder.

first layer, followed by continuous inverting pattern such as a Cushing or continuous Lembert stitch as illustrated previously (Fig. 8-5D). Some surgeons prefer two layers of inverting patterns (e.g., Lembert and Halsted). The suture material must be absorbable material such as catgut or one of the synthetic materials such as polyglycolic acid (Dexon), polyglactin 910 (Vicryl), or polydioxanone (PDS). No. 2/0 or 3/0 suture material is generally satisfactory for most foals. Tapered rather than cutting edged needles are recommended. Regardless of the pattern or material used for the closure, the important points are to invert the final layer and ensure a watertight closure. The bladder should be checked for leaks by distending it with saline solution. Any partial tears should be attended to immediately (by inverting suture lines) since these are also potential sources of leakage during the postoperative period.

We cannot overstress the need to attend to the urachal stump at its attachment to the body wall. If there is a urachal abscess, necrosis at this site will cause leakage during the postoperative period, requiring a second operation. For this reason we advocate either ligation or complete transection of the urachus as described in "Resection of the Diseased Urachus in Foals." The same suture pattern for the repair of the rent in the bladder can be used to oversew the stump of the urachus (Fig. 8-5D).

As repair of the bladder is progressing, an assistant (if available) should gradually remove the fluid from the abdominal cavity and begin replacing it with warm isotonic saline solution. This dialysis will aid in removing toxic urinary products (including potassium) while the operation is progressing.

The ventral midline closure is routine. We use no. 2 synthetic absorbable sutures in a simple interrupted pattern or a simple continuous pattern. In the subcutaneous layer, 2/0 or 3/0 simple continuous sutures of a synthetic absorbable material are recommended. The skin is closed with a nonabsorbable material of the surgeon's choice or stainless steel skin staples.

Postoperative Management

Despite large volumes of urine being frequently found in the abdominal cavity, peritonitis is unusual. If concurrent urachal abscessation has occurred, however, then septic peritonitis may pose a threat. In these cases, antibiotics are mandatory. We routinely provide a perioperative antibiotic coverage until 3 or 4 days after the operation. There are no controlled studies to show that antibiotics are essential to successful outcome of uncomplicated bladder rupture in foals.

Insertion of an indwelling catheter to keep the bladder decompressed has been recommended.[2-5] We do not use one for fear of trauma to the suture line. We feel that a meticulously placed watertight closure of the bladder wall is more important.

Intravenous fluids of normal saline solution should continue until urination is noticed. If the foal has been adequately hydrated before and throughout surgery, then a strong forceful urination will usually occur shortly after the foal recovers from the anesthesia and stands. Failure to do so may mean recurrence of the uroperitoneum (i.e., further unseen leaks in the bladder). Electrolyte balance should be monitored, and any corrections in therapy are made as necessary.

Comments

The prognosis for uncomplicated rupture of the urinary bladder is generally good if repair is attempted early and severe electrolyte abnormalities have not developed. Cases that have progressed for several days frequently suffer complications related to anesthetic management such as third degree atrioventricular block that is relatively resistant to atropine.[4] Surgical complications are usually due to failure to recognize additional leaks in the bladder or to attend to the urachus. Adhesions of bowel at the site of cystorrhaphy with subsequent stricture formation have been observed by one of us (AST). Leaks can also occur if the sutures in the bladder have been placed in unhealthy tissues, resulting in shredding of the tissue and separating of the suture line.

References

1. Behr, M.J., Hackett, R.P., Bentinck-Smith, J., et al.: Metabolic abnormalities associated with rupture of the urinary bladder in neonatal foals. J. Am. Vet. Med. Assoc., 178:263, 1981.
2. Kritchevsky, J.E., Stevens, D.L., Christopher, J., et al.: Peritoneal dialysis for presurgical management of a ruptured bladder in a foal. J. Am. Vet. Med. Assoc., 185:81, 1984.
3. Richardson, D.W., and Kohn, C.W.: Uroperitoneum in the Foal. J. Am. Vet. Med. Assoc. 182:267, 1983.
4. Richardson, D.W.: Urogenital problems in the neonatal foal. Vet. Clin. North Am. 1:179, 1985.
5. Walker, D.F., and Vaughan, J.T.: Bovine and Equine Urogenital Surgery. Philadelphia, Lea & Febiger, 1980.
6. Wellington, J.K.M.K.: Bladder defects in newborn foals (Letter). Aust. Vet. J. 48:426, 1972.

9

Removal of a Dentigerous Cyst (Aural Fistula)

A dentigerous cyst represents a special form of dental teratoma characterized by the presence of dental tissue at the base of a draining tract. The lesion appears as a fluctuant swelling at the base of the ear in a young horse, often accompanied by a discharging fistula that may open some distance up the margin of the pinna.[1] The tooth is usually associated with the temporal bone. When present, the condition is treated by complete removal of the tract and the cyst.

Anesthesia and Surgical Preparation

The operation is performed under general anesthesia with the horse in lateral recumbency and the affected side up. Prior to induction of anesthesia, the temporal area is clipped. Shaving and routine surgical preparation are performed after induction of anesthesia.

Surgical Technique

The skin incision is made over the central part of the lesion from the fistula craniad (Fig. 9-1A). The direction of the tract may be better defined if a probe can be placed through the fistula. Radiographs can also be used to ascertain the presence of a dental tissue and its position. The tract and the cyst are separated by blunt dissection at the base (Fig. 9-1B). The tooth is usually attached to the temporal bone and the attachments need to be cut or broken down, using an osteotome if necessary (Fig. 9-1C). This should be performed carefully, because the attachment can be firm and fracture in the temporal bone needs to be avoided. If possible, the cyst and its associated tract are removed unopened (Fig. 9-1C). Following removal, the cyst can be opened to confirm the presence of dental tissue.

373

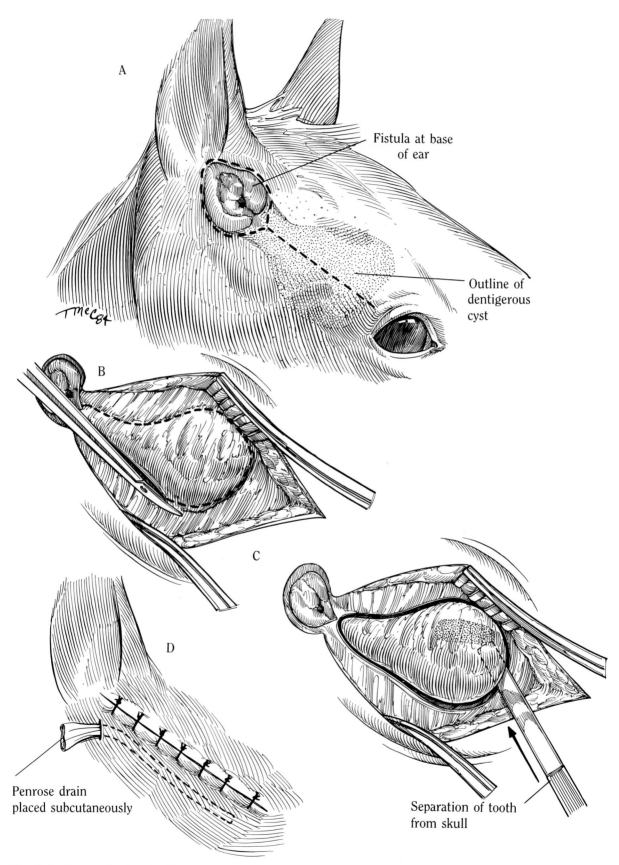

Fistula at base of ear

Outline of dentigerous cyst

A

B

C

D

Penrose drain placed subcutaneously

Separation of tooth from skull

FIG. 9-1. Removal of a dentigerous cyst.

The dead space left by removal of the cyst is closed as well as possible, using subcutaneous sutures of absorbable material, and a Penrose drain can be placed (Fig. 9-1D). The skin is closed with simple interrupted sutures of nonabsorbable material. A stent bandage using a 4-inch roll of gauze (Kling) may also be sutured over the incision to help prevent formation of a postoperative seroma.

Postoperative Management

The drain is removed at 4 to 5 days, and the skin sutures are removed at about 12 days. No other special care is necessary.

Reference

1. McIlwraith, C.W.: Equine digestive system. In The Practice of Large Animal Surgery. (P.B. Jennings, Ed.) Philadelphia, W.B. Saunders, 1984.

Appendix I

Equipment Required for Lag Screw Fixation

1. ASIF screw driver
2. 4.5-mm drill bit
3. 3.2-mm drill bit
4. 4.5-mm cortical bone tap
5. 4.5-mm tap sleeve
6. 3.2-mm drill guide
7. ASIF compressed nitrogen or similar drill
8. ASIF cortical bone screws (4.5-mm outside diameter)
9. Countersink
10. Depth gauge

Appendix II

Equipment Required for Bone Plate Application*

1. Countersink
2. Depth gauge
3. Tap handle and 4.5-mm taps (regular and extra long)
4. 6.5-mm cancellous tap
5. Standard screwdriver and screwdriver for quick coupling
6. Ruler
7. 8-mm hexagonal open-end wrench (for nuts)
8. Small air drill
9. Cortical and cancellous bone screw supplies
10. 4.5-mm drill bit—extra long (170 mm)
11. 4.5-mm drill bit (120 mm)
12. 3.2-mm drill bit—extra long (170 mm)
13. 3.2-mm drill bit (120 mm)
14. 2-mm drill bit
15. 6.5-mm cancellous tap sleeve
16. 3.5-mm tap sleeve
17. 4.5-mm tap sleeve and plate protector
18. Equine C-clamp
19. C-clamp
20. 3.2-mm drill sleeve
21. 22-mm wide-tipped Hohmann retractor
22. 18-mm narrow-tipped Hohmann retractor
23. Sharp hook
24. 35-mm wide-tipped Hohmann retractor
25. 43-mm narrow-tipped Hohmann retractor
26. Drill sleeve for tension device
27. Tension device—span 16 mm
28. Pin wrench
29. Socket wrench
30. Open-end and box wrench—11 mm
31. DCP neutral drill guide, green
32. DCP load drill guide, yellow
33. Bending irons (2)
34. Bending press

*Adapted from Fackelman, G.E., and Nunamaker, D.M.: Manual of Internal Fixation in the Horse. Berlin, Springer-Verlag, 1982.

35. Bending pliers for plates
36. Bending templates
37. 1.2-mm cerclage wire
38. Wire passer
39. Wire tightener with handle
40. Wire cutters
41. ASIF bone reduction forceps (large)
42. Verbrugge bone-holding forceps

Appendix II (continued)

Inventory of ASIF Dynamic Compression Plates

(Plate supply that would allow repair of most equine long-bone fractures)

	Narrow	Broad
8 hole	—	2
9 hole	2	2
10 hole	2	2
11 hole	2	2
12 hole	2	2
13 hole	—	2
14 hole	—	2
16 hole	—	2
18 hole	—	2

Appendix III

Equipment Required for Fiberglass Cast Application

Casting tape (4″, 5″, and 6″ widths)
Stockinette
Orthopedic felt
1 Towel clamp
Acrylic for the cap (e.g., Technovit)
Bailing wire
Hand drill and drill bit
Water at room temp. (70–75° F)

Appendix IV

Equipment Required for Arthroscopic Surgery

25° or 30° 4-mm Arthroscope
5-mm Arthroscopic sleeve
Sharp trocar and blunt obturator for insertion of sleeve
Fiberoptic cable
Fiberoptic light source
Video camera (optional)
Probe
Egress cannula
Biopsy cutting forceps (Storz)
McIlwraith arthroscopy rongeur (Scanlan)
Ferris-Smith intervertebral disc rongeurs, 4 × 10-mm cup (Scanlan)
5-mm ethmoid forceps (Scanlan)
Malleable fragment forceps (Scanlan)
Periosteal elevator
4-mm osteotome
Meniscotome
Curettes (2/0 and 1)
Curved curette (Scanlan)
Motorized burr (Dyonics or Wolf)

Index

Page numbers in **boldface** indicate figures; those followed by "t" indicate tables.